EASY PAEDIATRICS

Rachel U Sidwell
Consultant Dermatologist (Interest in Paediatric Dermatology)
Hemel Hempstead Hospital, Hemel Hempstead, UK

Mike A Thomson
Consultant Paediatric Gastroenterologist, Sheffield Children's Hospital
Foundation NHS Trust, Sheffield, UK

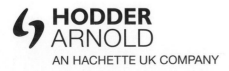
HODDER
ARNOLD
AN HACHETTE UK COMPANY

First published in Great Britain in 2011 by
Hodder Arnold, an imprint of Hodder Education, a division of Hachette UK
338 Euston Road, London NW1 3BH

http://www.hodderarnold.com

Hachette UK's policy is to use papers that are natural, renewable and recyclable products and made from
wood grown in sustainable forests. The logging and manufacturing processes are expected to conform to
the environmental regulations of the country of origin.

Whilst the advice and information in this book are believed to be true and accurate at the date of going
to press, neither the author[s] nor the publisher can accept any legal responsibility or liability for any
errors or omissions that may be made. In particular, (but without limiting the generality of the preceding
disclaimer) every effort has been made to check drug dosages; however it is still possible that errors have
been missed. Furthermore, dosage schedules are constantly being revised and new side-effects recognized.
For these reasons the reader is strongly urged to consult the drug companies' printed instructions, and
their websites, before administering any of the drugs recommended in this book.

British Library Cataloguing in Publication Data
A catalogue record for this book is available from the British Library

Library of Congress Cataloging-in-Publication Data
A catalog record for this book is available from the Library of Congress

ISBN-13   978-1-853-15826-1

1 2 3 4 5 6 7 8 9 10

Commissioning Editor: Joanna Koster
Project Editor: Sarah Penny
Production Controller: Jonathan Williams
Cover Design: Amina Dudhia

Cover image © Stockbyte/Getty Images

Typeset in 10 on 12pt Bembo by Phoenix Photosetting, Chatham, Kent
Printed in Italy

What do you think about this book? Or any other Hodder Arnold title?
Please visit our website: www.hodderarnold.com

Contents

Contents

Contributors

David John Atherton MA, MB, BChir, FRCP
Honorary Consultant in Paediatric Dermatology, Great Ormond Street Hospital for Sick Children NHS Trust, London, UK

Mike Berelowitz MB, BCh, MPhil, MRCPsych, FRCPsych
Consultant Paediatrician, Royal Free Hospital, London, UK

Nick Bishop MD
Professor of Paediatric Bone Disease, Sheffield Children's NHS Foundation Trust, Sheffield, UK

Siobhan Carr MSc, FRCPCH
Consultant Respiratory Paediatrician, St Bartholomew's and The Royal London Hospitals, London, UK

Robert C Coombes BSc, FRCPCH
Consultant Neonatal Paediatrician, Sheffield Children's Hospital NHS Trust, Sheffield, UK

Peter Cuckow FRCS(Paed)
Consultant Paediatric Urological Surgeon, Great Ormond Street Hospital for Sick Children NHS Trust and University College Hospital, London, UK

Claire Daniel BSc, FRCOphth
Consultant Ophthalmologist, Moorfields Eye Hospital NHS Foundation Trust, London, UK

James SA Green LLM, FRCS(Urol)
Consultant Urological Surgeon, Whipps Cross University Hospital, London, UK

Ian M Hann MD, FRCP, FCRPCH, FRCPath
Professor of Paediatric Haematology and Oncology, Great Ormond Street Hospital for Sick Children NHS Trust and UCL Institute of Child Health, London, UK

Simon Keady BSc (Hons), MRPharmS, Dip Clin Pharm, SP
Principle Pharmacist, UCLH Foundation Trust, London, UK

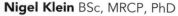

Nigel Klein BSc, MRCP, PhD
Professor of Immunology and Infectious Diseases, Great Ormond Street Hospital for Sick Children NHS Trust and UCL Institute of Child Health, London, UK

Melissa M Lees MRCP, DCH, MSc, MD, FRACP
Consultant in Clinical Genetics and Honorary Senior Lecturer, Great Ormond Street Hospital for Sick Children NHS Trust and UCL Institute of Child Health, London, UK

Ahmed F Massoud MRCP, MRCPCH, MD
Consultant Paediatrician and Endocrinologist, Northwick Park Hospital, London, UK

Anthony J Michalski FCRPCH, PhD
Consultant Paediatric Oncologist, Great Ormond Street Hospital for Sick Children NHS Trust, London, UK

Mike Potter MA, PhD, FRCP, FRCPath
Consultant Paediatric Haematologist, The Royal Marsden NHS Foundation Trust, London, UK

Robert J Sawdy BSc, MRCOG, PhD
Consultant Obstetrician and Specialist in Maternal and Fetal Medicine, Poole Hospital NHS Foundation Trust, Poole, UK

Rod C Scott MRCP, MRCPCH, PhD
Senior Lecturer in Paediatric Neurology, Ormond Street Hospital for Sick Children NHS Trust and UCL Institute of Child Health, London, UK

Rachel U Sidwell MRCP, MRCPCH, DA
Consultant Dermatologist (Interest in Paediatric Dermatology), Hemel Hempstead Hospital, Hemel Hempstead, UK

Mike A Thomson DCH, FRCP, FRCPCH, MD
Consultant Paediatric Gastroenterologist, Sheffield Children's Hospital Foundation NHS Trust, Sheffield, UK

Michael Wareing BSc, FRCS (ORL-HNS)
Consultant Otolaryngologist, St Bartholomew's and The Royal London Hospitals, London, UK

Nick Wilkinson MRCP, MRCPCH, DM
Consultant Paediatric Rheumatologist, Nuffield Orthopaedic Centre NHS Trust, Oxford, UK

Callum J Wilson DCH, Dip O&G, FRACP
Metabolic Consultant, Starship Children's Health, Auckland, New Zealand

Contributors

Paul JD Winyard MA, MRCP, MRCPCH, PhD
Senior Lecturer in Paediatric Clinical Science, Great Ormond Street Hospital for Sick Children
NHS Trust and UCL Institute of Child Health, London, UK

Rob WM Yates BSc, FRCP
Consultant Paediatric Cardiologist, Great Ormond Street Hospital for Sick Children NHS Trust,
London, UK

Contributors

Preface

This book has been written to help medical students navigate their way through the often complex, fascinating and rather different world of paediatrics in a user-friendly style. It is a thorough yet succinct introduction to the subject. We appreciate that medical students have a seemingly endless amount of knowledge to acquire in many different subjects, and therefore we wish to make the paediatric element as easy and smooth as possible. It has been written in an organised manner in a systems approach for ease of assimilating information, and employs the use of boxes, annotated diagrams and illustrations throughout.

The book is co-authored by sub-specialists within the different areas of paediatrics.

We hope the book provides a broad background knowledge, and may give inspiration to some to pursue the subject further.

We would like to thank all who helped with this book, in particular the specialists who have contributed to various chapters.

Finally we would like to thank the teams at Hodder Arnold and the Royal Society of Medicine Press for their positive and supportive approach.

Mike and Rachel, May 2011

To my little raisons d'être Charlie, Tilly and Amélie......

Rachel U Sidwell

To my four girls: Kay, Ella, Jess and Flo......

Mike Thomson

1 History and Examination

- Paediatric history
- Neonate
- Paediatric examination
- Further reading

PAEDIATRIC HISTORY

Taking a paediatric history and examination:

 The history is most often taken from the accompanying adult (dependent upon the child's age and condition). Note the accompanying adult(s), e.g. parent, nanny, grandparent, and from whom the history was taken

- Remember first to introduce yourself and to identify which child is the patient, referring to him/her by the correct gender
- It is often necessary to take parts of the history and examination 'out of order' depending on the condition and cooperation of the child
- Certain points should always be covered, e.g. immunization details (see paediatric history outline and examples below)

INFANT AND CHILD

Identification details

- Date and time
- Referral from
- Name
- Age and sex
- Accompanying adult(s)

Problem list

1. e.g. respiratory distress, vomiting jaundice
2. . . . .
3. . . . .

History of presenting complaint

Expand and clarify

- Duration?
- Are the symptoms intermittent or constant?
- Associated symptoms?
- Visits to GP/A&E?
- Treatment given?
- Travel, contacts (infectious diseases)

Systems review

Respiratory	Breathing difficulties, cough, hoarseness, noisy breathing, possibility of foreign body inhalation
Cardiovascular	Blue or white episodes, fainting, shortness of breath, palpitations, feeding difficulties and sweating (infants)
Gastrointestinal	Appetite, nausea, vomiting, mouth ulcers, weight loss, diarrhoea, constipation, stools – colour, blood, mucus
Genitourinary	Passing urine? Number of wet nappies in 24 h (infant), colour of urine, any stinging on passing urine (dysuria), nocturia
CNS	Headaches, migraines, learning difficulties, hearing, vision, fits, clumsiness
Musculoskeletal	Joint pain, swelling
Skin	Rashes, hair, nails, mucosal symptoms
Haematological	Bone pain, weight loss, infections, malaria, mouth ulcers, repeated infections

Past medical history

Pregnancy history	Any problems?
	Scans normal?
Birth history	Delivery:

- Normal vaginal delivery (NVD), assisted delivery, Caesarean section (emergency or planned)
- Problems at delivery
- Gestation

Newborn period:

- Birthweight
- Problems, e.g. jaundice, NICU admission

Nutrition	Breast fed/bottle fed
	Weaning

Previous medical problems, admissions, operations

Normal childhood infections

Developmental history

Enquire about each developmental area and milestones:

Infants	Developmental milestones, primitive reflexes and postural responses
Older child	Developmental milestones, educational and social difficulties

Vaccinations

Outline vaccines given and age. Are they up to date?

Family history (FH)

- Sketch family tree (see example below)
- Consanguinous parents?
- Inherited diseases, e.g. atopy, epilepsy, deafness
- Contagious disease?

Social history (SH)

- Parents (ages, working or unemployed, relationship, smoking)
- Any other carers, e.g. nanny, au pair, grandparents
- Home situation (financial or housing problems)
- School, nursery problems
- Friends (problems?)

Drugs

Regular medication and any given for current complaint (NB: include over-the-counter preparations).

Allergies

Any known allergy, plus *precise reaction* (if known).

Examination findings

Summary

Major symptoms and problems plus any relevant key additional information.

Differential diagnoses

List the main differential diagnoses in order of probability.

Plan

Outline a management plan consisting of:

■ Admit or not
■ Investigations to be done (tick these when done)
■ Monitoring
■ Treatment (including fluid management if necessary)

Sign this report at the end and print your name and give your position.

Example of initial history and examination in a child

28/08/10   21:55

Urgent referral via general practitioner

Mimi Sanderson
4 years 8/12   Female
With mother and father (history from both)

Problems

1. Sore throat
2. Fever
3. Vomiting

History of presenting complaint

Sore throat	For the last 2 days
	Painful to swallow
Fever	Unwell with fevers lasting 2 days
	Mother measured 38°C with home forehead thermometer
Vomiting	Today after some fluid
Appetite	Off food 2/7
	Not drinking much today
	Thirsty
	Passing urine less frequently than usual

Systems review

Respiratory	No cough, no dyspnoea
Cardiovascular	No palpitations
Gastrointestinal	As above
Genitourinary	No dysuria, no haematuria, passing urine, dark yellow
CNS	NAD

3

Past medical history

- NVD 38/40, normal pregnancy
- Birthweight 3.5 kg
- Breast fed until age 6 months
- Weaned normally onto solids aged 4–6 months
- Four previous episodes of tonsillitis this year

Developmental history

Normal developmental milestones

Vaccinations

- DPT, Hib and men C x 3 (2, 3, 4/12)
- Hib booster 12/12
- MMR 12/12

Family history

```
Dad _____ Mum
33              32
Asthma

 |_____|_____|
Fred      Tom        Mimi
8         6          4
Asthma    Well
```

- Family history of asthma (brother, father, paternal uncle)
- No recent travel
- No contacts

Social history

- Mother – 32 years, teacher
- Father – 33 years, engineer
- Doing well at school so far

Drugs

None

Allergies

None known

Examination

- Flushed, halitosis
- Temp. – 38.5°C (core)
- Lethargic
- Cervical lymphadenopathy
- No jaundice
- Capillary refill time 2 s
- Mucous membranes moist
- Eyelids slightly sunken

| Tonsils | Enlarged, bright red, white exudate |
| Cardiovascular | Pulse 140/min, tachycardic |

	Regular, strong
	HS I–II plus nil
	BP 120/60
Respiratory	AE good L=R
	No crackles or wheezes
Abdomen	Soft
	Non-tender
	No masses felt
	° LKKS
CNS	Grossly intact: alert, orientated, responding to commands

Summary

- 4 years 8/12 girl with 2 days unwell, sore throat, fever, off food and drink
- Worsening today, clinically 5% dehydrated

Diagnosis

Bacterial tonsillitis with poor fluid tolerance and intake

Differential diagnosis

Viral tonsillitis

Plan

- Throat swab
- FBC, U&E, creatinine
- Oral or NG fluids or, if not tolerated, IV fluids
- Fluid balance chart
- Regular oral analgesia
- Oral antibiotics if tolerated (if not IV)
- ENT review later in view of repeat attacks

C Thomson
Paediatric SHO

NEONATE

Identification details

- Date and time
- Referral from – postnatal wards, A&E, general practitioner
- Name
- Age/prematurity and sex
- Birthweight
- Accompanying adult(s)

Problem(s)

1. e.g. respiratory distress, vomiting, jaundice
2. ....
3. ....

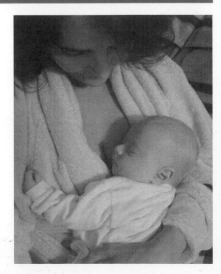

Figure 1.1 Newborn infant

History of presenting complaint

Expand and clarify

- Duration?
- Associated symptoms?
- Is the baby feeding?
- Fever?
- Any treatment given?
- Any visits to GP?

Maternal history

- Age and race
- Maternal medical problems, e.g. diabetes mellitus, epilepsy, medications
- Rhesus status, blood group
- Hepatitis B and C, HIV and syphilis serology
- Gravida, para

Pregnancy history

- Conception natural or assisted?
- Any problems?
- Ultrasound scans normal?
- Any other fetal investigations, e.g. chorionic villous sampling, amniocentesis

Delivery history

- Fetal distress
- Assisted labour (forceps, Ventouse, planned or emergency Caesarean section)
- Apgar scores at 1, 5 and 10 min

Neonatal history

- Breast or bottle fed
- Any feeding difficulties?
- Any other neonatal problems?

Family history/social history

- Parental situation, ages and occupations
- Immediate family tree (parents and siblings)

Examination findings

Pay particular attention to:

- Signs of birth trauma
- Handling
- Jaundice
- Fontanelle tension
- Non-specific signs of sepsis: lethargy, irritability, poor handling; poor feeding/suck; hypotonia; apnoeas; jaundice; temperature instability, core–peripheral temperature difference

Summary

Diagnosis

Differential diagnosis

Plan

- Admission to neonatal intensive care unit (NICU) or the ward?
- Investigations

- ■ Monitoring
- ■ Treatment

Example of initial history and examination in a neonate

24/04/05   05:05
Postnatal ward referral

Baby Moir
6 h old   34/40 premature Female
Birthweight 2.53 kg
History from mother

Presenting complaint
Respiratory distress

History of presenting complaint
- ■ Noticed rapid breathing last 1 h
- ■ Born LCSC for fetal distress
- ■ Apgars: 5 (1 min), 9 (5 min), 9 (10 min)
- ■ Breast fed x 1 with difficulty

Maternal history
- ■ 34 years, Caucasian
- ■ Diabetic
- ■ O Rh neg
- ■ Hep B, C, HIV and syphilis negative
- ■ G3, P2

Pregnancy history
- ■ Hyperemesis gravidarum – admitted at 16 weeks' gestation
- ■ Normal antenatal scans

Delivery history
Emergency LCSC for fetal distress

Neonatal history
As above

Family history/social history

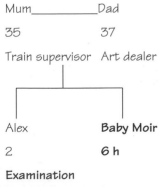

Mum_____Dad

35   37

Train supervisor   Art dealer

Alex   **Baby Moir**

2   **6 h**

Examination
- ■ Saturations 80% in air

- 92% head box oxygen
- Temp. – 38.5°C (core)
- Lethargic, sweaty
- Central cyanosis
- No jaundice
- Capillary refill time 3 s

Cardiovascular   Pulse 180/min
Regular, strong
HS I——II plus nil
BP 50/25

Respiratory   RR 65/min
Tracheal and suprasternal tug
Intercostal recession
Nasal flaring
AE reduced L=R
Bilateral diffuse crackles

Abdomen   Soft
Non-tender
No masses felt
° LKKS

CNS   Grossly intact

Summary

5 h old, premature infant with respiratory distress 1 h

Diagnosis

? Respiratory distress syndrome (RDS)

Differential diagnosis

- ? Transient tachypnoea of the newborn (TTN)
- ?? Pneumonia
- ?? Generalized sepsis
- ?? Cardiac defect
- ?? Intraventricular haemorrhage (IVH)
- ?? Other respiratory event

Plan

- Admit to NICU
- CXR
- BM stix
- FBC, U&E, blood sugar
- ABG
- Blood cultures
- Head box oxygen or assisted ventilation (dependent on capillary/arterial blood gas and trend in gases)
- Oxygen saturation monitor
- NG feeds 2–3 hourly (or IV if not tolerated)
- IV antibiotics

M Timble
Paediatric SHO

PAEDIATRIC EXAMINATION

Key points in the examination of infants and children are:

- Cooperation – try and obtain this if possible as it will make examination *much* easier
- Allow the child the time to get to know you
- Do examination in an unusual order if necessary (i.e. be *opportunistic* and not systematically rigid)
- Undress the child in stages to keep him/her calm
- Get the parent to help (undress, hold child) and wherever possible leave the child in a secure place (e.g. parental lap)
- Praise the child – age dependent
- Play with the child
- CNS examination is particularly age dependent

> **!** **NB: Listen to the heart first (crying helps breath sounds but not heart sounds to be heard) and check ENT last.**

Summary of examination

- General
- Cardiovascular system
- Respiratory system
- Abdomen
- Central nervous system
- Bones and joints
- Eyes
- Ear, nose and throat (NB: Do this last)

General

Is the child *well* or *sick*?	This is difficult to determine, but is learnt with experience:
	■ *Not too bad* – smiling, playing, or upset and does not allow examination
	■ *Unwell* – lethargic, not interacting, irritable, pale, allows examination
	■ *Very unwell* – grey, unrousable, severe respiratory distress
	If sick proceed to basic ABC and resuscitation as necessary (see ch. 26 Basic Life Support)
Level of consciousness	(as in APLS)
Interaction with parents	Signs of neglect?
	Playing normally?
Colour	Cyanosis (blue, grey) – distinguish if *central* (tongue) or *peripheral* (digits)
	Shock (pale, grey)
	Jaundiced
Peripheral perfusion	(Capillary refill time) and estimation of overall hydration state
Skin	Obvious rash, scars or bruising (especially linear or not overlying bony prominences)
Lymphadenopathy	Cervical, occipital
	Inguinal
	Axillary (rare)

Dysmorphic features
Nails   Clubbing, splinter haemorrhages
Measurements   Height, weight and head circumference (plot on growth chart)
     Temperature and BP (using *appropriately sized cuff*)
     Urine and stool (analysis and inspection. Inspect nappy)

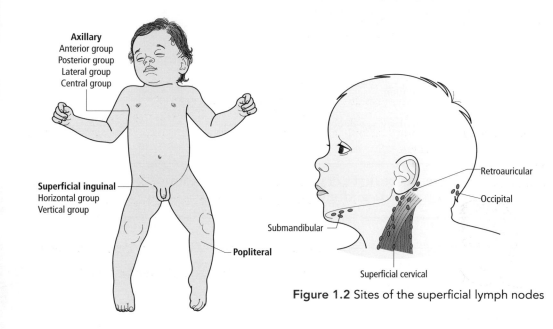

Figure 1.2 Sites of the superficial lymph nodes

Cardiovascular system

> **NB: As for other parts of the paediatric examination, cardiovascular examination may need to be opportunistic and not methodical in approach.**

Cyanosis   Distinguish if *central* (tongue) or *peripheral* (digits). NB: sensitivity – poor sign
Clubbing
Inspection   Chest symmetry:
    ■ Left chest prominence: chronic right ventricular hypertrophy
    ■ Right chest prominence: dextrocardia with ventricular hypertrophy
     Scars:
    ■ Median sternotomy (open heart surgery) (see Fig. 9.3)
    ■ Right or left lateral thoracotomy (see Fig. 9.3)
    ■ Groin scar (cardiac catheterization)
     Visible apex beat (*hyperdynamic*)
Pulse   **Rate** (beats/min) – tachycardic, bradycardic
     Volume, e.g. small volume in aortic stenosis, shock
     Character, e.g. bounding: sepsis, PDA
     Rhythm – regular, regularly or irregularly irregular (atrial fibrillation, ectopic beats, heart block)
     Check femorals – weak or absent = **coarctation**. NB: Radiofemoral delay cannot be detected in children <5 years of age

Palpation of precordium	Apex beat (4–5th intercostal space [ICS] mid-clavicular line): ■ *Displaced* (cardiomegaly, cardiac failure, dextrocardia) ■ *Hyperdynamic* Heaves (LVH or RVH) or thrills (palpable murmur)

NOW STOP AND THINK, THEN...

Auscultation (diaphragm then bell)	**Heart sounds** **Added sounds**, e.g. click **Murmur**: ■ Apex, parasternal border, pulmonary and aortic areas ■ Roll to left for mitral murmers, then back ■ Systolic, diastolic, continuous, maximal intensity ■ Grade (1–6), character, radiation, variation with respiration
Hepatosplenomegaly	Normal infant liver palpable 1–2 cm below costal margin (congestive cardiac failure, splenomegaly in SBE)
Blood pressure	

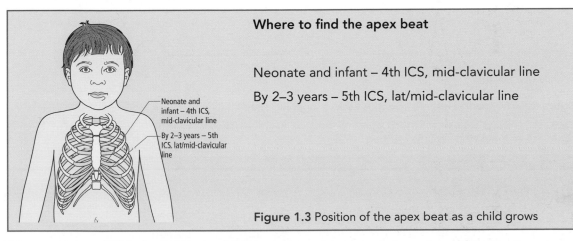

Where to find the apex beat

Neonate and infant – 4th ICS, mid-clavicular line

By 2–3 years – 5th ICS, lat/mid-clavicular line

Neonate and infant – 4th ICS, mid-clavicular line

By 2–3 years – 5th ICS. lat/mid-clavicular line

Figure 1.3 Position of the apex beat as a child grows

Measurement of blood pressure in children

■ Sphygmomanometer – stethoscope for older children, Doppler ultrasound in infants
■ Oscillometric (Dinamap) – unwell child, neonates, infants
■ Invasive – arterial line

Respiratory system

Peak expiratory flow (PEF)	In children > 5 years old
General inspection	Cyanosis Respiratory rate – tachypnoea, dyspnoea (for normal rates, see Table 1.1) Cough, snuffles, runny nose Stridor (inspiratory or expiratory) Hoarse voice **Respiratory distress** features: ■ Tachypnoea ■ Nasal flaring ■ Expiratory grunt ■ Intercostal, subcostal, suprasternal, sternal recession, tracheal tug ⎫ ■ Using accessory muscles (sternomastoid) ⎬ Dyspnoea ■ Difficulty feeding + talking ⎭

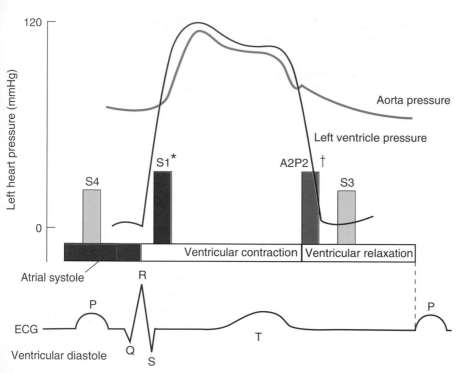

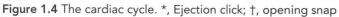

Figure 1.4 The cardiac cycle. *, Ejection click; †, opening snap

Table 1.1 Normal vital signs in children

Age	HR	RR	SBP	DBP
< 1	120–160	30–60	60–95	35–69
1–3	90–140	24–40	95–105	50–65
3–5	75–110	18–30	95–110	50–65
8–12	75–100	18–30	90–110	57–71
12–16	60–90	12–16	112–130	60–80

From: Duke J, Rosenberg SG (eds). *Anaesthesia Secrets*. St Louis: Mosby, 1996: 370.

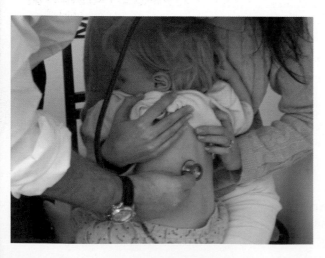

Figure 1.5 Chest examination in a relaxed child being cuddled by the mother

Inspection	Atopic facies (swollen eyelids, transverse nasal crease – allergic salute) Clubbing (*long term* cyanosis, e.g. cystic fibrosis) Chest deformity: ■ Pectus carinatum (pigeon chest – asthma), ■ Pectus excavatum (isolated congenital defect, Marfan) ■ Rib rosary (rickets) ■ Scars – tracheostomy, repair PDA, intercostal catheters Breathing pattern Symmetrical movement (asymmetrical in foreign body inhalation)
Palpation	Apex beat (*displaced in mediastinal shift*, e.g. tension pneumothorax) Parasternal area (*right ventricular heave*, e.g. pulmonary hypertension secondary to obstructive sleep apnoea) NB: Tracheal position is not useful in children
Auscultation	**Breath sounds** – quality, symmetry, transmitted sounds (from the upper airways to the chest) **Crackles**, e.g. pneumonia **Wheeze** – inspiratory or expiratory, e.g. asthma, bronchiolitis **Vocal resonance** (consolidation). NB: Not usually easy to identify NB: In severe asthma there are reduced breath sounds due to reduced air entry
Percussion	Hyperinflation (liver moves down) Consolidation (reduced resonance)

Abdomen

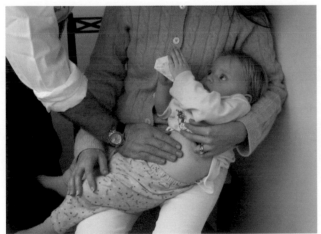

Figure 1.6 Abdominal examination – best done with the infant relaxed, which may not be possible in the conventional position

Inspection	Pallor (**anaemia**), jaundice, bruising, nutritional status, oedema, distension, scaphoid, hernia, ascites, stoma, scars (e.g. V–P shunt), striae, genitalia **Portal hypertension**: ■ Splenomegaly ■ Prominent abdominal wall veins (flowing away from the umbilicus, i.e. caput medusae) ■ Abdominal distension (ascites)
Palpation	Superficial then deep Clockwise from left iliac fossa Look for tenderness, pain, masses *Acute abdomen* – rebound tenderness, pain localized *Rigid abdomen* – perforation

Percussion	Hyperresonance (ileus, obstruction), masses, liver and spleen upper and lower borders
Auscultation	Bowel sounds, bruits
Liver	Palpate upwards from right iliac fossa. Normal = 1–2 cm below costal margin
	Hepatomegaly, small, tender, soft or hard
Spleen	Palpate upwards from right iliac fossa. Normal = 1–2 cm below costal margin
	Splenomegaly, tender
Kidneys	Large, bruits, tender, iliac fossa mass (renal transplant)
Inguinal hernia	Inspect, palpate and cough test
Testes	Both descended, tender, erythema, enlarged testes, enlarged scrotum
Genital exam	If necessary
Rectal exam	Not routine, though if indicated it must be done

Central nervous system

See Chapter 20. In brief:

- Postural reflexes and responses
- Movement and coordination
- Limbs
- Cranial nerves

Developmental assessment

See Chapter 2.

Check key milestones, primitive reflexes and postural responses.

Bones and joints

See Chapter 22.

If necessary:

Rash?	Butterfly, heliotrope, nodules, scleroderma, purpura
Joints	**Inspection** – joints involved, swelling, deformity, erythema, muscle wasting
	Palpation – tenderness, warmth, effusion
	Movement – active then passive if active restricted. Describe angle from neutral
Ligaments	

Eyes

- Squint (p. 410 [strabismus])
- Obvious deformity or injury
- Pupils:
  - Equal, size, outline
  - Direct and consensual light reflexes
- Fundi examination (lots of practice is the only way to be good at this)
- Slit lamp if eye problem
- Visual acuity if necessary (see p. 409 [visual acuity testing])
- Older children: visual fields as per adult examination

Ear, nose and throat

Throat (esp. tonsils) Positioning is crucial – get parent to hold child on lap facing you, one arm around child's arms, the other across the forehead

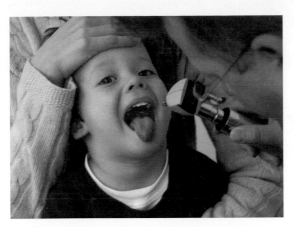

Figure 1.7 Throat examination – positioning is important: one hand holds the forehead and the other is across the child's arms. A tongue depressor is often necessary, but not in this case

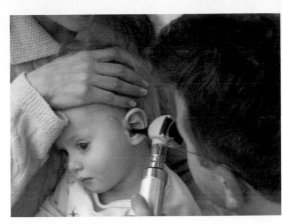

Figure 1.8 Ear examination – the infant is held with one hand across the head, and the other across the arms

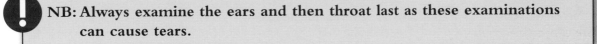

NB: Always examine the ears and then throat last as these examinations can cause tears.

	Use a tongue depressor only if necessary
	Enlargement, red, swelling, quinsy, pus
	Dental caries?
Ears	Positioning is crucial – use parent to hold child on lap
	External auditory meatus and pinna (otitis externa, pinna abnormalities)
	Auroscope examination (ear drum and internal auditory meatus)
	Hearing assessment (p. 112 [hearing assessment])
Nose	Coryzal signs?

FURTHER READING

Gill D, O'Brien N. *Paediatric Clinical Examination Made Easy*, 5th edn. London: Elsevier, 2006.

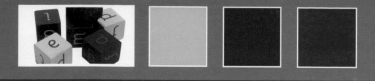

2 Development

- Developmental milestones
- Child health developmental assessment in the UK
- Primitive reflexes and postural responses
- Developmental delay
- Further reading

Child development can be divided into four areas:

Gross motor	Communication
Gross motor skills	Non-verbal communication
Primitive reflexes and postural responses	Speech and language
	Hearing

Fine motor	Psychological
Fine motor skills	Emotions
Vision	Behavioural
	Social

DEVELOPMENTAL MILESTONES

Development is assessed by checking key developmental milestones in the above four areas, i.e. skills that children should have learnt by a certain age. Continued developmental progress over time needs to be monitored.

> **!** **NB: The special senses, in particular hearing and vision, are crucial for development, so they must be checked first because difficulties with hearing or vision will result in associated developmental delay.**

DEVELOPMENTAL MILESTONES (NB: THE AGES ARE THE LATEST THAT THESE SKILLS SHOULD BE ACQUIRED BY)

Age	Fine motor	Gross motor	Language	Social skills
Newborn	Follows face and light to the midline	Tone – head lag Fetal position, symmetrical	Cries Startles to noises	Follows face
6 weeks	Smiles Follows face and objects to the midline	Head control on tummy (raises head) Better tone	Responds to mother's voice *Hello*	Smiles
3 months	Fixes and follows face through midline Hand regard Reaches	Pushes up with arms on tummy Head control good	Cries Laughs Babbles	Smiles
6 months	Palmar grasp Transfers from hand to hand	Sits unsupported (just) (back bent)	Babbles Turns towards quiet sounds *Blah blah*	Eats finger foods
9 months	Pincer grasp (9–14)	Sits well Pulls to stand Crawls	'Daddy' (non-specific) *Daddy*	Stranger awareness Understands 'no' Plays peekaboo *NO !*

Age	Fine motor	Gross motor	Language	Social skills
1 year	Releases objects	May walk (unsteady) or bottom shuffle	'Mummy' and 'daddy' (specific) + 3 other words *Daddy Mummy*	Waves bye-bye (from 10 months) Cup drinking
15 months	Scribbles	Walks well (most)	5–10 words	Drinking from cup
18 months	Scribbles Three-cube tower	Walks upstairs	5–10 words Names six body parts *Nose, eyes, mouth, hand, ears, hair*	Mimics Feeds with spoon Symbolic play
2 years	Circular scribbles Six-cube tower	Kicks Runs Kicks a ball	2–3 word sentences *I love you*	Undresses
3 years	Draws circle Bridge three cubes	Jumps	Says first name, colours, 3–4 word sentences *Charlie*	Dresses Has friend/ interactive play Buttons (50%)
4 years	Draws cross	Stands on one leg Hops	Good speech Says surname *Charlie Green*	Buttons (all)
5 years	Draws triangle	Bicycles	Good speech	Shoe laces

Variation

There is wide variability in the 'normal ranges'. This is particularly so with walking – normal children may walk from 11–18 months. If they bottom shuffle (instead of crawling), they generally walk late as bottom shuffling is so efficient.

Bladder and bowel control

This is also very variable. Bladder and bowel control is usually attained by 2 years of age in girls and by 3 years in boys. Nocturnal enuresis until 5 years is relatively common. Boys are notoriously slow. There is variation between countries, e.g. early in France.

CHILD HEALTH DEVELOPMENTAL ASSESSMENT IN THE UK

Scheduled developmental assessments are performed mostly by the GP or health visitor at home or in the surgery. This programme is developed to:

- Make sure the mother (and father) is coping well, and address any queries/concerns she has regarding her baby, e.g. breast feeding, colic
- Check on growth (plotted on growth charts)
- Check on vaccination programme
- Give health advice, e.g. weaning, practical tips, safety advice
- Screen for early detection of hearing or visual problems
- Screen for early detection of developmental delay
- Early detection of any other health problems

The visits are recorded in the child's developmental book ('red book'), which is kept by the parent. All other visits to doctors should be summarized in this book, so that a health summary is available with the parent should it need to be referred to.

DEVELOPMENTAL ASSESSMENTS (THIS DEVELOPMENTAL PROGRAMME IS VARIABLE)

Age	By whom	Assessment
Postnatal check (24 h)	In hospital by paediatrician or GP if at home	General examination (see ch. 4) Hips, heart, testes, hernias, ± hearing check Weight, length, head circumference (HC)
1 week check	Midwife	Weight, jaundice screen, Guthrie test
6 week check	GP in the surgery	General examination, hips, testes, hernias Weight, length, HC ± **Hearing check** using OAEs (see p. 112)

Age	By whom	Assessment
9 month check	Health visitor/GP	Developmental assessment, any concerns Weight, length, HC **Hearing test** using distraction testing (see p. 114)
2–2½ year check	Health visitor	Developmental assessment, any concerns Weight, height, HC
3–4 years (pre-school)	Health visitor	Weight, height, developmental assessment
5 years (school)	School nurse	Vision and hearing, weight, height Examination if any concerns

AGE GROUPS

Fetus	*In utero*
Neonate	0–1/12
Infant	1/12–1 year
Toddler	1–3 years
School child	4–16 (18) years
Teenager	12–19 years

NB: Preterm infants are age-corrected until age 2 years.

PRIMITIVE REFLEXES AND POSTURAL RESPONSES

Primitive reflexes are present from birth and asymmetry or persistence for longer suggests neurological deficit.

PRIMITIVE REFLEXES

Reflex	Usual age to disappear (months) (all variable)	Description	
Sucking reflex	6–8 weeks	Automatic suck if object placed in mouth	
Rooting reflex	6–8 weeks	Stroke cheek and mouth opens and moves towards it	
Palmar grasp	3–4	Stroke palm and it closes	
Plantar grasp	12–18	Stroke sole and it closes	
Moro reflex	4–5	Sudden neck extension – extension, abduction then adduction of the arms and flexion of fingers, wrists and elbows	
Stepping reflex	2	When held and 'walked', the feet move in a stepping sequence	
Asymmetrical tonic neck reflex	6	In a supine infant, turning the head laterally – extension of the arm and leg on the side to the turn, and flexion of both on the side away from the turn (like an archer)	

The **Babinsky reflex** is initially upgoing (but hard to elicit because of the plantar reflex) and becomes downgoing from around 1 year.

POSTURAL RESPONSES

Reflex	Appears (months)	Disappears	Description
Forward parachute	5–6	Stays for life	When held prone by the waist and lowered, arms and legs extend
Landau reflex	3–6	1 year	When held prone, legs, spine and head extend
Lateral propping reflex	7	Stays for life	When sitting and pushed sideways, arms extend to prevent a fall

DEVELOPMENTAL DELAY

Developmental delay may be:

Specific   Affecting one or more particular areas of development only, or
Global   All areas of development affected

There is, however, inevitable overlap between the different developmental areas, such that a problem in one area will affect another, e.g. low intelligence results in language delay, and motor delay in cerebral palsy can result in speech delay.

It may also be:

- *Mild, moderate* or *severe*
- A *gradual* steady developmental delay from birth, e.g. genetic, lack of stimulation, chronic illness
- *New onset* after previously normal development, e.g. new-onset deafness or visual impairment, unhappy social situation, autism, neurodegenerative condition. This may manifest as a *slowing down* of development, an *arrest* of development or in some cases developmental *regression*

Motor delay

- Gross motor
- Fine motor

! NB: Retention of primitive reflexes beyond the normal age to lose them is a feature of motor delay.

Communication (speech, language and non-verbal communication) delay

- **Speech delay** is delay in speech articulation, e.g. incomprehensible speech, stammering, dysarthria
- **Language delay** is delay in language *comprehension* (receptive) and/or *expression*
- **Non-verbal communication** is an important part of language and pre-language development
- Social development is also affected

! NB: Always check hearing and vision thoroughly if developmental delay is present.

ASSESSMENT

Developmental delay is generally initially suspected by the parents or detected by the health visitor or GP. Full assessment and management of developmental delay includes input from:

- Neurodevelopmental paediatrician
- Speech and language therapist
- Physiotherapists, occupational therapist
- Teacher, psychologist
- Social worker and health visitor

CONCERNING SIGNS IN DEVELOPMENT

- No social smiling by 2 months
- Not sitting alone by 9 months
- Not crawling by 1 year
- Not walking by 18 months
- No speech by 18 months
- Hand preference development < 1 year (this usually develops at 18–24 months)

History and examination

The history should include the onset, natural history and area(s) of delay, in addition to a general personal and family history. In particular, the following should be assessed:

- Full neurological examination including cerebellar signs
- Dysmorphic features
- Head circumference
- Vision
- Hearing

Investigations

These are led by the history and examination findings and may include:

Bloods	Thyroid function tests
	Chromosome analysis including fragile X
	Antenatal infection screen
	Metabolic screen (see p. 279)
	White cell enzymes
Imaging	Cranial USS, CT or MRI brain
EEG	
Other	Nerve conduction studies, EMG, nerve and muscle biopsy, CPK

LEARNING DISABILITY

Learning disability is impairment of cognitive function. This may range from mild to profound, and is often part of a global delay. A comprehensive assessment is used to assess severity in addition to the intelligence quotient (IQ):

Moderate	Learning disability = IQ 50–70
Severe	Learning disability = IQ 20–50
Profound	Learning disability = IQ < 20

- A significant proportion of school-age children are assessed as having learning disability
- Child may have associated delay in other areas
- Most cases of severe disability have an organic cause; no cause is found in around one-quarter
- These children are formerly assessed by a paediatric team, and their disability and needs are identified and reported in a **Statement of Special Educational Needs**. Any special services outlined can then be offered to the child. These statements need regular review (see ch. 27)
- A specialist individual home education programme prior to nursery, known as **Portage**, may be arranged

Dyslexia

Dyslexia is difficulty in learning to read despite adequate intelligence, conventional instruction and sociocultural opportunity. Diagnosed by finding a significant discrepancy between reading achievement and intellectual ability (IQ test scores may be done).

Management

- Multidisciplinary involvement with teachers, psychologists and paediatricians
- Counselling to deal with the frustrations that it causes the child is helpful
- Specific remedies include visual training (ocular tracking exercises) and sensory–motor integration therapy, though evidence for their efficacy is lacking

Causes of developmental delay

Motor

- Normal, e.g. delay in walking in commando crawlers or bottom shufflers
- Neurological disorder, e.g. cerebral palsy
- Neuromuscular disorder, e.g. Duchenne muscular dystrophy
- Any cause of global developmental delay

Communication (speech, language and non-verbal)

- Hearing disorder
- Visual disorder
- Lack of stimulation
- Articulation defect – neuromuscular disorder, physical abnormality, e.g. cleft palate
- General developmental delay
- Autism
- Communication is also affected by general intelligence and motor function

Global

- Genetic low intelligence
- Lack of stimulation
- Chronic illness
- Psychological upset
- Genetic disorder or syndrome, e.g. Down syndrome; metabolic disorder, e.g. phenylketonuria; brain abnormality, e.g. hydrocephalus
- Antenatal disorder – congenital infection; teratogens
- Birth asphyxia
- Prematurity
- Hypothyroidism
- Neurological insult – head trauma; meningitis, encephalitis; metabolic, e.g. hypoglycaemia

Clinical scenario

A 10-month-old boy is seen in a paediatric outpatient clinic because the health visitor has agreed with the mother that he is not yet sitting properly and is not particularly interested in his surroundings.

On pulling to sit he has a tendency to be pulled along the examination couch and fall backwards. He will not support his own weight on supported standing. His asymmetrical tonic neck reflex is pronounced to the right and not present to the left. He has a flexed posture of his left upper limb at rest and does not seem to move this arm.

1. What is the most likely neurological diagnosis?
2. What should be done?

He has also had significant problems in establishing feeding and will only take milk from a bottle in small amounts with a number of aspiration-like events. His weight and length are therefore progressing poorly and he is moving downwards across the centiles.

3. What nutritional approach might be recommended, which would also protect his airway?

ANSWERS

1. The most likely diagnosis is right hemiparesis with possible diplegia accounting for the increased lower limb tone.
2. Referral to multidisciplinary developmental team.
3. The use of PEG.

FURTHER READING

Sheridan M, Sharma A, Cockerill H. *From Birth to Five Years: Children's Developmental Progress*, 3rd edn. New York: Taylor & Francis, 2007.

Slater M, Lewis M. *Introduction to Infant Development*, 2nd edn. New York: Oxford University Press, 2006.

Hall D, Williams J, Elliman D. *The Child Surveillance Handbook*, 3rd edn. Abingdon: Radcliffe, 2009.

Further reading

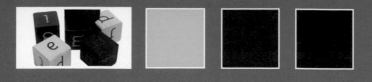

3 Genetics

- Clinical applications of genetics
- Genetic mutations
- Genetic disorders
- Inheritance patterns
- Dysmorphology
- Further reading

CLINICAL APPLICATIONS OF GENETICS

Genetics is a rapidly advancing and fascinating field of medicine, which has particular relevance in paediatrics. Increasingly, medical genetics is becoming central to the understanding of many diseases, not just rare disorders. A large proportion of paediatric admissions are due to genetic diseases, as are a large proportion (50%) of paediatric deaths.

The role of a **clinical geneticist** is to help individuals or families with, or at risk of developing, a genetic disorder to live and reproduce as normally as possible. This will include:

- Drawing a family pedigree
- Making or confirming a diagnosis using clinical skills and investigations, with genetic testing where appropriate
- Discussing the natural history of the disorder and relevant management
- Discussing the risks to other family members of developing or passing on the disorder
- Options for screening and prenatal diagnosis

GENETIC SCREENING

Genetic screening is the search in a population for persons possessing certain genotypes (variations of a specific gene) that:

- Are known to be associated with disease or predisposition to disease, or
- May lead to disease in their offspring

Disorders such as thalassaemia are amenable to population screening as the test can be performed by a buccal smear or blood test; the carrier frequency is common in specific populations; gene carriers themselves are not at increased risk of disease; and a specific prenatal test can be offered to couples identified to be at risk.

Genetic carrier testing is the search in at-risk individuals for a specific genotype known to be associated with disease in that family.

PRENATAL DIAGNOSIS

This involves both **screening tests** that give a probability of disease and **diagnostic tests** that give a definite diagnosis. An example of a screening test is antenatal nuchal USS, which identifies a pregnancy at increased risk of Down syndrome, where definitive testing via chorionic villus biopsy or amniocentesis may be offered. Diagnostic tests include DNA analysis of a fetal sample looking for DNA changes known to be associated with disease in that family, e.g. analysis of the cystic fibrosis gene in a CVS sample, where both parents are known to be carriers of the disorder.

Reasons for antenatal testing

- To reassure parents in a normal pregnancy
- To identify an affected fetus in a high-risk family
- To allow parents to make an informed decision regarding continuation of the pregnancy where an anomaly is identified
- To enable optimal medical management (*in utero* and after birth), e.g. arrange for the baby with a congenital cardiac anomaly to be born in a hospital where the cardiologist is aware of and able to manage the problem

Prenatal screening tests

- Nuchal USS (11–14 weeks)
- Fetal anomaly USS (20–24 weeks)

Prenatal diagnostic tests

- Chorionic villus sampling (CVS) (11–14 weeks)
- Amniocentesis (> 16 weeks)
- Percutaneous umbilical blood sampling (> 20 weeks)

Testing of genetic disorders in at-risk families

- Heterozygote screening in at-risk families, e.g. cystic fibrosis gene analysis
- Pre-symptomatic testing in adult-onset disorders, e.g. Huntington disease, breast cancer
- Carrier testing for at-risk relatives in X-linked disorders, e.g. Duchenne muscular dystrophy
- Family history of chromosomal disorder, e.g. translocation

GENE THERAPY

This is the treatment of genetic disease via **genetic alteration** of cells of individuals with a genetic disease. Although this is an exciting area which may in the future provide treatment for genetic disorders, success to date has been limited. Many clinical trials are in progress. Most techniques involve inserting a functioning normal gene into somatic cells to programme the cell to produce the normal gene product. Currently, gene therapy is being used in somatic cells and *not* in germline cells (which could result in the future generation being affected).

Examples of diseases in which gene therapy is being investigated

Disease	Gene inserted	Somatic cells into which gene is inserted
Cystic fibrosis	CFTR	Airway epithelial cells
Duchenne muscular dystrophy	Dystrophin	Muscle
Haemophilia B	Factor IX	Hepatocytes and skin fibroblasts

GENETIC MUTATIONS

A **mutation** is a change in the DNA sequence which leads to an alteration of gene function:

- Mutations in germline cells (cells that produce gametes) generally result in genetic diseases
- Mutations in somatic cells (normal body cells) may result in cancer

A **polymorphism** is a variation in DNA sequence, found with a frequency of at least 1% in the normal population.

- Genes differ among individuals due to polymorphisms
- Corresponding DNA sequences between two chromosomes are called **alleles**
- If someone has the same mutation on both alleles of a chromosome pair, they are **homozygous** for that mutation
- If the mutation is only present on one allele, the individual is **heterozygous**
- A **locus** is the position of a gene on a chromosome
- The **genotype** is the alleles present at a given locus in an individual

A mutation may be large – resulting in major alteration of the structure of chromosome(s) or their number – and visible under the light microscope (see p. 31). Alternatively, it may be submicroscopic, affecting a single gene only as a result of several different mechanisms (see below), and is studied by **molecular genetic techniques**.

Single gene mutations

- **Insertions** or **deletions** of one or more base pairs, e.g. the most common cystic fibrosis mutation, ΔF508 (three base-pair deletion at position 508 of the CFTR gene)
- **Point mutations** may cause one amino acid to change to another (**missense mutation**), or produce a stop codon (**nonsense mutation**) such that no protein product is produced
- **Whole gene duplications**, e.g. Charcot–Marie–Tooth disease (three copies of PMP22 encoding myelin)

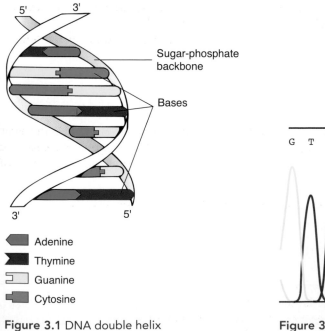

Sugar-phosphate backbone

Bases

5'   3'

3'   5'

◄ Adenine
► Thymine
▭ Guanine
▭ Cytosine

Figure 3.1 DNA double helix

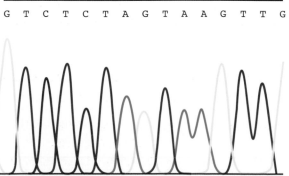

G T C T C T A G T A A G T T G

Figure 3.2 DNA sequence

- **Promotor mutations** (affinity of RNA polymerase to a promotor site is altered)
- **Splice site mutations**
- **Expanded repeats**, e.g. Fragile X syndrome

Causes

Spontaneous mutations	Occur naturally during DNA replication
Induced mutations	Caused by mutagens:

- Ionizing radiation, e.g. X-rays, nuclear bombs
- Non-ionizing radiation, e.g. UV light
- Chemicals, e.g. nitrogen mustard, aflatoxin B1

Certain diseases have defective **DNA repair**, and consequently have a high rate of tumour formation, e.g. xeroderma pigmentosa, Fanconi anaemia, ataxia telangiectasia, Bloom syndrome.

Karyotype and chromosome banding

Karyotype is the name given to the result of chromosome analysis, giving information on the number of chromosomes present. Structural chromosomal rearrangements may be identified. Staining techniques bring out the chromosome **bands** and these are visible under the light microscope.

Normal karyotypes   46, XX (female)
46, XY (male)

GENETIC DISORDERS

Genetic disorders are broadly classified into:

Chromosomal disorders	Entire chromosomes or large segments of them are altered (duplicated, missing, translocated, etc.), e.g. trisomy 21 syndrome
Single gene disorders	Single genes are altered, e.g. cystic fibrosis, Tay–Sachs
Multifactorial disorders	Disorders due to a combination of genetic and environmental factors, e.g. cleft lip and palate
Mitochondrial disorders	Disorders caused by alterations in the cytoplasmic mitochondrial DNA, e.g. MELAS, MERRF

CHROMOSOMAL DISORDERS

Chromosomal abnormalities

These are changes that are large enough to be seen by looking at the chromosomes under the light microscope. They are studied by **cytogenetic techniques**. They are due to either changes in the *number* of chromosomes (e.g. trisomy) or large changes within the structure of chromosomes (*chromosomal rearrangements*).

Incidence 1 in 150 live births; 50% of first trimester abortions and 20% of second trimester.

Abnormalities of chromosome number

Polyploidy	Extra *whole sets* of chromosomes:

- Triploidy (69, XXX) ⎫
- Tetraploidy (92, XXXX) ⎬ Lethal in humans ⎭

Aneuploidy	Missing or extra *individual* chromosomes:

- Monosomy (only one copy of a particular chromosome)
- Trisomy (three copies of a particular chromosome)

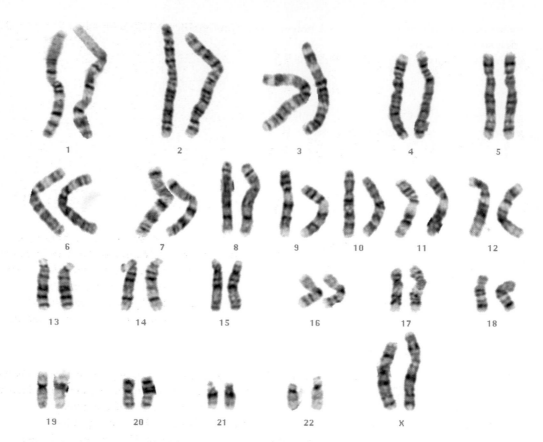

Figure 3.3 Banded karotype of a normal female (courtesy of the North East London Regional Cytogenetics Laboratory)

Down syndrome (trisomy 21)

This is the most common autosomal trisomy.

Clinical features are:

General	**Hypotonia** (floppy babies), small stature, hyperflexible joints
CNS	Developmental delay, Alzheimer disease (later)
Craniofacial	Brachycephaly, mild microcephaly, upslanting palpebral fissures (Mongolian slant to eyes), **epicanthic folds**, myopia, acquired cataracts, **Brushfield spots** (speckled irises), small ears, mixed hearing loss, glue ear, small nose, **protruding tongue**, dental hypoplasia, short neck (risk of atlanto-axial subluxation with anaesthetics)
Skin	Loose neck folds (infant), dry skin, folliculitis in adolescents
Hair	Soft, fine; straight pubic hair
Hands and feet	Short fingers, 5th finger clinodactyly, **single palmar crease** (present in 1% of normal population), wide gap between 1st and 2nd toes (sandal gap)
Cardiac	CHD (40%): AVSD, VSD, PDA, ASD; valve prolapse > 20 years
Respiratory	Increased chest infections
Genitalia	Small penis and testicular volume. Infertility common
Blood	Increased incidence of leukaemia
Endocrine	Increased incidence of hypothyroidism

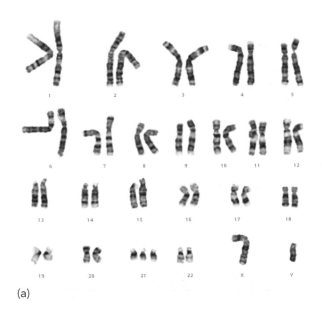

(a)

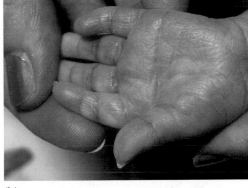

(b)

Figure 3.4 Down syndrome. (a) Karyotype (courtesy of the North East London Regional Cytogenetics Laboratory). (b) Single palmar crease. Also note short phalanges and metacarpals, and hypoplasia of the mid-phalanx of the little finger with clinodactyly

There are several mechanisms of trisomy 21:

1. **Non-disjunction** (95%). Karyotype: 47, XY + 21. This occurs where the two chromosome 21s do not separate at meiosis. The extra chromosome is maternal in 90% of cases, and the incidence increases with maternal age (see Table 3.1). Non-disjunction is the commonest cause of aneuploidy
2. **Robertsonian translocation** (4%). Common karyotype: 46, XY,–14,+ t (14q21q). Here a chromosome 21 is translocated onto another chromosome (14, 15, 21 or 22). This may arise as a new event in the child or occur when one of the parents carries a balanced translocation. The risk of recurrence is:
    - 10–15% if the mother is a translocation carrier
    - 2.5% if the father is a translocation carrier
    - 100% if a parent has the translocation 21:21
    - < 1% if neither parent has a translocation
3. **Mosaicism** (1%). These children have some normal cells and some trisomy 21 cells. Karyoptye: 47, XY + 21/46, XY. This occurs from non-disjunction occurring during mitosis *after* fertilization

Table 3.1 Risk of Down syndrome with maternal age

Maternal age	Approximate risk
All ages	1 in 650
30	1 in 1000
35	1 in 365
40	1 in 100
45	1 in 50

Edwards syndrome (trisomy 18)
Karyotype: 47, XY, + 18

Clinical features are:

General   Low birthweight, fetal inactivity, single umbilical artery, skeletal muscle and adipose hyopoplasia, mental deficiency

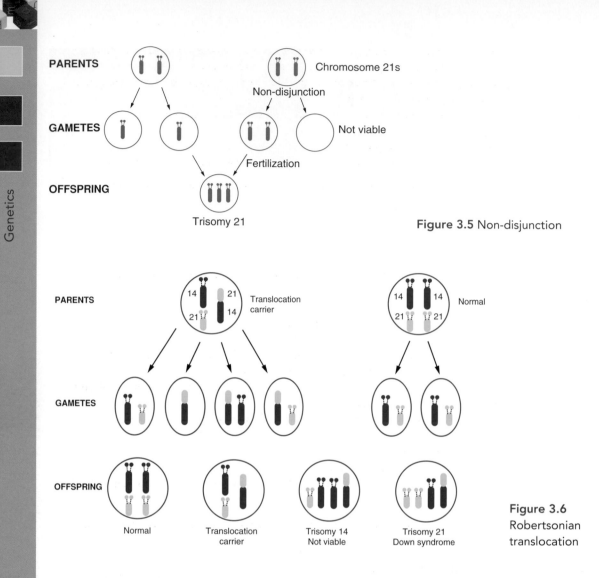

PARENTS

Chromosome 21s

Non-disjunction

GAMETES

Not viable

Fertilization

OFFSPRING

Trisomy 21

Figure 3.5 Non-disjunction

PARENTS

14 21 Translocation carrier
21 14

14 14 Normal
21 21

GAMETES

OFFSPRING

Normal

Translocation carrier

Trisomy 14 Not viable

Trisomy 21 Down syndrome

Figure 3.6 Robertsonian translocation

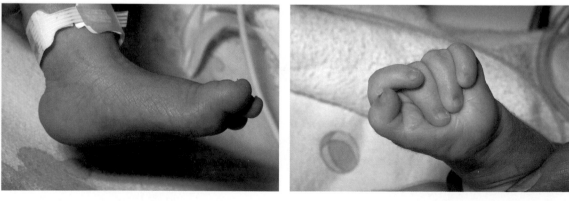

(a)

(b)

Figure 3.7 Edwards syndrome. (a) Rocker bottom feet. (b) Clenched fist in ulnar deviation with index finger overlying third finger and little finger overlying ring finger. Also note the short thumb, absence of distal crease over ring finger and little finger, and hypoplasia of little finger nail

Craniofacial	Narrow bifrontal diameter, short palpebral fissures, low-set abnormal ears, small mouth, micrognathia, epicanthic folds, cleft lip and/or palate
Hands and feet	**Overlapping of index finger** over 3rd and 5th finger over 4th. Clenched hand, small nails, **rocker-bottom feet**
Trunk and pelvis	Short sternum, small nipples, inguinal or umbilical hernia, small pelvis
Genitalia	Cryptorchidism (male)
Cardiac	VSD, ASD, PDA, bicuspid aortic + pulmonary valves
Other organs	Right lung malsegmentation or absence, renal and gastrointestinal abnormalities

50% die within the first week and only 5–10% survive the first year. Recurrence risk is low unless parental translocation is present.

Turner syndrome (monosomy of the X chromosome)
Karyotype: 45, X0.

This is generally a sporadic event. Mosaicism is well-recognized and usually results in milder manifestations.

Clinical features are:

General	**Short stature**, loose neck folds in infants
CNS	Visuospatial difficulties, hearing impairment
Gonads	**Ovarian dysgenesis** with hypoplasia or absence of germinal elements (90%)
Lymph vessels	**Congenital lymphoedema** (puffy fingers and toes)
Craniofacial	Abnormal ears (often prominent), narrow maxilla, small mandible, **short webbed neck**, low posterior hair-line
Skeletal	**Broad chest** with **wide-spaced nipples, cubitus valgus**
Nails	**Narrow hyperconvex nails**
Skin	Multiple pigmented naevi
Renal	Horseshoe kidney, double renal pelvis
Cardiac	Bicuspid aortic valve (30%), coarctation of the aorta (10%), aortic stenosis, mitral valve prolapse

These children may be given growth hormone (and oestrogen replacement if necessary at adolescence).

Klinefelter syndrome
Karyotype: 47, XXY. Estimated to affect 1 in 500 males.

Clinical features are very variable. Klinefelter syndrome may be identified as an incidental finding or may present with behavioural difficulties or as infertility in an adult.

Skeletal	Tall and slim, long limbs, low upper:lower segment ratio, mild elbow dysplasia
Genitalia	Relatively small penis and testes in childhood, most enter puberty normally, primary infertility secondary to azoospermia, reduced secondary sexual characteristics, gynaecomastia (33%)
CNS	Mild learning difficulties

Testosterone therapy may be given.

47, XYY syndrome
Incidence 1 in 840 males. Most cases are phenotypically normal.

Clinical features may include:

CNS	Mild learning difficulties, poor fine motor coordination, speech delay, behavioural problems (hyperactivity, temper tantrums)
Growth	Accelerated growth in mid-childhood

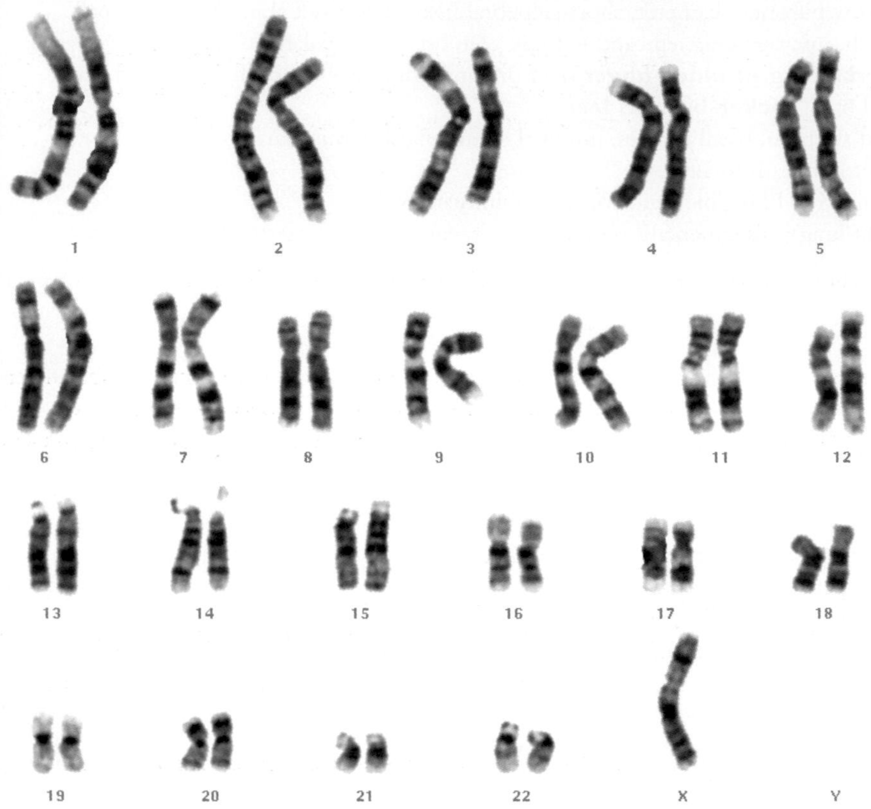

Figure 3.8 Turner syndrome karyotype (courtesy of the North East London Regional Cytogenetics Laboratory)

Craniofacial	Prominent glabella, large ears
Skin	Teenage acne
Skeletal	Long fingers and toes, mild pectus excavatum

CHROMOSOMAL REARRANGEMENTS

These are not whole but *partial* chromosome abnormalities, and may result from a number of types of chromosome mutation.

Translocations

This is the interchange of genetic material between non-homologous chromosomes. There are two types:

1. **Reciprocal translocations**. Two breaks on different chromosomes occur and so genetic material is exchanged between the two chromosomes. A carrier of a *balanced* translocation is usually of normal phenotype because they have the normal chromosome complement. However, their offspring may have an *unbalanced* translocation resulting in a partial trisomy or monosomy, e.g. 6p trisomy, 4p monosomy

2. **Robertsonian translocation** (results in altered chromosome numbers – see Down syndrome above). The long arms of two acrocentric chromosomes fuse together to make one long chromosome, and their short arms are lost. This only occurs between chromosomes 13, 14, 15, 21 and 22 because these are acrocentric (have very small short arms that contain no essential genetic material). It can result in Down syndrome for the offspring of a carrier of the Robertsonian translocation

Deletions

Deletion of a portion of the chromosome occurs, e.g. cri du chat syndrome (46, XY, del [5p]). Microdeletions (smaller deletions now visible microscopically using new techniques such as high-resolution banding and FISH, or by molecular techniques) include Williams syndrome and DiGeorge syndrome (chromosome 22 microdeletion).

Duplications

Two copies of a portion of the chromosome are present, e.g. Charcot–Marie–Tooth disease.

DiGeorge syndrome

This is due to a microdeletion of 22q. The syndrome overlaps with velocardiofacial syndrome or Shprintzen syndrome, and is now more commonly known as the **22q11 microdeletion syndrome**, which covers the spectrum of abnormalities. The features result from a fourth branchial arch development defect (3rd and 4th pharyngeal pouches).

Clinical features are:

Thymus	Hypoplasia/aplasia, cellular immunity defect
Parathyroids	Hypoplasia/absence, hypocalcaemia and neonatal fits
Cardiac	Aortic arch anomalies (right-sided aortic arch, interrupted aortic arch, truncus arteriosus, VSD, TOF)
CNS	Learning difficulties
Growth	Short stature
Craniofacial	Absent adenoids, cleft palate, prominent nose, long maxilla, small mandible, ear abnormalities

Williams syndrome

This is due to a microdeletion of the chromosomal region 7q11.23, including the elastin gene.

Clinical features are:

Craniofacial	Medial eyebrow flare, depressed nasal bridge, epicanthic folds, periorbital fullness, blue eyes, **stellate pattern iris**, prominent lips (fish-shaped), full cheeks

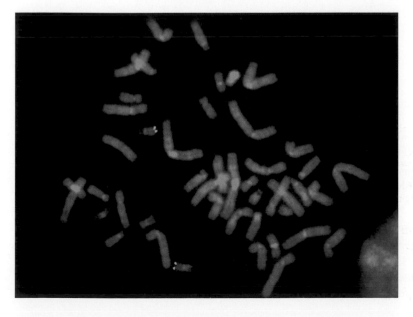

Figure 3.9 DiGeorge syndrome. Microdeletion of 22q demonstrated by a FISH study. The green dots are probes close to the telomeres of the long arm (q) of chromosome 22, and the red dots show the region of chromosome 22 which is deleted in children with DiGeorge syndrome. The lower chromosome 22 is showing no red signal and so is deleted for the DiGeorge syndrome region (courtesy of the North East London Regional Cytogenetics Laboratory)

CNS	Mental retardation, friendly manner, **'cocktail party' speech**, hypersensitivity to sound
Skeletal	Short stature, hypoplastic nails, scoliosis, kyphosis, joint limitations
Cardiac	Supravalvular aortic stenosis, peripheral pulmonary artery stenosis, VSD, ASD, renal artery stenosis
Renal	Nephrocalcinosis, pelvic kidney, urethral stenosis

SINGLE GENE DISORDERS

Single gene traits are also termed Mendelian traits after Gregor Mendel, the Austrian monk who derived some basic genetic principles from his experiments with peas in the 19th century. Inheritance of single gene disorders is based on the principles that genes occur in pairs (alleles), that only one allele from each parent is passed to the offspring, and that an allele may act in a *dominant* or *recessive* manner. Many exceptions and factors complicate this pattern.

A **pedigree** of relatives (as far back as possible) is constructed to understand the inheritance of a particular condition.

Autosomal disorders

Autosomal disorders are diseases caused by genes on any of the autosomes.

Examples of autosomal disorders

Autosomal dominant	Autosomal recessive
Marfan syndrome	Cystic fibrosis
Achondroplasia	Galactosaemia
Noonan syndrome	Phenylketonuria
Otosclerosis	Congenital adrenal hyperplasia

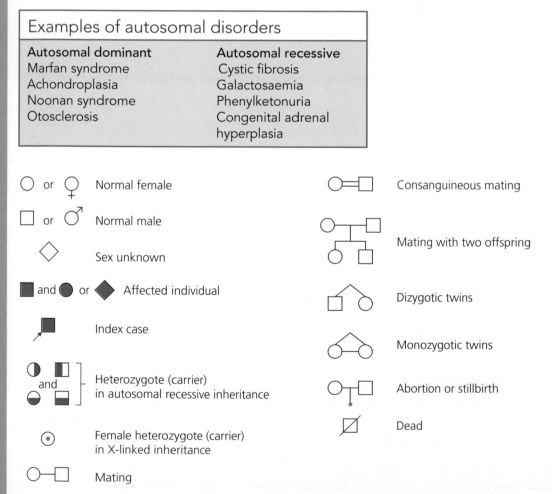

Figure 3.10 Pedigree symbols

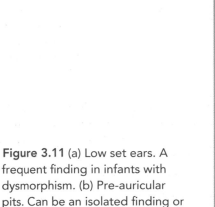

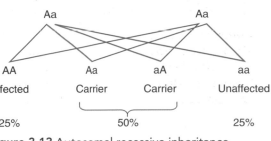

Figure 3.11 (a) Low set ears. A frequent finding in infants with dysmorphism. (b) Pre-auricular pits. Can be an isolated finding or associated with deafness and certain syndromes

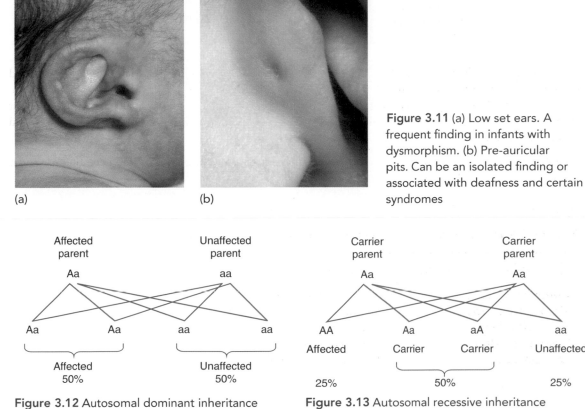

Figure 3.12 Autosomal dominant inheritance

Figure 3.13 Autosomal recessive inheritance

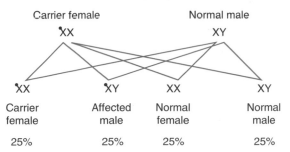

Figure 3.14 X-linked recessive inheritance

X-linked inheritance

X-linked disorders are diseases caused by mutations on the X chromosome. They are usually recessive (although rare dominant conditions exist). The Y chromosome is very small and contains few known genes.

MITOCHONDRIAL DISORDERS

Mitochondria contain their *own* chromosomes, which are *maternally derived*. A few diseases are the result of mitochondrial mutations, e.g. the mitochondrial cyopathies that have a screening test for a raised fasting lactate, which have characteristic (not strictly Mendelian) inheritance through the maternal line.

Characteristics of autosomal disorders

Autosomal dominant	**Autosomal recessive**
A single allele exerts an effect (so both heterozygotes and homozygotes manifest the disease). NB: Homozygote state may be lethal	Both alleles need to carry a mutation for the disease to manifest, i.e. homozygotes only
	A heterozygote for a recessive condition is an asymptomatic carrier (both parents of an affected individual)
Often structural defects	Often metabolic conditions
Vertical transmission pattern, i.e. seen in in successive generations	Horizontal transmission pattern, i.e. seen in multiple siblings but not parents
Offspring of an affected parent have a 50% chance of inheriting the disease	Offspring of affected parent have a 25% chance of inheriting the disease and a 50% chance of being an asymptomatic carrier
	Consanguinuity increases chances of disorder being expressed

Examples of X-linked disorders

X-linked recessive	**X-linked dominant**
Haemophilia A Colour blindness Duchenne muscular dystrophy G6PD deficiency	Familial hypophosphataemic rickets Incontinentia pigmentii II

Characteristics of X-linked recessive disorders

- Affect males
- Carrier females *may* be affected (usually mildly)
- Sons of female carriers have a 50% chance of being phenotypically affected
- Daughters of female carriers have a 50% chance of being carriers
- No father-to-son transmission
- Daughters of affected males have a 100% chance of being carriers

MULTIFACTORIAL INHERITANCE

Phenotypes affected by genetic and environmental factors are multifactorial. Many quantitative traits are multifactorial, e.g. height. Many diseases are inherited in a multifactorial fashion, e.g. pyloric stenosis, cleft lip and palate, and neural tube defects.

Recurrence risks are based on empirical data (observed occurrences), e.g. risk of cleft lip with or without cleft palate is 1 in 700 live births; recurrence risk after one affected child is 3–4% and after two affected children is around 10%.

INHERITANCE PATTERNS

Many factors alter inheritance patterns, but two important ones are **imprinting** and **premutation** (triple repeat disease).

IMPRINTING

Genomic imprinting is the differential activation of genes dependent on which parent they are inherited from. Diseases inherited in this way include Beckwith–Wiedemann syndrome (IGF2 gene at 11p15.5, maternal copy imprinted; some cases caused by paternal uniparental disomy), Prader–Willi syndrome and Angelmann syndrome.

Prader–Willi syndrome and Angelmann syndrome

These syndromes both result from loss of a gene at chromosome 15q11–13. *Failure* to inherit the active gene causes the syndrome.

The absence of the active gene may result from:

- *New mutation* – normal parental chromosomes, gene deletion in gametes
- *Uniparental disomy (UPD)* – normal parental chromosomes, but child inherits both copies from one parent and none from the other, so effectively there is a deletion of one parental copy

Failure to inherit the *paternal* copy leads to Prader–Willi syndrome (paternal deletion or maternal UPD). Failure to inherit the *maternal* copy leads to Angelmann syndrome (maternal deletion or paternal UPD).

Clinical features are:

Prader–Willi syndrome	Neonatal hypotonia, learning difficulties, obsession with food, obesity, micropenis
Angelmann syndrome (happy puppet syndrome)	Ataxia, severe learning difficulties, happy personality, epilepsy, characteristic facies (broad smile)

PREMUTATION (TRIPLET REPEATS)

Some diseases are caused by an expansion of the number of triplet repeats (repeats of a three base pair code seen within a gene). Triplet repeats are found at many places across the genome and the normal number of

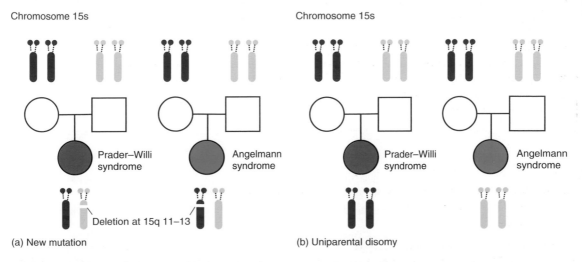

(a) New mutation

(b) Uniparental disomy

Figure 3.15 Imprinting

repeats may vary between individuals. However, a repeat number above a certain size may make the gene unstable (**premutation**) and more likely to expand further, to a size that interferes with the function of the gene (full mutation). An example of this is fragile X syndrome.

Fragile X syndrome (FRAXA)

- An X-linked dominant condition with premutation occurring in the mother
- Relatively common (1 in 1250 males and 1 in 2500 females). (The term fragile X comes from the fact that the X chromosome has a fragile site and may develop breaks when cultured in a medium devoid of folic acid)
- The gene (FMR 1) contains a CGG repeat at one end. Normal individuals have 5–50 copies of this repeat; those with fragile X syndrome have > 200 repeats. Individuals with an intermediate number of repeats (50–200) carry a premutation and are seen in *normal transmitting males* and their *female offspring*
- An expansion in the number of repeats occurs when a premutation is passed through the *female line*, and may result in a larger premutation or in the full mutation size
- When an allele containing repeats the size of a premutation passes through the male line it does not expand, but is passed stably
- Most males with a full expansion will have clinical signs of the condition. About one-third of females with a full mutation will be clinically affected

Clinical features are:

Learning difficulties	Milder in females
Dysmorphic facies	Large ears, long face
Other	Macro-orchidism (large testes), hypermobile joints

DYSMORPHOLOGY

This is the study of abnormal physical development during embryogenesis, resulting in congenital defects. Four pathogenic processes may occur:

Malformation	Primary defect resulting from intrinsic abnormal development during embryogenesis, e.g. polydactyly, cleft lip and palate
Dysplasia	Primary defect involving abnormal organization of cells into tissues, e.g. haemangioma
Deformation	Secondary alteration of previously normal body part by intrinsic or extrinsic mechanical forces, e.g. arthrogryposis may be caused by extrinsic factors such as oligohydramnios or intrinsic factors such as a primary muscle disorder in the fetus
Disruption	Secondary defect resulting from breakdown of an originally normal developmental process. Causes include teratogens and transplacental infection

Human teratogens

Drug	Potential effect	Critical period
Warfarin	Nasal hypoplasia	6–9 weeks
	Bone defects (chondrodysplasia punctata)	
	Intracerebral and other fetal haemorrhage	> 12 weeks
Carbamazepine	Neural tube defects	< 30 days
	Cardiac defects	
	Hypospadias	

Sodium valproate	Neural tube defects Cardiac defects Hypospadias Skeletal defects	< 30 days
Isotretinoin	Spontaneous abortion Hydrocephalus and other CNS defects Cotruncal heart defects Small or missing thymus Micrognathia	All pregnancy
Cocaine	Placental abruption Intracranial haemorrhage Premature delivery Omphalocoele Vascular events, e.g. bowel atresia secondary to necrosis	> 12 weeks
Lithium	Polyhydramnios Pulmonary hypertension Ebstein anomaly and other cardiac defects	All pregnancy
Alcohol	Fetal alcohol syndrome (rare in the UK): ■ Craniofacial – long philtrum, flat nasal bridge, mid-facial hypoplasia, micrognathia, upturned nose, ear deformities, eye malformations, cleft lip and palate ■ CNS – microcephaly and developmental delay, growth retardation ■ Other – cardiac, renal and limb abnormalities	< 12 weeks

Clinical scenario

A ten-year-old girl is referred to the general paediatrician locally due to parental concern regarding her growth. The paediatrician notes that she is below the 0.4th centile for height and has broadly spaced nipples with a low neck line and what appears to be a webbed neck.

1. What is the most likely diagnosis?
2. What might be heard on cardiac auscultation?
3. What two hormones might be useful in this situation?

ANSWERS

1. Turner's syndrome would be the most likely diagnosis
2. Ejection systolic murmur. NB: check for absent femorals
3. Growth hormone and oestrogen

FURTHER READING

Jorde L, Carey J, Bamshad M, White, R. *Medical Genetics*, 3rd edn. London: Elsevier, 2006.

Jones K. *Smiths Recognizable Patterns of Human Malformations*. London: Elsevier, 2005.

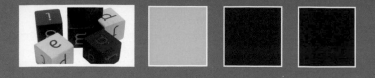

4 Neonatology

- ■ Pregnancy
- ■ Fetal medicine
- ■ Congenital infections
- ■ Delivery
- ■ Normal newborn
- ■ Birth injuries
- ■ Neonatal definitions and statistics
- ■ Intrapartum and postnatal infections
- ■ Neonatal intensive care
- ■ Abnormal growth *in utero*
- ■ Prematurity
- ■ Neonatal problems in term babies
- ■ Further reading

PREGNANCY

ANTENATAL SCREENING AND DIAGNOSIS

Blood and urine tests		
Sample	**Timing**	**Details**
General maternal blood tests	< 12 weeks	Blood group and antibodies (Rhesus and other red cell antigens) FBC Rubella, syphilis and hepatitis B + HIV serology Haemoglobinopathy screening (sickle and thalassaemia)
	26 weeks	Oral glucose tolerance test or random blood sugar (some centres)
	28, 34 weeks	Rhesus antibodies if Rh negative (at the same time as IM anti-D)
	34 weeks	FBC
Maternal urine	Regularly	Dipstick for glucose, leucocytes, nitrites and protein

Ultrasound scans

8–12 weeks	**Dating scan** (crown–rump length)
11–14 weeks	**Nuchal scan** – nuchal fold thickness measured In Down syndrome ↑ – 77% sensitive for 5% false-positive rate. Improved to 92% by combining results of serum PAPP-A and inhibin levels sampled at similar gestation (the **combined test**), and up to 97% if presence/absence nasal bones included Gives an individual risk for Down, trisomy 13 and 18, and aids prediction of other genetic syndromes Also acts as a dating scan, early anomaly scan and allows early diagnosis of twins and assessment of uteroplacental circulation and cervical integrity (length)
20–24 weeks	**Anomaly scan** – detailed scan to look for fetal growth and biometry consistent with gestational dates, and major congenital malformations Neural tube defects > 98% accuracy
> 20 weeks	**Growth scans** – done only if concern about fetal growth or well-being Biparietal diameter (BPD) Head circumference (HC) Femur length (FL) Abdominal circumference (AC)

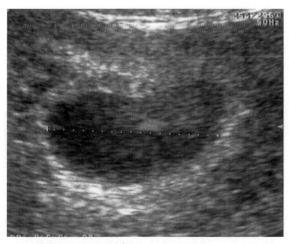

Figure 4.1 Early dating scan (8 weeks)

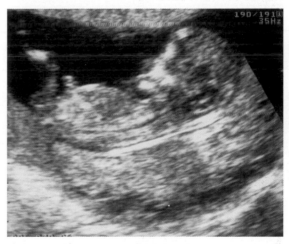

Figure 4.2 Nuchal scan (12 weeks)

Disorders diagnosable by ultrasound at 20 week anomaly scan

Anencephaly	Hydrops fetalis	Limb defects
Encephalocoele	Gastroschisis	Cleft lip
Holoprosencephaly	Exomphalos	Congenital heart disease
Hydrocephalus	Renal agenesis	Skeletal abnormalities
Polycystic kidneys	Hydronephrosis (not a disorder as such)	Diaphragmatic hernia

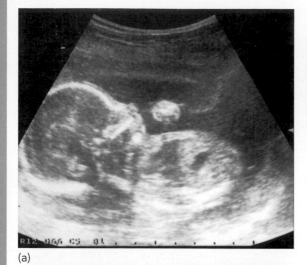

(a)

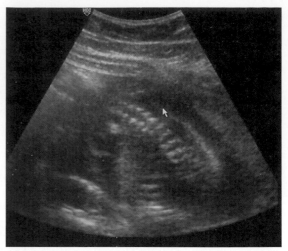

(b)

Figure 4.3 Anomaly scan. (a) Normal. (b) Spina bifida. (c) Cystic hygroma

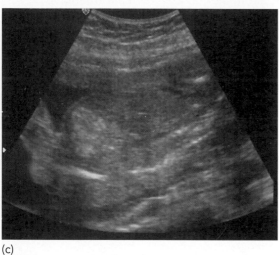

(c)

Invasive tests

Chorion villous sampling

- 11–14 weeks – performed earlier than amniocentesis
- 1% procedure-related risk (overall 1.5%) of miscarriage
- Chorionic villous cells sampled
- Can check:
  - **Chromosome analysis** PCR – 24 h result informing on major trisomies and sex chromosome aneuploidies (see genetics). Full karyotype reporting in 10–14 days of cell culture
  - **Enzyme analysis** inborn errors of metabolism
  - **Congenital infection** viral particle DNA using PCR

Amniocentesis

- 16 weeks onwards
- 1% procedure-related risk (overall 1.5%) of miscarriage
- Tests as for CVS using fetal cells in amniotic fluid

Fetal blood sampling

- \> 20 weeks
- Used to confirm suspicions of severe fetal anaemia or thrombocytopaenia

Future screening methods

Non-invasive techniques are being developed. These include:

- Diagnostic techniques using fetal DNA obtained from *fetal cells* in the maternal circulation or *free fetal DNA* in maternal plasma
- Three-dimensional USS
- Fetal MRI scanning } Looking for structural anomalies

FETAL MEDICINE

Fetal medicine is concerned with the antenatal detection, pregnancy management and treatment (where applicable) of fetal disorders. This includes:

- Antenatal screening (see above) and additional diagnostic tests where indicated, including interventional tests, e.g. CVS, and counselling of options should they be abnormal
- Genetic counselling
- Treatment during pregnancy (see below) and termination of pregnancy where appropriate

FETAL THERAPY	INDICATION
Multiple fetal pregnancy reduction	Triplets and other higher multiples
Selective termination	Abnormality in multiple pregnancy
Laser ablation/multiple amniocentesis/selective fetocide	Severe twin–twin transfusion syndrome
Shunting for megacystis	Posterior urethral valves, pleural effusion
Fetal blood sampling	Intravascular transfusion (alloimune red cell and platelet disorders)
	Diagnosis of fetal karyotype, infection, genetic, metabolic, biochemical abnormality
	Rarely for intrauterine therapy, e.g. antiarrhythmic drugs in persistent fetal tachycardia
Amniodrainage	Polyhydramnios (prevents preterm labour and unstable lie)
Amnioinfusion	Diagnostic: confirms ruptured membranes, better visualization of certain defects, e.g. renal agenesis
Needle aspiration of cysts	Megacystis, ovarian, lung, bowel
Laser ablation of tumours	Sacrococcygeal teratomas, cardiac rhabdomyomas

HIGH-RISK PREGNANCIES

Pregnancies are classified as high risk due to:

- Pre-existing maternal disease
- Antenatally detected fetal disorder, or
- Pregnancy complications/indications

MULTIPLE PREGNANCY

- Twin, triplet and higher multiple pregnancies are associated with specific increased risks to both the mother and the fetuses
- Establishing chorionicity (indirectly aids zygosity testing) in the first trimester gives best results

High-risk pregnancies		
Maternal diseases	**Fetal disorders**	**Pregnancy complications**
Chronic disease, e.g. diabetes mellitus, heart disease, renal disease, asthma	**Identified genetic abnormality**, e.g. Down syndrome, cystic fibrosis	Multiple pregnancy
Nutritional disorders resulting in excessively low or high BMI and deficient dietary intake	**Fetal structural abnormality** diagnosed via antenatal USS, e.g. spina bifida, renal abnormality	Oligo- or poly-hydramnios
Maternal alloimmune disease	**Fetal arrhythmia**	Antepartum haemorrhage Pregnancy-induced hypertension and pre-eclampsia (toxaemia of pregnancy)

- Growth discordance affects all twins (monochorionic twins more so)
- Regular scanning in pregnancy is required – dichorionic: 4 weekly; monochorionic: 2 weekly

Monozygotic (identical)	Incidence 3.5 in 1000 pregnancies
	Single fertilized egg
	May be:
	   ■ Single chorion and amnion
	   ■ Mixed (separate amnion, but monochorionic), or
	   ■ Separate chorion and amnion
	Risk of twin–twin transfusion syndrome. A monoamniotic pregnancy may also lead to fatal cord entanglement and locked twins at delivery

Dizygotic (non-identical)	Familial, variable rate, 1 in 66 spontaneous rate Two separately fertilized eggs Dichorionic placenta

Associated risks

- Prematurity
- IUGR, discordant growth
- Asphyxia
- Second twin particularly at increased risk of asphyxia, trauma and respiratory distress syndrome (RDS)
- Monozygotic twins – increased congenital anomalies; if single chorion and amnion – twin–twin transfusion syndrome, cord entanglement, discordant growth
- Increased fetal and maternal mortality

Twin–twin transfusion syndrome

This is a difference in haemoglobin > 5 g/dL between monochorionic twins, i.e. they share the same placenta. If untreated, death of both twins occurs in > 90%; if treated, both twins survive in 66%. Essentially one twin has the majority of the placental blood flow (and nutrients), and hence grows larger and is plethoric, while the other twin is anaemic and smaller. It is the *large plethoric twin* who is at higher risk because diminished blood flow through smaller vessels (secondary to high haematocrit) can cause multiorgan damage.

Features of anaemic and plethoric twin

Anaemic twin	Plethoric twin
IUGR	May have IUGR
Preterm delivery	Preterm delivery
Severe anaemia	Cardiac failure and hypertension
Hydrops fetalis	CNS – apnoeas and seizures Gastro – necrotizing enterocolitis Renal – renal vein thrombosis Other – hypoglycaemia, hypocalcaemia, jaundice

Antenatal treatments include amnioreduction (repeated removal of amniotic fluid) and septostomy, or selective fetal reduction.

MATERNAL DISEASES ASSOCIATED WITH MALFORMATIONS AND NEONATAL DISORDERS

- Maternal illnesses have a *general impact* on fetal growth and well-being, e.g. pre-eclampsia, chronic renal disease
- They can cause **fetal malformations**, e.g. maternal diabetes, **fetal damage, premature delivery** or **temporary neonatal disease** due to maternal transfer of IgG antibodies (IgG will cross the placenta), e.g. autoimmune thrombocytopaenia. Sometimes, a transient transfer of antibodies can result in permanent consequences for the infant, e.g. congenital heart block in maternal lupus

Examples of impact of maternal illness on the infant

Maternal illness	Malformation/disorder
Diabetes mellitus	Macrosomia organomegaly, transient neonatal hypoglycaemia
	Caudal regression syndrome (sacral agenesis)
	Doubled risk of any congenital anomaly
	Renal vein thrombosis, CHD, hypertrophic subaortic stenosis
Placental antibody transfer	
Rhesus disease	Fetal anaemia
Lupus erythematosis	Neonatal lupus, congenital heart block
Hyperthyroidism	Transient neonatal thyrotoxicosis
Autoimmune thrombocytopaenia	Transient neonatal thrombocytopenia
Myasthenia gravis	Transient neonatal disease and arthrogryphosis

CONGENITAL INFECTIONS

Vertical transmission (from mother to child) may be:

- Transplacental
- Intrapartum (cervical secretions, haematogenous), or
- Postnatal (breast milk, saliva, urine)

Congenital infections

Cytomegalovirus	Herpes simplex virus (HSV)
Rubella	*Neisseria gonorrhoea*
Toxoplasmosis	*Listeria monocytogenes*
Varicella	Group B streptococcus
HIV	*Escherichia coli*
Chlamydia trachomatis	Hepatitis A, B and C
Malaria	Parvovirus B19
Syphilis	

Common features

Features that would arouse suspicion of a congenital infection are:

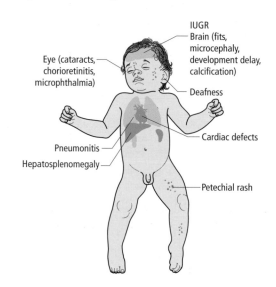

Figure 4.4 Common features of congenital infection

Congenital infection may also result in miscarriage or stillbirth.

> **!** **NB: Some common features of congenital infection have specific antenatal scan features.**

CYTOMEGALOVIRUS

- Most common congenital infection in the UK (approximately 2000 live births/year)
- 50% of fetal infections are asymptomatic, around 5% will have clinical infection at birth, others presenting later. Up to 10% develop neurological sequelae (mainly deafness)
- Primary maternal cytomegalovirus (CMV) infection during pregnancy is associated with a worse prognosis

Diagnosis

Urine   CMV culture; blood CMV–specific IgM (↑)

Clinical features

Brain	**Cerebral periventricular calcifications ('c' shape, aide memoire)**
	Sensorineural deafness (can be progressive)
	Developmental delay (mild or severe)
	Microcephaly, encephalitis
Skin	**Petechial rash**
Lungs	**Pneumonitis**
Liver	**Hepatosplenomegaly, jaundice**
Eyes	Chorioretinitis, optic atrophy
Teeth	Dental defects
Other	**IUGR**

TOXOPLASMOSIS

- Intracellular parasite, acquired from raw meat, unwashed vegetables and fruit, and cat faeces (kittens with primary infection can be high excretors)
- Incidence of primary maternal infection during pregnancy is 1 in 1000
- Risk of infant infection is inversely related to gestational age at the time of primary maternal infection – from 15% risk (first trimester) to 65% (third trimester)
- Severity of disease in the infant is dependent on the gestation. Most severe at 24–30 weeks. Overall > 10% have clinical features
- Infection particularly affects the developing brain. Most have no *apparent symptoms*, but intracranial calcification is often present with neurological consequences

Clinical features

Brain	**Cerebral calcifications, diffusely scattered dense, round lesions, basal ganglia curvilinear streaks**
	Seizures
	Hydrocephalus, microcephaly, encephalitis
	Developmental delay (mild or severe)
Eyes	**Chorioretinitis, cataract**
Liver	**Hepatosplenomegaly, jaundice**
Blood	**Anaemia**
Lungs	Pneumonitis

CONGENITAL RUBELLA

This is now very rare (only 6 cases reported in the UK in the last 5 years). Risk and severity are dependent on gestation at maternal infection, highest < 8 weeks' gestation.

Clinical features

Brain	**Sensorineural deafness**
	Psychomotor delay (mild or severe)
	Progressive degenerative brain disorder
Eyes	**Cataracts, corneal opacities, glaucoma, microphthalmia**
Skin/haem	**Petechial rash, thrombocytopenia**
Cardiac	PDA, pulmonary artery stenosis, aortic stenosis, VSDS

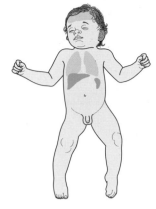

Figure 4.5 Clinical features of cytomegalovirus

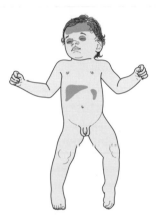

Figure 4.6 Clinical features of toxoplasmosis

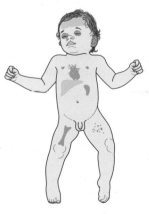

Figure 4.7 Clinical features of congenital rubella

Liver	**Hepatosplenomegaly**, hepatitis
Bone	**Radiolucent bone lesions**
Lung	Pneumonitis
Other	**IUGR**

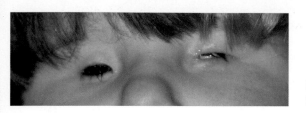

Figure 4.8 Microphthalmia (courtesy of Dr J. Uddin)

VARICELLA

Congenital varicella syndrome is extremely rare, and can occur with primary maternal infection during pregnancy. **Maternal infection around delivery** (< 5 days pre–2 days after), however, may cause *severe* chicken pox illness in the infant (high titres of virus with no maternal antibodies yet made to protect the infant). These infants are given varicella immune globulin (VZIG) as post-exposure prophylaxis and also often aciclovir.

Indications to give VZIG to baby

- Maternal infection < 5 days pre–2 days post delivery
- < 28 weeks' gestation or < 1000 g, regardless of maternal history (little antibody crosses placenta before third trimester)
- Other babies on the ward who may have been exposed if < 28 weeks' gestation or mother non-immune

---

PARVOVIRUS B19

This can cause fetal anaemia, hydrops fetalis and stillbirth (see ch. 5)

LISTERIA MONOCYTOGENES

This may be acquired transplacentally or by ascending infection. Acquired from unpasteurized cheeses and milk products, soft cheeses, chicken, raw vegetables, uncooked meats, over-the-counter reheated foods.

Clinical features

It may present in different ways.

- Premature delivery, abortion or stillbirth; maternal flu-like illness
- Meconium passed *in utero* in premature delivery (this would not normally happen)
- Pneumonia, meningitis, septicaemia
- Disseminated infection (fits, generalized rash, hepatosplenomegaly)
- Hydrocephalus is a common sequel

Treatment

IV ampicillin and gentamicin.

DELIVERY

RESUSCITATION

A minority of infants do not establish respiration rapidly after birth (they are 'flat'), and they need immediate assessment and intervention. **APGAR scores** are performed on all babies directly after birth (at 1, 5 and 10 min after birth, and longer if necessary) in order to assess their condition. These are, however, a poorly predictive indicator of later adverse outcome. Five parameters are assessed, each scoring 0–2, and the total (out of 10) gives the Apgar at that time.

A good Apgar score may read: 7 at 1 min, 8 at 5 min and 10 at 10 min.

Table 4.1 Apgar score

Physical sign	Score		
	0	1	2
Appearance	Pale	Blue extremities	Pink
Pulse	Absent	< 100 bpm	> 100 bpm
Grimace on suction	None	Grimace	Cry, cough
Activity	Flaccid	Some limb flexion	Active
Respiratory effort	Absent	Irregular	Regular

Basic resuscitation

- Start the clock
- Dry and stimulate the baby and keep him/her warm (warm towel, overhead heater) (infants of 3 kg lose 1°C/min in ambient theatre temperature)
- Bag and mask ventilation
- External cardiac massage

Advanced resuscitation

- Endotracheal intubation
- Drug therapy
- Blood or other fluids via umbilical venous catheter
- Transfer baby to NICU

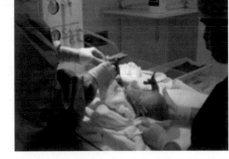

Figure 4.9 Newborn infant on resuscitaire

NORMAL NEWBORN

NEONATAL EXAMINATION

All infants should be given a general examination within 24 h of birth, usually at the hospital by the paediatrician, or if at home, by the GP.

- Always wash hands carefully first
- In general it is easiest to work from the head down
- Listen to the heart, then the lungs whenever the baby is quiet
- Do the hip examination last because this will probably make the baby cry

High-risk deliveries

Fetal/delivery
- Instrumental delivery – hypoxia, intracranial bleed, fractures, cervical and brachial plexus injury, shoulder dystocia
- Breech vaginal delivery
- Caesarean:
  - Dependent on indication
  - Direct fetal laceration/trauma
  - Head may be stuck in second stage with breech
- Acute fetal hypoxia (fetal distress)
- Difficult airway, e.g. face presentation, hypertonus, laryngomalacia, tumour
- Meconium stained liquor
- Big baby/small baby/preterm baby
- Abnormal baby
- Multiple pregnancy

Maternal conditions
- Pyrexia
- Diabetic
- Severe pre-eclampsia/toxaemia
- Drug misuse
- Any severe chronic illness, e.g. cardiac disease, renal failure
- Autoimmune disorder with placental antibody transfer, e.g. Rhesus disease

Measurements	Gestational age, weight, (length), head circumference
General	Appearance (dysmorphic), posture, movements
Skin	Colour (cyanosis, jaundice, anaemic, plethoric), birth marks
Head	Fontanelles (normal size, pressure, fused sutures), head shape
Face	Features of dysmorphism
Ears	Size, formation, position
Mouth	Size, other abnormality (cleft lip/palate), neonatal teeth
Palate	Inspect and palpate (cleft palate), sucking reflex checked
Eyes	Red reflex, discharge, colobomas, size
Neck	Any swellings (cystic hygroma, sternomastoid 'tumour')
Respiratory	Respiratory movements, rate, auscultation
Cardiovascular	Auscultation, femoral pulses
Abdominal	Palpation (masses)
Genitalia	Inspection (malformations, ambiguous genitalia), testes (both descended fully)
Anus	Patent. NB: Meconium normally passes within 48 h of birth (and within 24 h in 95%). Most units ask surgeons to review if no meconium by 24 h
Back	Check spine (any midline defects)
Muscle tone	Observation and hold baby prone
Reflexes	Moro reflex
Hips	Check for congenital dislocation of the hips. Enquire if breech or family history of risk factors (see p. 445), in which case a hip USS is arranged

Neonatal hip examination

- Baby should be relaxed when this is carried out
- *Pelvis is stabilized* with one hand, and the middle finger of the other hand is placed over the greater trochanter and the thumb around the femur. The hip is *flexed*. Then:
- **Barlow manoeuvre** to check if the hip is *dislocatable*. The femoral head is gently pushed downwards. If dislocatable, the femoral head will be pushed out with a clunk

■ **Ortolani manoeuvre** to see if the hip is *dislocated and can be relocated* into the acetabulum. The hip is abducted and upward pressure applied by the finger on the greater trocanter. If the hip were dislocated, it would clunk back into position

> **!** **NB: Insignificant mild *clicks* due to ligaments may be heard.**

VITAMIN K

Prophylactic vitamin K is recommended for all newborns to prevent haemorrhagic disease of the newborn. It is given shortly after birth, either IM (one dose) or orally – one dose if bottle feeding; after birth, at 1 week and at 6 weeks if breast feeding.

Haemorrhagic disease of the newborn

■ Due to low vitamin K–dependent clotting factors at birth (immature liver, low gut bacteria) and a further fall in breast-fed babies (breast milk is a poor source of vitamin K)
■ Rare (< 10 cases/year in the UK)
■ Presents as bleeding on day 2–6; usually mild, but may be catastrophic
■ Late presentation (rarely) may occur up to 6 weeks
■ If bleeding occurs, give vitamin K IV, fresh frozen plasma, and blood and plasma as needed. Also check for liver disorder

GUTHRIE TEST

This is a biochemical screen to detect some metabolic defects and is performed on all infants at the end of the first week of life via a blood test (usually a heel prick sample).

Tandom mass spectroscopy is used to detect rare metabolic conditions. It is often also used anonymously to determine prevalence of HIV within a population.

Diseases screened for by Guthrie test	
Disease	**Compound/test**
Phenylketonuria	Phenylalanine
Hypothyroidism	TSH level
Non-universal:	Immunoreactive trypsinogen
Cystic fibrosis	
Haemoglobinopathies and sickle	

BIRTH INJURIES

HEAD INJURIES

Caput succadeum	Very common. Bruising and oedema of the presenting part of the head
Chignon	Bruising from Ventouse suction cap
Cephalohaematoma	Bleed beneath the periosteum due to torn veins. It resolves spontaneously over a few weeks
	Complications:
	■ Neonatal jaundice

- Underlying skull fracture (present in 20% but rarely needs treatment)
- Associated intracranial haemorrhage
- Eventual calcification (leaving permanent bump on head)

NERVE INJURIES

Erb's palsy

- 1 in 2000 deliveries. Common injury to upper nerve roots of brachial plexus (C5, 6±7)
- Often follows shoulder dystocia
- **'Waiter's tip'** position (arm in adduction, elbow extended, internally rotated, forearm pronated and wrist flexed)
- Phrenic nerve involvement also in a few (causing ipsilateral diaphragmatic paralysis), a pneumothorax, fractured clavicle and/or Horner syndrome

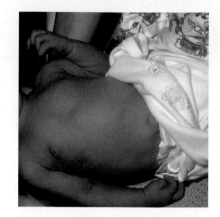

Figure 4.10 Features of Erb's palsy

Facial nerve palsy

- Mostly lower motor neurone damage due to a forceps injury or secondary to prolonged pressure on maternal sacral promontory
- Few are upper motor neurone secondary to brain injury

These two lesions can be difficult to distinguish clinically; both result in an asymmetrical face when crying and an inability to close the eye on the affected side.

Management

Physiotherapy is given to prevent contractures. If there is no improvement at 2–3 months, refer to a specialist unit. For facial nerve injury, eye patching and artificial tears are needed if eye closure incomplete.

MUSCLE INJURIES

Sternomastoid tumour

- Injury to the sternocleidomastoid muscle
- May be from traumatic delivery or secondary to position *in utero*
- Manifests as a firm **swelling** within the sternomastoid muscle and a **torticollis**
- Swift and regular physiotherapy (taught to parents) results in resolution of the swelling over a few weeks. The preferential turning of the head to one side only can result in plagiocephaly and permanent postural deformity

BONE INJURIES

Clavicle fracture

- Most common delivery injury (particularly among large babies with impacted shoulders, e.g. baby of diabetic mother)
- Often not detected
- Heals on its own but may need analgesia

NEONATAL DEFINITIONS AND STATISTICS

Definitions

Embryo	< 9 weeks' gestation
Fetus	9 weeks' gestation–delivery
Abortion	Fetal death and expulsion from the uterus < 24 weeks' gestation
Stillbirth	Fetal death and expulsion from the uterus > 24 weeks' gestation
Term	37–42 weeks
Neonate	Infant < 28 days old
Low birth weight (LBW)	Infant ≤ 2500 g at birth
Very low birth weight (VLBW)	Infant ≤ 1500 g at birth
Extremely low birth weight (ELBW)	Infant ≤ 1000 g at birth
Small for gestational age (SGA)	Birthweight < 10th centile
Large for gestational age (LGA)	Birthweight > 90th centile
Appropriate for gestational age (AGA)	Birthweight between the 10th and 90th centiles
Stillbirth rate	Number of stillbirths/1000 deliveries
Perinatal mortality rate	Number of stillbirths + deaths within the first 7 days/1000 deliveries
Neonatal mortality rate	Number of deaths of liveborn infants within 28 days of birth/1000 live births
Post-neonatal mortality rate	Number of deaths between 28 days and 1 year/1000 live births
Infant mortality rate	Number of deaths between birth and 1 year/1000 live births

UK birth statistics

Total UK births	650 000/year	
Perinatal mortality rate (PNM)	6–10/1000	
Survival figures (of those admitted to NICU)	24 weeks' gestation	45%
	26 weeks' gestation	73%
	28 weeks' gestation	90%

INTRAPARTUM AND POSTNATAL INFECTIONS

Infections which may be acquired during delivery

- Sepsis (causes of neonatal sepsis and meningitis – Group B β-haemolytic streptococcus, *Esherichia coli*, *Staphylococcus epidermidis*)
- Conjunctivitis (see p. 416)
- Herpes simplex
- Umbilical infection (*E. coli*, *Staph. aureus*)
- HIV infection
- *Chlamydia trachomatis*
- Gonococcal infection

GROUP B β-HAEMOLYTIC STREPTOCOCCUS

There is increasing pressure to establish a mother's Group B streptococcus status before delivery and to give intrapartum prophylaxis with penicillin or clindamycin for colonized mothers.

■ Colonization of the vagina with group B β-haemolytic streptococcus occurs in approximately 30% of women
■ At least 10% of babies will become colonized during delivery. 1% of colonized babies develop Group B streptococcus sepsis, with about a 10% mortality (70 deaths in UK/year)
■ Risk factors for sepsis are maternal pyrexia, premature rupture of membranes, or if the infant is preterm and inadequate labour prophylaxis was given, when the infant should be treated

Group B streptococcal neonatal infection causes *serious* disease with:

■ *Early* lethargy, poor feeding, temperature instability, irritability, apnoeas, jaundice. Then features of sepsis and shock, meningitis and pneumonia
■ *Late-onset* disease from 48 h

Investigations
■ FBC, CRP and septic screen (blood culture in particular)
■ CXR (diffuse or lobular changes)
■ Check maternal high vaginal swab result

Treatment
IV antibiotics, e.g. gentamicin and penicillin.

> ❗ **NB: Any neonate in whom serious infection is suspected should be covered for Group B β-haemolytic streptococcus.**

NEONATAL HERPES SIMPLEX INFECTION

■ Rare but increasing. UK incidence is approximately 1.65 in 100 000 live births
■ Acquired from the birth canal during delivery (in most cases the mother is asymptomatic). Primary maternal infection during pregnancy is rare
■ Primary maternal infection – up to 50% of infants infected; recurrent maternal infection – 3% infants infected
■ Increased risk of neonatal infection with prolonged rupture of membranes (> 6 h)
■ Infection may be localized skin vesicles only, or widespread vesicles develop within the first week of life and rapid CNS involvement develops (meningoencephalitis)
■ Infection in neonates may be severe (mortality 80% untreated)
■ *Treatment* is with IV aciclovir

UMBILICAL INFECTION

Omphalitis is umbilical stump infection; **funisitis** is umbilical cord infection.

■ Usually due to *Staph. aureus* or *E. coli*
■ May lead to portal vein infection thrombosis and subsequent portal hypertension
■ *Management* – swab umbilicus (M, C & S); gentle cleansing; IV antibiotics if signs of spread (cellulitis around umbilicus)

NEONATAL INTENSIVE CARE

The neonatal intensive care unit (NICU) is a specialist unit that provides care to premature and sick neonates.

Thermal stability

Incubators provide a stable warm environment designed to be thermoneutral, i.e. neither too hot, requiring the neonate to expend energy to keep cool, nor too cool, requiring the neonate to expend energy to keep warm.

Monitoring

Heart rate	
Respiratory rate	
Temperature	Ambient and that of infant
Blood pressure	Via umbilical artery or peripheral arterial line or BP cuff (less accurate)
Oxygenation	Pulse oximetry (O_2 saturation)
	Transcutaneous (O_2 tension)
CO_2 levels	Transcutaneous (CO_2 tension)
Blood gases	Transcutaneous, via arterial line or capillary analysis from heel prick samples

Blood gases — Acidosis:
  - **Respiratory acidosis** (high CO_2), e.g. underventilated
  - **Metabolic acidosis** (low bicarbonate), e.g. sick infant

Alkalosis
  - **Respiratory alkalosis** (low CO_2), e.g. overventilated
  - **Metabolic alkalosis** (high bicarbonate)

Bloods	Regular samples (heel prick, venous or via arterial line) to monitor blood gases and blood glucose

Ventilation

Ambient oxygen	(Room air) or oxygen via head box/in incubator may be sufficient
Continuous positive airway pressure (CPAP)	Continuous flow of oxygen via nasal cannulae, face mask, or endotracheal tube (ETT). This keeps the terminal bronchials open in expiration and prevents them from collapsing
Intermittent positive pressure ventilation (IPPV)	Paralysis and sedation may be needed if the baby is struggling and 'fighting' the ventilator. There are different types of IPPV:

  - Continuous mandatory ventilation (CMV) – full ventilation
  - Intermittent mandatory ventilation (IMV) – only occasional breaths given by the ventilator. Used to wean a baby who is making some respiratory effort off the ventilator
  - Patient triggered ventilation (PTV) – ventilator assisted ventilation triggered by baby initiating the breath. Used to wean babies off the ventilator

High frequency oscillatory ventilation (HFOV)	Very high frequency rate (10 Hz or 600/min) ventilation via ETT. This is useful in infants with severe lung disease, e.g. meconuim aspiration syndrome
Extracorporeal membrane oxygenation (ECMO)	Extracorporeal circuit oxygenates the blood outside of the body. Used only in severe cases and if other ventilatory methods fail, and particularly useful for meconium aspiration syndrome in which the lungs are very stiff and for a ventilation–perfusion mismatch. It can only be used on infants > 2.5 kg and is only available in a few UK centres. Complications and contraindications include intracranial haemorrhage (heparinization is necessary for ECMO)

Nitric oxide

This is a specific vasodilator acting particularly on the pulmonary artery smooth muscle. Therefore used in persistent pulmonary hypertension of the newborn (PPHN) to decrease pulmonary hypertension.

Circulatory support

- IV fluids given as 10% dextrose with added electrolytes (Na, K and Ca)
- Daily amount of fluid (ml/kg/day) increases over the first few days of life, and then stabilizes
- Extra fluid is needed by premature infants and those receiving phototherapy
- Inotropes, e.g. dopamine and dobutamine, given if needed (if the mean arterial pressure is low)

Feeding

Enteral feeds	Breast or formula milk
	Given by breast or bottle (usually able to feed if > 34 weeks' gestation), or bolus nasogastric feeds if unable to feed
	NB: Special formulae exist for premature infants who require a very high calorie intake
Total parenteral nutrition (TPN)	Used if enteral feeds are not tolerated or contraindicated, e.g. extreme prematurity, NEC
	Given via umbilical venous catheter (UVC) or a peripheral long line
	High calorie feed individually prepared to provide each infant's nutritional requirements (fat, carbohydrate, protein, elements, iron, calcium and trace metals)
	Complications – sepsis, cholestasis, microemboli

Supplements

Children's vitamin drops	Started when enteral feeds commenced until age 5 years
Iron	Give oral supplements if birthweight < 2.5 kg or < 36 weeks' gestation, from 6 weeks of age until on solid food

ABNORMAL GROWTH *IN UTERO*

INTRAUTERINE GROWTH RETARDATION

Growth may be restricted *in utero* for many reasons. IUGR is sometimes defined as growth < 3rd centile and sometimes < 10th centile. The term should be reserved for those infants who have not reached their genetic potential. These babies may be:

Asymmetrical Weight on lower centile than head circumference due to relative sparing of the brain
Due to placental failure late in pregnancy
Rapid weight gain after birth
Causes:
- Pre-eclampsia
- Multiple gestation
- Maternal cardiac or renal disease
- Uterine malformation

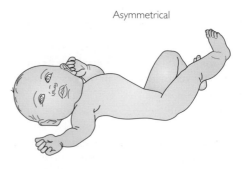
Asymmetrical

Figure 4.11(a) Intrauterine growth retardation

Symmetrical	Head and body equally small

Results from prolonged intrauterine growth failure

Fetus is usually normal, although may be abnormal

Postnatal growth is also poor

Causes:

- Maternal drug misuse, smoking, malnutrition, chronic illness
- Chromosomal disorder
- Congenital infection

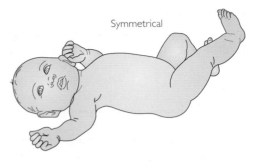

Symmetrical

Figure 4.11(b) Intrauterine growth retardation

Associated problems

- Hypoglycaemia due to small fat and glycogen stores. Need frequent feeds
- Hypothermia (large surface area:weight ratio and not much fat insulation)
- Infection
- Hypoxic–ischaemic encephalopathy
- Hypocalcaemia
- Polycythaemia

LARGE FOR GESTATIONAL AGE

Large for gestational age (LGA) is newborn weight > 90th percentile.

Causes

- Diabetic mother
- Familial, i.e. large parents
- Beckwith–Wiedemann syndrome

Associated problems

- Hypoglycaemia (hyperinsulinism)
- Birth trauma (difficult delivery)
- Hypoxic ischaemic encephalopathy (difficult delivery)
- Polycythaemia

PREMATURITY

Prematurity is birth at < 37 weeks' gestation.

The following conditions are not exclusive to premature neonates, but they are associated with prematurity. PDA is a particular problem of prematurity and is described in Chapter 9.

RESPIRATORY DISORDERS
Features of respiratory distress in a neonate

- Tachypnoea (RR > 60/min)
- Expiratory grunting
- Nasal flaring
- Recession (intercostals, subcostal and suprasternal)
- Cyanosis

Specific problems associated with prematurity

Temperature	Thermal instability. Temperature regulation mechanisms not fully developed and low body fat
Lungs	Apnoeas, RDS, pneumothorax, pulmonary haemorrhage, bronchopulmonary dysplasia (BPD)
Cardiac	Patent ductus arteriosus (PDA) (see p. 151), persistent pulmonary hypertension of the newborn (PPHN) (see p. 160)
CNS	Apnoeas, hypoxic ischaemic encephalopathy (HIE), intracranial haemorrhage, lack of primitive reflexes, e.g. sucking
Gastrointestinal	Intolerance of enteral feeds, gastro-oesophageal reflux, necrotizing enterocolitis (NEC)
Liver	Jaundice
Kidneys	Inability to concentrate urine, inability to excrete acid load
Immunity	Immature immune system, with susceptibility to infections
Eyes	Retinopathy of prematurity (see p. 418)
Metabolic	Hypoglycaemia, electrolyte imbalances, e.g. hypocalcaemia, osteopaenia of prematurity
Haematological	Iron-deficiency anaemia, physiological anaemia
Surgical	Inguinal and umbilical hernia

Investigations

- Oxygen saturation (pulse oximetry and blood gas)
- Chest transillumination with cold light (? pneumothorax)
- Pass nasogastric tube (if choanal atresia or oesophageal atresia suspected)
- CXR
- Nitrogen washout test to differentiate cause of cyanosis
- Infection screen (blood, urine, CSF, gastric aspirate for bacterial and viral culture; umbilical, ear and throat swabs). Also check maternal high vaginal swab result
- Other bloods – FBC, haematocrit and serology

Respiratory distress syndrome

Respiratory distress syndrome (RDS) is a specific disease due to **insufficient surfactant**:

- Neonate's lungs are non-compliant or 'stiff'
- A low alveolar compliance leads to hypoxia and acidosis and, if severe, causes PPHN

Surfactant

Surfactant lowers surface tension and increases compliance in alveoli leading to alveolar collapse. It is a phospholipid composed of lecithin and sphingomyelin, made by type II pneumocytes. The lecithin:sphingomyelin (LS) ratio is altered in RDS (less lecithin, LS ratio low, < 2).

Predisposing factors

- Prematurity
- Hypoxia, acidosis, shock, asphyxia
- Second twin, antepartum haemorrhage, diabetic mother

Protective factors

- Prolonged intrauterine stress, e.g. IUGR
- Maternal steroids

Clinical features

- Respiratory distress from 6 h of age
- Worsens over 2–3 days, then improves over 1–2 weeks
- CXR – fine reticular 'ground glass' appearance, air bronchograms

Management

- Surfactant replacement. Administered via the endotracheal tube. There are different formulations, and more than one dose may be necessary
- Ventilatory support – oxygen, CPAP or positive pressure ventilation as needed
- Antibiotics if infection is suspected
- Minimal handling

Complications

- Pneumothorax
- Intraventricular haemorrhage
- Bronchopulmonary dysplasia (late)

Prevention

If early delivery is planned, maternal oral dexamethasone is commenced 48 h prior to delivery.

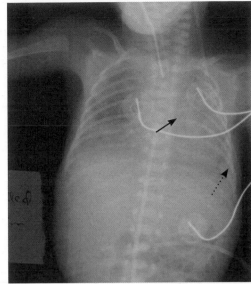

Figure 4.12 Chest X-ray of respiratory distress syndrome showing an air bronchogram (arrow) on a background of ground glass appearance (dotted arrow)

Pneumothorax

Causes

- Idiopathic (in 1% of term babies)
- Secondary to ventilation (especially if 'stiff' lungs in RDS or meconium aspiration)

Clinical features

- Mostly asymptomatic
- If large, causes respiratory distress (see above)

> **!** **NB: Rapid deterioration suggests a tension pneumothorax.**

Diagnosis

- Chest transillumination with fibre-optic 'cold' light. (This does not damage infant's skin)
- CXR

Management

Insertion of chest drain (anterior axillary line, 4th intercostal space)

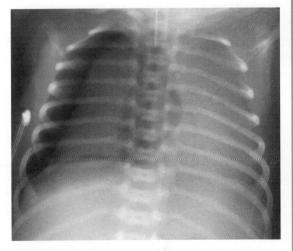

Figure 4.13 Right-sided tension pneumothorax with mediastinal shift. (Reproduced with permission from Greenough A. and Milner AD. Neonatal Respiratory Disorders, Second Edition. 2003. Hodder Arnold.)

Pulmonary haemorrhage

This is haemorrhagic pulmonary oedema due to elevated pulmonary capillary pressure from acute left ventricular failure or lung injury.

Associations

- Prematurity, RDS, asphyxia
- Pneumonia, acute cardiac failure (PDA), coagulopathies

Presentation

Frothy pink sputum (in ET tube if ventilated) and acutely unwell neonate

Management

- Ventilation
- Antibiotics
- Correct any coagulation defect

Bronchopulmonary dysplasia

Bronchopulmonary dysplasia (BPD) is a condition of chronic lung damage with persistent X-ray changes. It is defined as an oxygen requirement either on day 28 of life or at 36 weeks' gestation. It occurs after severe RDS and other neonatal lung disease.

Clinical features

- Chest hyperinflation, intercostal and subcostal recession
- Crackles on auscultation
- Oxygen requirement
- Chest X-ray – 'honeycomb lung' (cystic pulmonary infiltrates in reticular pattern); areas of emphysema and collapse, and fibrosis and thickening of the pulmonary arterioles

Management

- Steroids and diuretics if ventilator dependent. Steroids may have an adverse effect on long term neurodevelopmental outcome
- Bronchodilators if wheezy
- May need long-term home oxygen

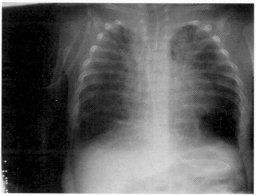

Figure 4.14 Chest X-ray of an infant with bronchopulmonary disease showing hyperexpanded lungs with diffuse fibrosis. A nasogastric tube is *in situ*

Apnoea

Apnoea is cessation of breathing for > 20 s. It may be accompanied by **bradycardia** and **cyanosis**.

Causes

- Central factors (chemoreceptor or respiratory centre failure)
- Airway obstruction
- Reflex protective mechanisms

Premature neonates have poorly developed central chemoreceptors and respiratory centres and therefore frequently have apnoeas.

Management

- Treat the underlying cause

Central	Obstructive	Reflex
Prematurity (usually resolves by 36 weeks)	Choanal atresia	Gastro-oesophageal reflux*
Hypoxia	Laryngeal nerve palsy	
Metabolic disturbance, e.g. hypoglycaemia	Foreign body	Vagal response, e.g. suctioning, physiotherapy
Sepsis	Pierre–Robin sequence (see p. 120)	
Hyper- and hypothermia		
Intracranial haemorrhage		
Convulsions		
Drugs, e.g. maternal intrapartum narcotics		

*Not proven as a cause

- Acute episode – stimulation, manual ventilation if necessary, apnoea monitoring
- Recurrent episodes:
    - CPAP, methylxanthines, e.g. caffeine, theophylline
    - Intubation and ventilation if severe
    - Resuscitation skills for the parents
    - Home apnoea monitor if parents wish, or hypoventilation syndrome

NEUROLOGICAL DISORDERS

Hypoxia–ischaemia

Hypoxia is insufficient arterial oxygen concentration; **ischaemia** is insufficient blood flow to the cells.

Fetal hypoxia–ischaemia can occur as an intrauterine or intrapartum event (a minority of cases are due to birth asphyxia). After birth, hypoxia may result from several causes, including severe shock, failure to breathe adequately and severe anaemia.

Intrauterine hypoxia may be *chronic*, presenting as **IUGR**, or *acute*, presenting with **fetal distress**. Intrapartum hypoxia may be *acute* or *acute on chronic*.

Signs of fetal distress

- Fetal bradycardia, reduced beat-to-beat variability, late decelerations (type II dips – recovery of heart rate after the end of the contraction)
- Reduced fetal movements
- Meconium

Causes

Maternal	Pre-eclampsia, eclampsia, acute hypotensive episode
Placental	Placental abruption, cord prolapse, chronic insufficiency (many causes, e.g. pre-eclampsia)
Fetal	Prematurity, postmaturity, obstructed labour

Hypoxia–ischaemia can result in damage to all organs, but initially there is preferential sparing of the brain at the expense of other organs. The effects of hypoxia–ischaemia in the different organs are:

Kidneys	Acute tubular necrosis
Gut	Necrotizing enterocolitis
CNS	Hypoxic–ischaemic encephalopathy (HIE)

Heart	Ischaemic changes
	Heart failure
Lungs	RDS
	Pulmonary haemorrhage
	PPHN
Metabolic	Metabolic acidosis
	Hypoglycaemia
	Hyponatraemia

Hypoxic–ischaemic encephalopathy

- Disturbance of neurological behaviour due to ischaemic damage to the brain
- Areas affected are the 'watershed zones' between the major arteries (those most susceptible to hypoperfusion). The condition can result in **cortical and subcortical necrosis** and cysts, and **periventricular leukomalacia (PVL)**. (In premature infants intraventricular haemorrhage occurs)
- Classified as *mild*, *moderate* or *severe*
- Infants are floppy after birth, with seizures and irregular breathing, and may become hypertonic over a period of days
- Mild disease generally resolves over a few days, but in severe HIE there is a 50% mortality and an 80% risk of cerebral palsy

Periventricular haemorrhage

The term periventricular haemorrhage (PVH) encompasses several types of intracranial haemorrhage:

- Neonates develop PVH as a result of an unstable circulation
- Risk factors include prematurity, RDS, IPPV (ventilation)
- Graded I–IV (most severe)
- Diagnosis and grading is made on cranial ultrasound scan
- Complications include hydrocephalus, porencephaly and cerebral palsy

CARDIAC DISORDERS

Patent ductus arteriosus

PDA is a particular problem of prematurity and is described in Chapter 9.

GASTROINTESTINAL DISORDERS

Necrotizing enterocolitis

Necrotizing enterocolitis (NEC) is a disease of bowel wall inflammation, ulceration and perforation. It has many causes and may be secondary to an **ischaemic or hypoxic insult** to the gut. There is mucosal damage leading to bacterial invasion and gastrointestinal gangrene and perforation.

Risk factors

- Prematurity
- Hypoxia
- Sepsis
- Hypovolaemia
- Hyperosmolar feeds
- Exchange transfusion
- Venous and umbilical catheters

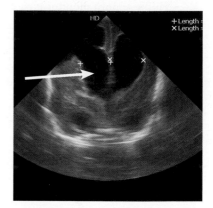

Figure 4.15 Cranial ultrasound scan of a 28 week premature infant showing bilateral dilated ventricles (arrow) secondary to a periventricular haemorrhage

Clinical features

General   Apnoeas, lethargy, vomiting, temperature
                 instability, acidosis and shock
Abdominal   Shiny distended abdomen, bile aspirates, rectal
                 fresh blood
AXR   Fixed loops of bowel, **pneumatosis
                 intestinalis** (intramural gas), portal vein gas,
                 pneumoperitoneum

There is a 10% mortality, higher if perforation occurs.

Complications

Short term   Perforation, obstruction, gangrenous bowel,
                 intrahepatic cholestasis, sepsis, DIC
Long term   Stricture, short bowel syndrome (due to
                 resection of diseased bowel)

Management

1. Manage shock, acidosis, electrolyte disturbance, anaemia,
   clotting disorder and ventilate if necessary
2. Systemic antibiotics
3. Gastrointestinal decompression (NG tube with aspiration)
4. Give parenteral nutrition only until gut has recovered
5. Surgical intervention if surgical complication occurs

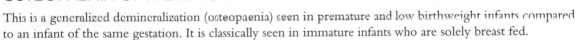

Figure 4.16 Abdominal X-ray of necrotizing enterocolitis

OSTEOPAENIA OF PREMATURITY

This is a generalized demineralization (osteopaenia) seen in premature and low birthweight infants compared to an infant of the same gestation. It is classically seen in immature infants who are solely breast fed.

Causes

■ Mineral deficiency, particularly phosphate, due to placental insufficiency and/or
■ Inadequate phosphate levels in breast milk or low phosphate feeds

Risk factors

■ VLBW
■ Severe IUGR and prematurity
■ Inadequate milk intake or insufficient phosphate in feeds
■ Chronic lung disease
■ Drugs – steroids, long term diuretics

Clinical features

■ Asymptomatic, diagnosed on long bone X-ray. Clinical rickets is rare, but rib fractures are not uncommon in babies with chronic lung disease
■ Calcium normal, phosphate ↓, PTH ↑, alkaline phosphatase ↑

Treatment

■ Low birthweight formula (contain increased phosphate)
■ Supplement breast milk with phosphate

NEONATAL JAUNDICE

Most neonates develop some jaundice in the first few weeks of life because they have a:

- Relative polycythaemia
- Shortened red cell lifespan (70 days as compared to 120 days in adults)
- Relative immaturity of the liver
- Most neonatal jaundice is due to **unconjugated (UC) bilirubin** and is *physiological*. Conditions involving haemolysis, e.g. Rhesus disease, excessive neonatal bruising, result in more pronounced jaundice, sometimes severe, and premature and unwell infants also develop more severe jaundice
- **Conjugated (C) hyperbilirubinaemia** is *always pathological*, and has many rare causes (see p. 204)
- Conjugated bilirubin is not toxic to the brain
- When levels of unconjugated bilirubin are high, they exceed the albumin-binding capacity of the blood and exist as **free unconjugated bilirubin**. This is harmful to the baby. It is lipid soluble and therefore can cross the blood–brain barrier where it causes neurotoxicity (known as kernicterus)
- **Kernicterus:**
  - *Immediate effects* – lethargy, irritability, increased tone, opisthotonus
  - *Long term effects* – sensorineural deafness, learning difficulties and choreoathetoid cerebral palsy
- Premature infants, sick neonates and those with low albumin levels are at increased risk

Causes of unconjugated neonatal jaundice

- Physiological
- Breast milk jaundice
- Excessive neonatal bruising, e.g. after Ventouse delivery
- Haemolytic disease:
  - Blood group incompatibility (Rhesus or ABO)
  - Red cell shape abnormality, e.g. spherocytosis, elliptocytosis
  - Red cell membrane instability, e.g. glucose-6-phosphate dehydrogenase deficiency, pyruvate kinase deficiency
- Sepsis (UC and C)
- Hypothyroidism (UC and C)
- Congenital hyperbilirubinaemias (UC and C), e.g. Gilbert disease, Crigler–Najar types I and II
- Metabolic disease (UC and C), e.g. galactosaemia, fructosaemia

Causes of neonatal jaundice related to time

< 24 h of birth:	Haemolytic disease Congenital infection sepsis	
24 h–2 weeks:	Physiological jaundice Prematurity Hypothyroidism Haemolysis Congenital hyperbilirubinaemias	Breast milk jaundice Sepsis Galactosaemia Bruising
> 2 weeks:	Breast milk jaundice Sepsis Haemolysis	Neonatal hepatitis Biliary atresia Choledochal cyst

Physiological jaundice

- Seen in 65% of term babies and 80% of premature babies
- Commences after 24 h and lasts 5–7 days

- Due to immature fetal liver, postnatal haemolysis and shorter red cell lifespan in infants
- Phototherapy is needed if serum bilirubin level is high

Breast milk jaundice

This is a diagnosis of exclusion that is poorly understood. It lasts for several weeks, requires no treatment, and breast feeding should continue. It is necessary to investigate the infant to rule out other causes.

Management

1. Baseline investigations to assess the severity, type and possible cause of jaundice:
   - Serum bilirubin (SBR)
   - Blood group, Coombs' test and FBC
   - Bilirubin conjugated and unconjugated fractions (conjugated is < 20% of total in unconjugated hyperbilirubinaemia and > 20% in conjugated hyperbilirubinaemia)
   - Urine (microscopy, culture and sensitivities)
2. If the SBR exceeds a certain level, treatment is commenced with phototherapy (or exchange transfusion if very rapidly increasing levels). Charts which act as guidelines for the level of bilirubin to commence phototherapy or exchange transfusion have been developed, and vary for different gestations and weights, and for sick babies (see chart)

Phototherapy

Phototherapy does not remove the bilirubin, but the UV radiation converts the harmful unconjugated bilirubin into water-soluble bilirubin, which can be excreted by the body.

- Whole baby under phototherapy lamp 24 h a day
- Undressed to increase skin exposed to UV
- Eyes are covered to prevent damage (cataracts)
- Extra fluid (30 ml/kg/day) given to prevent dehydration

Exchange transfusion

In this time-consuming procedure repeated small aliquots of the infant's blood are removed via peripheral arterial line, or umbilical artery or vein, and replaced with O Rh negative blood (or infant's ABO type if mother same group) which will not haemolyse. Complications include acidosis, hypoxia, apnoeas and bradycardias, thrombocytopacnia and NEC.

Haemolytic jaundice due to Rhesus or ABO incompatibility

- Due to high levels of haemolysis, resulting in too large a bilirubin load for the immature fetal liver
- Jaundice develops within first 24 h and rapidly rises
- Mixing of blood with just a few fetal red cells entering the maternal circulation can result in maternal antibodies developing to the fetal cells if they have a different antigenic component
- This mixing usually occurs at delivery or, if there is a placental bleed, may occur during pregnancy. The antibodies are therefore usually formed after the first pregnancy and so it is subsequent pregnancies that are affected as the antibodies cross the placenta
- Anti-D injections (as this is the most common form) are therefore given during pregnancy to Rhesus negative women to 'mop up' any fetal red cells in the maternal circulation and prevent antibodies developing

Clinical features

- Jaundice
- Anaemia

Management

1. Cord blood is taken for Hb, PCV (to assess severity), fetal blood group, maternal antibodies, Coombs' test and bilirubin level
2. Phototherapy
3. Regular 6-hourly serum bilirubin, Hb and PCV levels
4. Exchange transfusion if the bilirubin level becomes high enough
5. Intrauterine exchange transfusions can be done in fetal medicine units in very severe cases

Rhesus incompatibility	ABO incompatibility
Maternal antibodies to Rhesus C, D or E antigen (usually anti-D)	Maternal antibodies to red cell A or B antigens develop
Mother is blood group Rhesus negative, the baby Rhesus positive	Mother is Group O, the baby group A, B or AB
If severe, the infant can become profoundly anaemic and develop hydrops fetalis	Rarer but more severe than Rhesus incompatibility

NEONATAL PROBLEMS IN TERM BABIES

RESPIRATORY DISORDERS

Transient tachypnoea of the newborn

- Due to excessive retained fetal lung fluid
- Self-limiting condition
- Seen in 1–2% of newborns
- Elective Caesarean section (as no stress and fluid not squeezed out of lungs during delivery), birth asphyxia and infant of diabetic mother are all predisposing factors

Clinical features

- Respiratory distress from birth, resolving over the first 24 h
- CXR – generalized streakiness, fluid in the fissures and pleural effusions

Treatment

- Oxygen (ambient, CPAP if necessary, rarely ventilation needed)
- Antibiotics until pneumonia and sepsis excluded

Meconium aspiration syndrome

Meconium is present in 10% of deliveries.

Inhaled meconium can produce:

- Airway plugging with distal atelectasis, air leaks and secondary pneumonia
- Chemical pneumonitis (meconium is toxic to lung tissue)
- Hypoxia, respiratory and metabolic acidosis, and PPHN if severe

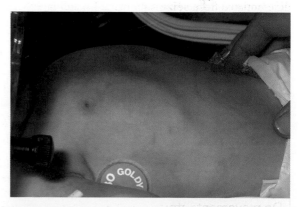

Figure 4.17 Meconium aspiration. Note chest hyperinflation

Clinical features

- Respiratory distress from birth, worsening
- Hyperinflated chest (due to air trapping)
- Severe acidosis
- Signs of cerebral irritation
- CXR – hyperinflation and diffuse patchy opacification

Management

- Respiratory support (high ventilatory pressures or high frequency oscillatory ventilation may be needed)
- Antibiotics and physiotherapy
- Management of PPHN (see below)

Persistent pulmonary hypertension of the newborn

In persistent pulmonary hypertension of the newborn (PPHN) there is a failure of the pulmonary vascular resistance to fall after birth, and blood is therefore shunted away from the lungs via the ductus arteriosus (right to left) and the foramen ovale. This results in **central cyanosis.**

Predisposing factors

- Hypoxia–ischaemia
- Metabolic disturbance/acidosis
- Severe lung disease, e.g. severe RDS, meconium aspiration syndrome
- Hypothermia

Clinical features

- Oxygen tension (and saturation) is low and there is little improvement with 100% oxygen therapy because little blood is entering the lungs
- Can be difficult to distinguish clinically from cyanotic congenital heart disease, but the CXR shows a normal heart and oligaemic lung fields, and echocardiogram shows a structurally normal heart

Management

PPHN is managed with positive pressure ventilation or HFOV, and inhaled nitric oxide (a vasodilator), prostacyclin IV or tolazoline IV. ECMO may be necessary if ventilation fails.

NEONATAL CONVULSIONS AND JITTERINESS

Neonates fairly commonly show signs of '**jitteriness**' with rapid fine shaking of the limbs, which must be differentiated from **seizures** (which have different causes and management).

Neonatal seizures are not always obvious and may present, for example, simply as apnoeas.

Differentiating jitteriness from seizures

	Neonatal jitteriness	Neonatal seizures
Predominant movement	Rhythmic movements of limbs	Multifocal, altered tone Apnoeas
Conscious state	Alert or asleep	Altered
Eye movements	Normal	Eye deviation occurs
Do movements stop when the limb is held?	Yes	No

Causes

Jitteriness	Hypoglycaemia
	Hypocalcaemia
	Sepsis
	Drug withdrawal (maternal drug addict)
Seizures	Asphyxia
	Infection (sepsis, meningitis, congenital)
	Metabolic disturbance (glucose $\downarrow$, Ca $\downarrow$, Mg $\downarrow$, Na $\uparrow$ or $\downarrow$)
	CVA, subarachnoid haemorrhage
	Pyridoxine deficiency or other inborn error of metabolism
	Congenital brain anomalies

Investigations

- Infection screen (blood, CSF and urine microscopy and culture, and serology)
- Electrolyte disturbance (urea and electrolytes including magnesium and calcium)
- Metabolic screen (glucose, and metabolic work-up if indicated)
- USS brain
- EEG

Treatment

- Treat the cause, e.g. give IV glucose, IV antibiotics or IV pyridoxine
- Give anticonvulsants for seizures if necessary, e.g. phenobarbitone, phenytoin

HYDROPS FETALIS

Hydrops fetalis consists of severe oedema, ascites and pleural effusions at birth.

Causes

- Immune – severe intrauterine anaemia, e.g. severe disease of the newborn (Rhesus or other blood group incompatibility)
- Non-immune – severe anaemia, e.g. fetomaternal haemorrhage
  Congenital infection, e.g. parvovirus B19
  Cardiac failure, e.g. uncontrolled fetal SVT
  Hypoproteinaemia, e.g. maternal pre-eclampsia
  Congenital malformations, e.g. anomalies of lymphatics – lymphangiectasia

HYPOGLYCAEMIA

Normal newborns can have intermittent low blood glucose levels but hypoglycaemia is frequently seen in small and premature infants, and also in sick neonates. There is no accepted universal definition; however, blood glucose levels < 2.6 mmol/L at any age are hypoglycaemic. Persistent neonatal hypoglycaemia is unusual.

State	Cause
Transient neonatal hypoglycaemia	Substrate deficiency – prematurity, IUGR, asphyxia, hypothermia, sepsis
	Hyperinsulinism – diabetic mother, gestational diabetes
Persistent neonatal hypoglycaemia	Hyperinsulinism – persistent hyperinsulinaemic hypoglycaemia of infancy (PHHL, nesidoblastosis), Beckwith–Wiedemann syndrome
	Metabolic disorder – galactosaemia, organic acidaemia, e.g. maple syrup urine disease

Clinical features

- Asymptomatic
- Apnoeas, jitteriness, seizures, lethargy, hypotonia

Management

■ Check BM stix (to gauge immediate level) and blood glucose (for accuracy)
■ Give oral milk feed, then hourly feeds with monitoring of blood glucose levels
■ If symptomatic or unable to feed, give 10% glucose bolus intravenously and then 10% glucose infusion, with frequent blood glucose monitoring
■ If the glucose remains low, a 15–20% glucose infusion may be necessary

Clinical scenario

A boy is born at 38 weeks' gestation weighing 5.4 kg. He is immediately jittery and has a blood sugar on testing of 1.8 mmol/l.

1. What is the most likely diagnosis?
2. What treatment is needed?

Subsequently he is noted to have a heart murmur and is going dusky.

3. What might be the cause of such a situation?

On further detailed history taking it transpires that his mother is addicted to cocaine.

4. How would this have some input to his health issues?

ANSWERS

1. The most likely diagnosis is neonatal hypoglycaemia secondary to maternal gestational diabetes mellitus –take particular note of excessive birthweight
2. Rapid administration of glucose enterally, or preferably intravenous dextrose
3. Cyanotic congenital heart disease, which is higher in incidence in infants of mothers with gestational diabetes mellitus
4. There are further risk factors for jitteriness with withdrawal symptoms and for congenital heart disease

FURTHER READING

Creasy RK, Resnik R, Iams JD *et al. Creasy and Resnik's Maternal-Fetal Medicine – Principles and Practice (6th edition).* Philadelphia: Saunders. 2008

D'Alton ME, Norwitz E and McElrath TF. *Maternal-Fetal Medicine (Cambridge Pocket Clinicians).* New York: Cambridge University Press. 2007.

Kumar S. *Handbook of Fetal Medicine.* Cambridge: Cambridge University Press. 2010.

Lissauer T, Fanaroff A. *Neonatology at a Glance*, 2nd edn. Oxford: Blackwell, 2011.

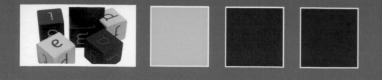

5 Infectious Diseases

- The febrile child
- Serious infections
- Common viral infections
- Bacterial infections
- Tropical infections
- Vaccination schedules
- Further reading

Acquiring various infectious diseases is an inevitable part of childhood. The commoner infectious diseases are outlined in this chapter. Many of the more organ-specific infectious diseases are discussed in the relevant specific chapters. For congenital infections see ch. 4.

THE FEBRILE CHILD

Fever can hamper the growth of certain organisms and can accelerate some immune responses. However, high fever can also impair the immune response and result in febrile convulsions. Management of the febrile child includes a thorough history and examination to help elucidate the cause.

Important points to ask about in the history
<ul><li>Symptoms of current illness</li><li>Contacts with others with febrile illness or infectious disease</li><li>Contact with animals and insects</li><li>Immunization status</li><li>Travel abroad e.g. shigella, malaria</li><li>Dietary history, e.g. unpasteurized milk consumption – listeria, brucellosis</li><li>Age (age-related infections)</li><li>Season</li><li>Congenital heart disease?</li><li>Immunocompromised state? e.g. chemotherapy, congenital immunodeficiency, HIV</li></ul>

Important points to note in the examination
<ul><li>Degree of fever (in infants a core temperature > 38°C is regarded as fever)</li><li>General clinical state and vital signs (see below)</li><li>Rash?</li></ul>

- Lymphadenopathy? Hepatosplenomegaly?
- Localizing signs? e.g. tonsillar exudate, joint tenderness, chest signs, abdominal mass or tenderness
- Heart murmur
- Features of immunodeficiency? (see ch. 6)

The majority of children with a fever will have a self-limiting viral infection. It is important, however, to distinguish those with a more serious cause. There is no single clinical or laboratory finding that will distinguish viral from bacterial infection, and so it is necessary to develop an *impression* of the child as a whole and *frequently* to reassess to observe the development of the situation. Features that help distinguish a bacteraemia are listed below.

Fever can be divided into:

- Fever with localizing signs, i.e. able to localize infection
- Fever without localizing signs

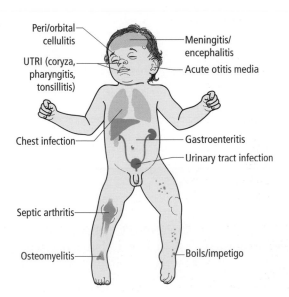

Peri/orbital cellulitis

UTRI (coryza, pharyngitis, tonsillitis)

Meningitis/encephalitis

Acute otitis media

Chest infection

Gastroenteritis

Urinary tract infection

Septic arthritis

Osteomyelitis

Boils/impetigo

Figure 5.1 Common localizations of infection

Management

Fever with localizing signs

Investigate and treat as appropriate for that condition

Fever without localizing signs (origin unknown)

- It is most important to recognize that all infections are *dynamic*, as such a child who has a mild fever and looks well may be in the early stages of a septicaemic illness. *Regular review* by family, primary or secondary health care workers is imperative (see p. 80)
- It is important not to miss a **bacteraemic illness**. Features suggestive of bacteraemia are listed below; however, these are non-specific features and none is diagnostic

- Children who are clinically ill are investigated (with CRP and FBC; blood, throat, urine, stool ± CSF cultures ± CXR) and then either commenced empirically on antibiotics, or observed with antibiotics only given if the exact cause of illness is found or sepsis becomes apparent
- If a fever persists for more than a few days with no cause found, causes of prolonged fever should be looked for (see below). In particular, Kawasaki disease should be considered in children under 5 (see p. 401)

Features suggestive of an unwell child (not necessarily a bacterial infection, but think of it in this context). NB: These features have a low sensitivity and specificity

Symptom/sign/test	Observation
Temperature	Markedly elevated (> 39°C)
	Hypothermia (neonates and impending severe sepsis)
Pulse rate	Tachycardia/bradycardia
Colour	Pale or mottled
Capillary refill time	Prolonged
Peripheries	Cool
Tone	Floppy
Responsiveness	Intermittent or unresponsive
WCC	> 15 x 10^9/L or < 2.5 x 10^9/L
ESR, CRP	Elevated

Causes of prolonged fever	
Viral	CMV, EBV, HHV 6, HIV
Bacterial	TB, bacterial endocarditis, osteomyelitis, abscess, salmonella, spirochaetes, brucellosis
Other infections	Malaria, chlamydia, toxoplasmosis, rickettsia, fungal infections
Non-infectious causes	**Kawasaki disease** (> 5 days fever), collagen vascular disease (JIA, SLE), malignancy (leukaemia), inflammatory bowel disease, familial Mediterranean fever (gene test available)

SERIOUS INFECTIONS

SEPSIS

Most pathogens are intercepted at their primary site of entry by the host first-line defence mechanisms. If microorganisms manage to break through this first line of defence and invade the bloodstream, and if the host does not rapidly resolve the infection, bacterial proliferation can ensue. This results in a systemic **host inflammatory response**, which, together with the virulent properties of the invading organism, causes the features of sepsis to develop.

- Enterotoxins from staphylococci and streptococci can cause toxic shock syndrome, even with localized infection, due to their virulence
- Viruses (particularly herpesviruses, enteroviuses and adenoviruses) can cause disease clinically similar to bacterial sepsis in children and neonates particularly

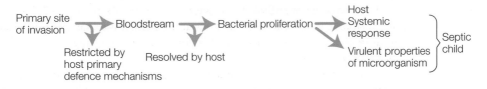

Figure 5.2 Pathway of sepsis

In **septic shock** there is persistent hypotension despite adequate fluid resuscitation and/or hypoperfusion after adequate inotrope or pressor support.

Common causes

Neonates (< 3 months age)	Children > 3 months of age	Immunocompromised
Group B streptococcus *Escherichia coli* Other Gram-negative bacteria *Listeria monocytogenes* *Staphylococcus aureus*	*Streptococcus pneumoniae* Group A streptococcus *Neisseria meningitidis* *Haemophilus influenzae* type b *Staphylococcus aureus* *Salmonella* spp.	As for children plus: Gram-negative organisms Fungi Opportunistic infections

Clinical features

Clinical features depend upon the organism, child's age and pre-existing health, and duration of illness. Early bacteraemia can be difficult to diagnose, with few or no specific features. For this reason **frequent reassessment** of the child for progression or lack of improvement is essential.

Non-specific early features	Lethargy, irritability, hypotonia, poor feeding, nausea and vomiting, mottled skin
Cardiovascular	Tachycardia/bradycardia, poor peripheral perfusion, prolonged capillary refill time, peripheral oedema, decreased urine output
Other organs	Respiratory, gastrointestinal, neurological derangement
Rash	Petechial rash, meningococcal (see below), erythroderma, mucosal erythema and oedema (toxic shock syndrome)

Management

Frequent reassessment of the patient is mandatory. Initially there are usually a small number of invading organisms, but these multiply (often logarithmically), resulting in rapid clinical deterioration. Therefore, *the most important management aspect is recognition of sepsis as early as possible* and initiation of antibiotics and supportive treatment.

Investigations

- Source of infection:
  - Blood cultures, urine microscopy and culture
  - Other samples, e.g. throat swab, LRT secretions if ventilated, lumbar puncture if suspected meningeal involvement (and no contraindication)
  - CXR
  - **Rapid analysis** can be done using **PCR** to detect bacteria, viruses and fungi on blood, and on urine and CSF samples to identify an organism
- Indicators of infection – WCC, inflammatory markers, e.g. CRP
- Other – coagulation profile, FBC, U&E, creatinine, glucose, LFTs, blood gas

Treatment	*Initial resuscitation* (ABC) as necessary
	Appropriate antibiotic therapy as soon as possible. (Choice depends upon likely pathogen, resistance, and patient factors, e.g. immunosuppression, neonates, sickle cell disease)

Supportive measures for septic shock (see p. 464):

- Fluid management (of hypovolaemia due to fluid maldistribution): continuous CVP monitoring, urine output; plasma, blood and other fluids as necessary
- Mechanical ventilation (as capillary leak into lungs)
- Inotropic support (for myocardial depression)
- Vasopressors (peripheral vasodilatation)
- Management of DIC (coagulation pathways dysregulated)

Adjuvant therapy – new treatments involving administering antagonists of host-derived inflammatory mediators are being developed

MENINGITIS

Meningitis is an acute infection involving the meninges. It is usually a result of bacterial or viral infection, but may be caused by fungal or other microbial agents.

Common causes of bacterial meningitis

Neonates	2–3 months	3 months–5 years	> 5 years
Group B β-haemolytic streptococcus *Escherichia coli* *Staphylococcus aureus* *Listeria monocytogenes*	As for neonates *Neisseria meningitidis*	*N. meningitidis* (meningococcus) *Streptococcus pneumoniae* (pneumococcus) *Haemophilus influenzae* type b (uncommon since Hib vaccine)	*N. meningitidis* *Strep. pneumoniae*

Causes of viral meningitis

- Enteroviruses (cause > 80%, especially coxsackie A and B and echovirus)
- Adenovirus
- Mumps
- EBV, CMV, VZV, HSV
- HIV

Clinical features

These depend on the age of the child, and in young infants are *non-specific*, with the classic features of meningitis in adults often not apparent. It is important therefore to maintain a high index of suspicion.

Some of the following features may be present:

Neonate	Non-specific features of lethargy, apnoeas, poor feeding, temperature instability and shock
	Respiratory distress, irritability, a high-pitched cry, seizures and a bulging fontanelle may also be present
	Rash (occasionally)
Infant	Fever, lethargy, irritability, poor feeding, vomiting
	Bulging fontanelle, shock, seizures, coma
	Rash

Older child
(> 18 months)

Fever, headache, vomiting, drowsiness, rash, shock, seizures (late), papilloedema (rare)

Features of **meningeal irritation:**

■ Headache
■ Photophobia
■ Neck stiffness
■ **Kernig sign** (pain on lower leg extension with hip flexed)
■ **Brudzinski sign** (involuntary flexion of knees and hips with neck flexion) – useful in infants

Tuberculous meningitis

This is rare and presents *insidiously*. Symptoms of headache, anorexia, focal neurology, seizures and cortical blindness are typical. Only later do classical signs of meningeal irritation develop.

Rash

A petechial rash is classically associated with **meningococcal septicaemia** and can lead to necrotic areas of skin. It may also be seen in pneumococcal and *Haemophilus influenzae* infections (see below).

Glass test

A petechial rash can be identified by pressing a glass to the affected skin: if the rash does *not* blanch it is petechial. This is a useful test for parents to know.

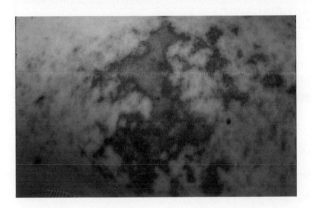

Figure 5.3 Petechial rash

Causes of petechial rash

Infections	Other
Meningococcal infection (sepsis, meningitis)	Henoch–Schönlein purpura (buttocks, thighs and sock line)
Haemophilus influenzae infection (sepsis, meningitis)	Idiopathic thrombocytopaenic purpura
Streptococcus pneumoniae (sepsis, meningitis)	Anaphylactoid purpura
Rikettsial infection, e.g. Rocky Mountain spotted fever, ehrlichiosis	Leukaemia
Viral infection (EBV, CMV, atypical measles, enteroviruses)	DIC
Malaria	Vigorous coughing or vomiting, e.g. pertussis (face, neck and upper chest)
	Attempted strangulation (face and neck)

Management

- *Commence treatment with antibiotics immediately* on suspicion (including in the community prior to arriving in hospital)
- General investigations – glucose, blood gas, FBC, clotting, U&E and creatinine, CRP. An elevated CRP indicates infection
- Source of infection – **blood** and **urine** samples, a **throat swab** and a **lumbar puncture** (unless contraindicated) for microscopy and culture, and a **CXR**
- Rapid analysis can be done using **PCR** to detect bacteria and viruses on blood, urine and CSF samples and to identify an organism
- Lumbar puncture findings can help differentiate bacterial from viral meningitis (see below), and identify the infecting organism
- Treatment:
  - Intravenous broad-spectrum antibiotics commencing *immediately* (prior to LP results)
  - Supportive measures (as for sepsis, p. 80)
  - Use of steroids is controversial for meningitis but generally empirically given. For *H. influenzae* most authorities give 0.6 mg/kg/day dexamathasone for at least 48 h (but it may only have the effect of decreasing post-meningitis deafness rate)
  - There is no specific treatment for viral meningitis other than aciclovir for HSV or VZV infection

> **NB: If in doubt about whether bacterial or viral, treat as *bacterial* until culture results at 48 h. Neonates and young infants have a low threshold for the use of empirical aciclovir.**

Table 5.1 Lumbar puncture findings (excluding neonatal period)

	Normal	Bacterial	Viral	TB
Appearance	Clear	Turbid	Clear	Viscous or clear
Lymphocytes (/mm³)	< 5	< 50	10–100	100–300
Polymorphs (/mm³)	Nil	> 200	Nil	0–200
Protein (g/L)	0.2–0.4	0.5–3	0.2–1.0 (N or ↑)	0.5–6.0
Glucose	> 1/2 serum	< 1/2 serum	> 1/2 serum (N)	< 1/3 serum

This is a guide only as lymphocytosis may predominate in early or partially treated bacterial meningitis and in neonates.

> **NB: In a bloody tap the RBC:WBC ratio can reach around 400:1, similar to peripheral blood.**

Complications

- SIADH
- Cerebral – seizures, subdural effusion (may be chronic in onset), abscess, infarction, hydrocephalus
- Deafness – due to VIIIth cranial nerve involvement (hearing test at follow-up is mandatory)

Prevention/prophylaxis

- Oral rifampicin therapy for 2 days is given to all contacts of meningococcal meningitis, and for 4 days if there is an unvaccinated infant under 4 years in the household. It is also given to all close contacts in *H. influenzae*

Contraindications to lumbar puncture

- Neurological:
  - Signs of raised intracranial pressure (papilloedema, bradycardia, hypertension [see p. 365]): may result in cerebral herniation (very rare if fontanelle still open)
  - Impaired consciousness
  - Focal neurological signs
  - Focal or prolonged seizures
- Cardiopulmonary compromise
- Local skin infection overlying the lumbar puncture site
- Coagulopathy or thrombocytopaenia

- Both *H. influenzae* and meningococcus C are now routinely vaccinated against
- A vaccine for the more common meningococcus B has yet to be developed
- Notifiable disease

ENCEPHALITIS

Encephalitis is inflammation of the brain parenchyma. It is usually due to direct viral invasion, although can be secondary to a post-infectious immune response or a slow virus infection (as in SSPE). Viral encephalitis and viral meningitis are caused by the same organisms and form a continuum.

Causes of viral encephalitis

- HSV 1 and 2 – treated with aciclovir, 70% mortality untreated; predeliction for temporal lobes
- VZV – treated with aciclovir; post-infectious cerebellar ataxia is a complication
- HHV 6
- Mumps – deafness common (VIIIth nerve damage)
- Measles
- Rubella
- Enteroviruses – echovirus, coxsackie virus
- HIV 1

Clinical features

- Insidious onset compared to meningitis
- Generalized features of fever, headache, vomiting, lethargy, behavioural change, decreased conciousness
- Signs of meningeal irritation (uncommon in young infants)
- Seizures (often difficult to control)
- **Focal neurological signs**
- Features of raised intracranial pressure
- Neurological sequelae are common (cognitive and motor deficits, epilepsy, behavioural change)

Management

- Investigations as for meningitis, in particular blood serology, viral cultures (CSF, throat and stool), and PCR for specific pathogens
- Neuroimaging with MRI scan may show areas of inflammation
- EEG is done to check generalized brain activity and to look for any localized damage, e.g. temporal slow wave activity in HSV
- Antiviral agents are given intravenously and supportive care is given as necessary

COMMON VIRAL INFECTIONS

HERPES VIRUSES

- Human herpes viruses (HHV) are DNA viruses; eight known currently
- Cause a primary infection and then *remain latent* and can cause reinfection later on
- Reinfection can be triggered by stress, illness, sunlight and immunosuppression

The herpes viruses	
Herpes virus	**Disease(s)**
HHV: HSV 1 and 2	Primary infection – gingivostomatitis, keratoconjunctivitis, herpetic Whitlow Reinfection – cold sores
HHV 3: VZV	Primary infection – chicken pox (varicella) Reinfection – shingles (zoster)
HHV 4: EBV	
HHV 5: CMV	Infectious mononucleosis
HHV 6	Roseola infantum (exanthem subitum)
HHV 7	Disease very similar to HHV 6
HHV 8	Associated with Kaposi sarcoma, an endothelial malignancy seen in certain populations and the immunocompromised

Herpes simplex virus (HSV; HHV 1)

Common infection that is usually asymptomatic.

Transmission	Direct contact. Babies often infected by kisses from an adult with a cold sore
Incubation	2–15 days

Two viral types exist (NB: these can overlap):

HSV 1	Transmitted mainly via saliva and the cause of most childhood infections
HSV 2	Transmitted mainly via genital secretions or via vaginal delivery (see p. 48) and the primary cause of genital herpes

The *primary infection* causes a severe vesicular rash wherever the primary innoculation was:

- **Mouth infection** is **gingivostomatitis** (most common primary infection). If severe, swallowing is painful and nasogastric or intravenous fluids may be required. Fever for 2–3 days, healing in 1 week. Peak age 1–3 years
- **Skin infection**, e.g. **herpetic Whitlow** (infection on finger)
- **Eye infection** (**keratoconjunctivitis**) can result in corneal scarring, and ophthalmological review by the ophthalmologist is important

Dormancy occurs in the local sensory nerve dorsal root ganglia, with *reinfection* via that nerve root, e.g. **cold sore** (herpes labialis) from trigeminal nerve ganglia infection.

Serious HSV infection

CNS infection	**Encephalitis** – temporal lobe damage, 70% mortality if untreated **Meningitis**
Eczema herpeticum	Widespread severe herpes infection that occurs in children with eczema
Immunocompromised child	Severe infection, may become disseminated (very serious)
Neonatal infection	See p. 48

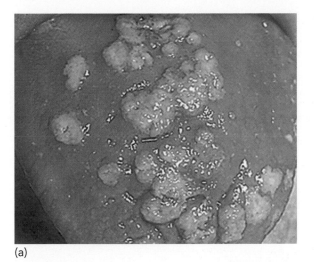

(a)

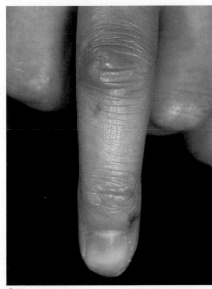

(b)

Figure 5.4 HSV infection. (a) Primary HSV stomatitis.
(b) Herpetic Whitlow

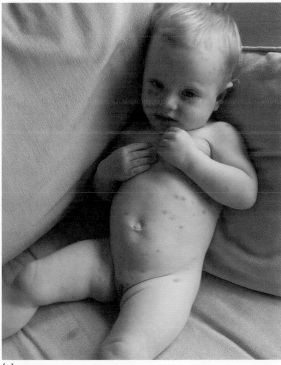

(a)

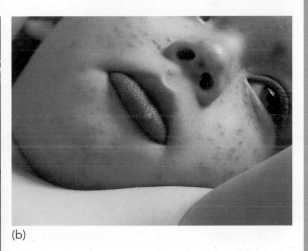

(b)

Figure 5.5 (a) A 1-year-old infant at the onset of
the chicken pox rash. Note the truncal distribution
of the vesicular rash. (b) A 3-year-old boy with a
chicken pox lesion on his tongue

Treatment
Aciclovir (oral in mild infections, intravenous in severe infections)

Varicella zoster virus (VZV; HHV 2)

This causes both chicken pox (varicella) and shingles (zoster).

Varicella (chicken pox)

Transmission   Airborne or contact
Incubation   14–21 days. The child is infectious for 5 days after onset of the rash

Clinical features

- Mild prodromal illness with fever lasting 2–3 days (not in young children)
- Peak age 2–8 years
- Rash – face, scalp and trunk, spreads *centrifugally*
- Macules → papules → vesicles → pustules → crusts. NB: *All stages are seen at once* on the skin

Congenital infection can affect the fetus (see p. 48), in third trimester.

Complications

Several complications can occur in previously healthy children.

Superinfection of skin   Pustules, crusts, or bullous lesions, prolonged fever. Usually *Staph. aureus* or streptococcal infection
Pneumonia   Common in adults (30%), CXR dramatic
Encephalitis   Recovery good. Acute truncal cerebellar ataxia (post-infectious)
Purpura fulminans   Vasculitis in skin and subcutaneous tissues, can result in skin necrosis
Other   Thrombocytopaenia, hepatitis, arthritis, stroke
Immunocompromised   Severe disseminated haemorrhagic disease. High mortality

Zoster (shingles)

- Occurs from reactivation of dormant VZV, usually from the dorsal root or cranial ganglia
- Although thought to be due to immunocompromise, it is commonly seen in normal children
- Lesions are identical to varicella, itchy and slightly painful but usually restricted to < 3 dermatomes
- Infection of the geniculate ganglion can cause ear pinna vesicles and facial nerve palsy (**Ramsay–Hunt syndrome**)

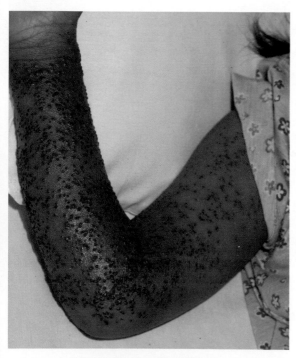

Figure 5.6 Haemorrhagic chicken pox

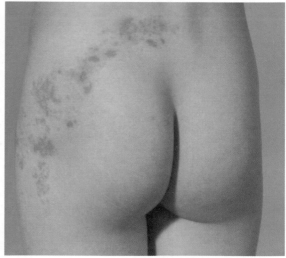

Figure 5.7 Shingles rash

Treatment

This is not required except in severe disease, for ophthalmic infection and if immunocompromised (treat with intravenous aciclovir).

Prophylaxis

Zoster immunoglobulin (ZIG) passive immunization is given to:

- Immunocompromised children exposed to VZV, e.g. bone marrow transplant patients, congenital immunodeficiency, on immunosuppressives or high-dose steroids in previous 3 months
- Neonates of mothers infected with varicella from between 5 days pre–2 days post delivery

VZV vaccine is currently not routinely used in the UK. High-risk individuals such as adults may be offered the vaccine.

Cytomegalovirus (CMV; HHV 3)

Transmission	Saliva, breast milk, genital secretions or blood, and transplacental
	Most children are infected when toddlers, and half of adults have positive serology, i.e. IgG to CMV

Clinical features

Healthy individuals	Usually asymptomatic
	May cause a similar clinical picture to EBV with fever, malaise but tonsillitis and lymphadenopathy less obvious
	Liver involvement is common, with raised LFTs
Immunocompromised	Severe infection including encephalitis, retinitis, pneumonitis, gastrointestinal infection, atypical lymphocytes, hepatitis
Congenital infection	See p. 48

> ❗ **NB: CMV screening is important in organ transplant patients as it may be introduced via the donated organ or blood transfusions.**

Investigations

Blood count	Lymphocytosis with atypical lymphocytes. Sometimes neutropaenia
Serology	Primary infection (IgM), previous infection (IgG)
Urine	For CMV DEAFF (signifies active replication)
CMV PCR	On blood and other secretions
Tissues	Intranuclear 'owl's eye' inclusions on microscopy, direct immunofluorescence and viral culture

Treatment

- None required in healthy individuals
- Ganciclovir, foscarnet or cidofovir if immunocompromised

Epstein–Barr virus (EBV; HHV 4)

This produces infectious mononucleosis (glandular fever), often in adolescents. It is often asymptomatic in young children.

Transmission	Aerosol, saliva
Incubation	20–30 days

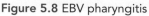

Clinical features

The virus particularly infects **B lymphocytes**.

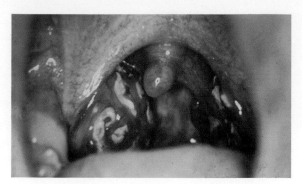

Figure 5.8 EBV pharyngitis

- Fever, headache
- Tonsillopharyngitis, palatal petechiae
- Generalized lymphadenopathy
- Maculopapular rash
- Splenomegaly (tender), hepatomegaly, hepatitis (jaundice)
- Thrombocytopaenia, haemolytic anaemia, atypical T lymphocytes, mononuclear cells
- Arthropathy
- Symptoms last 1–3 months
- May produce depression and malaise for *many months*
- Gastrointestinal dysmotility

> **!** **NB: A generalized bright red rash occurs if ampicillin is given (90% of cases).**

Complications

- Meningitis, encephalitis
- Myelitis, Guillain–Barré syndrome
- Myocarditis
- Mesenteric adenitis
- Splenic rupture

> **!** **NB: Burkitt lymphoma, nasopharyngeal carcinoma and lymphoproliferative disease in the immunocompromised are thought to be caused by EBV infection.**

Diagnosis

- Atypical lymphocytes in the blood (> 10% large T cells)
- Paul–Bunnell reaction positive (heterophile antibodies that agglutinate sheep RBCs). (Non-specific, false positives seen with leukaemia, non-Hodgkin lymphoma, hepatitis)
- Monospot test positive (heterophile antibodies to horse RBCs; unreliable < 5 years due to false negatives)
- EBV IgM may be detected (75–90% by end of third week)
- EBV PCR
- Other serology (EBV VCA, EBV NA)

Treatment

Treatment is not usually required except in the rare cases of lymphoproliferation where monoclonal antibodies to the B-cell antigen CD20 are used.

Roseola infantum (exanthem subitum; HHV 6)

Almost all children have been infected in infancy and around one-third are symptomatic.

> **!** **NB: Roseola infantum is a common cause of febrile convulsions in children < 2 years (approximately one-third).**

Transmission   Droplet
Incubation   9–10 days

Clinical features

- High fever and malaise, cervical lymphadenopathy
- Few days later, red macular rash over face, trunk and arms lasting 1–2 days
- *Sudden* improvement after the rash
- Red papules on soft palate
- Febrile convulsions
- Rarely, meningitis, encephalitis, hepatitis

Treatment

There is no specific treatment.

ENTEROVIRUSES

These include polio virus, coxsackie A and B, echoviruses and rhinoviruses. They cause a variety of illnesses including hand, foot and mouth disease, myocarditis, encephalitis and the common cold.

Hand, foot and mouth disease

This is a mild disease which can be caused by coxsackie A or B, and enterovirus 71.

Transmission   Via droplet, direct contact or the faecal–oral route

Clinical features

- Mild disease lasting about a week, usually in pre-school children
- Fever
- Vesicles in the oropharynx and on the palms and soles
- May also be a more generalized maculopapular rash
- Resolves spontaneously
- In X-linked agammaglobulinaemia (see ch. 6), enteroviruses can cause extensive cerebral infections

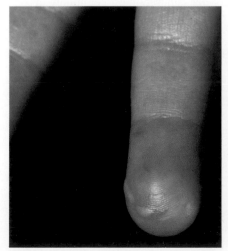

(a)

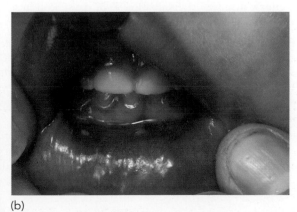

(b)

Figure 5.9 Hand, foot and mouth disease.
(a) Hand. (b) Mouth

Polio

This infection is now very rare in the UK and is usually only seen in immunocompromised patients who have received live vaccine. It has yet to be eradicated in all developing countries.

The clinical effect of polio varies from subclinical infection to a mild febrile illness to paralysis. Certain factors predispose to paralytic polio (exercise early in the illness, male gender, trauma and surgery).

Transmission   Faecal–oral route
Incubation   7–14 days

Clinical features

Subclinical infection (95%)   Asymptomatic
Abortive poliomyelitis (5%)   Fever, myalgia, sore throat
Non-paralytic poliomyelitis (2%)   Above with meningeal irritation
Paralytic poliomyelitis (0.1%)   Above, then asymmetrical paralysis:
- *Spinal* poliomyelitis (thorax, diaphragm, trunk, limbs)
- *Bulbar* poliomyelitis (motor cranial nerve palsies)

Treatment

Therapy is purely supportive.

Polio vaccines

New intramuscular vaccine given as part of five-component infant vaccination
Sabin – live vaccine. Oral polio vaccine (a bitter purple liquid), part of vaccination programme
Salk – killed vaccine. Intramuscular (given only to the immunocompromised)

PARVOVIRUS B19

This virus attacks the erythroid precursors and leads to transient arrest of erythropoiesis.

Transmission   Respiratory route, blood, vertical transmission
Incubation   Variable

It produces various clinical syndromes:

1. **Slapped cheek disease Erythema infectiosum (fifth disease)**   Incubation 4–21 days. Seen in school-age children, most commonly in spring
Fever, malaise, headache, myalgia. Then after 1 week, very red cheeks, and then a macular erythema over the trunk and limbs with central clearing of the lesions resulting in a *lacy pattern* which may recur over weeks
2. **Asymptomatic infection**   Common
3. **Arthropathy**   Usually transient, older children may develop arthritis
4. **Immunocompromised**   Chronic infection with anaemia
5. **Transient aplastic crisis**   Occurs in children in states of chronic haemolysis, e.g. in sickle cell anaemia, thalassaemia and spherocytosis
6. **Congenital infection**   Severe anaemia with hydrops fetalis (see p. 48)

MEASLES

This is a potentially serious illness and can be fatal. Incidence has been reduced with the MMR vaccine; however, the incidence is now rising again as the MMR vaccine uptake is poor. (A vaccine coverage of >90% is required to prevent epidemics.)

Transmission	Droplet (coughing, sneezing)
Incubation	7–14 days
	Infectious from pre-eruptive stage until 1 week of the rash appearing

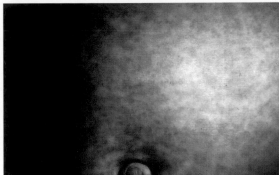

Figure 5.10 Measles rash on the trunk

Clinical features

| Pre-eruptive stage | Child unwell with high fever, conjunctivitis, cough and coryzal symptoms. **Koplik's spots** (pathognomonic small white spots on buccal mucosa and gums around 2nd molar) |
| Eruptive phase | Fine red maculopapular rash beginning behind ears and on face and spreading down the whole body |

Complications

- Common in *malnourished* children with vitamin A deficiency (developing countries)
- Otitis media
- Secondary bacterial pneumonia, bronchitis
- Hepatitis, diarrhoea, myocarditis
- Post-measles blindness secondary to keratitis (seen in developing countries)
- Encephalomyelitis (post-infectious)
- Subacute sclerosing panencephalitis (SSPE): a rare progressive dementia occurring several years after measles infection in < 1 in 100 000 cases. This is not caused by vaccine strains

Management

Treatment is symptomatic only. Human pooled immunoglobulin and ribavirin can be given within 6 days of exposure (given to the immunocompromised and young infants).

MUMPS

This generally results in mild illness in children, but in adults it can be severe. It is vaccinated against as part of the MMR.

Transmission	Droplet (respiratory) and direct contact, mostly in the winter and spring
Incubation	14–21 days
	Infectious for 6 days pre–9 days post the parotid swelling

Clinical features

- Prodrome of fever, headache, earache and anorexia. Usually asymptomatic
- Painful salivary gland swelling – parotid and sometimes also submandibular. This is usually bilateral, though unilateral in one-third
- Trismus may occur

Complications

- Meningeal signs
- Encephalitis (1 in 5000)
- Transient hearing loss
- Epididymo-orchitis (in 20% after puberty)
- Other organs – pancreatitis, oophoritis, myocarditis, arthritis, mastitis, hepatitis

Management

Diagnosis is clinical, and there is no treatment. The virus can be isolated from urine, saliva, throat swab or CSF (in mumps meningitis), and a rise in antibody titre can be looked for in sera (as in rubella) in complicated cases.

RUBELLA (GERMAN MEASLES)

This is a common and generally mild, often asymptomatic illness. Its importance lies in the potentially devastating consequences of maternal infection during pregnancy as it can be teratogenic (see p. 48). For this reason vaccination is part of the MMR. The dramatic reduction in congenital rubella is largely due to the decreased risk of young mothers being exposed to infectious children.

Transmission   By droplet (respiratory), most common in the winter and spring
Incubation   14–21 days
               Infectious for < 7 days from the onset of the rash

Clinical features

< 5 years old   Generally asymptomatic
> 5 years old   Low grade fever, conjunctivitis and lymphadenopathy (especially suboccipital and post-auricular)
                Forcheimer spots (palatal petechiae)
                Splenomegaly
                < 7 days fine pink maculopapular rash firstly on face, then whole body. Lasts 3–5 days

Complications (rare)

- Arthritis (small joints)
- Myocarditis
- Thrombocytopaenia
- Encephalitis
- Congenital rubella syndrome (see p. 48)

Management

Diagnosis is clinical but can be confirmed if a pregnant woman may have been exposed. This is done by taking acute and convalescent (after 7 days) serum to check for rubella-specific IgM levels which should rise. No treatment is available or necessary.

The viral exanthems	
First disease	Measles
Second disease	Scarlet fever
Third disease	Rubella
Fourth disease	Dukes disease (term no longer used, a rubella variant circa 1900)
Fifth disease	Slapped cheek disease (erythema infectiosum, parvovirus B19)
Sixth disease	Roseola infantum (HHV 6)

Approximate viral incubation times mnemonic	
CRUMPS (**c**hicken pox, **r**ubella, m**umps**)	= 14–21 days
Most other	= 7–10 days

BACTERIAL INFECTIONS

STAPHYLOCOCCAL INFECTIONS

Staphylococci are part of the normal flora of the skin, upper respiratory and gastrointestinal tracts. The coagulase-positive *Staphylococcus aureus* is responsible for most infections, and 25% of the population are asymptomatic carriers. The clinical diseases are caused by either direct bacterial invasion or the toxins produced.

Diseases caused by staphylococcal infection		
	Bacterial invasion	**Toxin mediated**
Skin	Boils, impetigo (p. 295), cellulitis (p. 417) Staphylococcal scarlet fever	Bullous impetigo (p. 288), SSSS (p. 296)
General	Septicaemia	Toxic shock syndrome (TSS)
Gut	Enterocolitis	Food poisoning
Bones	Septic arthritis (p. 406), osteomyelitis (p. 406)	
Eyes	Orbital cellulitis, preseptal cellulitis (p. 413)	
Lungs	Pneumonia	
CNS	Meningitis	
Cardiac	Acute endocarditis (p. 165)	

Toxic shock syndrome

This severe infection is due to exotoxins, e.g. toxic shock syndrome toxin (TSST-1) usually from *Staph. aureus*. The focus of infection is usually minor, e.g. a boil. There is an association with tampon use.

Diagnostic features

- Fever > 38.9°C
- Conjunctivitis
- Diffuse tender pale red rash followed by desquamation
- Hypotension
- Vomiting and diarrhoea
- Toxic effects in other systems (≥ 3 required for diagnosis) – myalgia, renal impairment, drowsiness, thrombocytopaenia, mucous membrane involvement

Management

The management is IV antibiotics, IVIG and supportive therapy with IV fluids, cardiovascular support, ventilation and renal dialysis as necessary.

STREPTOCOCCAL INFECTIONS

Streptococcal infections are usually due to Group A β-haemolytic streptococci (GAS, *Strep. pyogenes*). 15–20% of healthy children have asymptomatic pharynx carriage of GAS. Some infections are due to *Strep. pneumoniae* (a non-β-haemolytic streptococcus). In neonates infection is usually due to Group B β-haemolytic streptococcus (GBS). *Strep. viridans* (a group of non-β-haemolytic streptococci) cause infective endocarditis (see p. 165).

The clinical diseases are due either to direct bacterial invasion, toxins or post-infectious immune response.

Diseases caused by streptococcal infection

	Bacterial invasion	Toxin-mediated	Post-infectious
Skin	Impetigo (see p. 295) Cellulitis	Scarlet fever	Erythema nodosum
Respiratory	Otitis media, tonsillitis, pneumonia, mastoiditis, sinusitis		
Bone	Osteomyelitis (usually *Staph.*)		Arthritis
CNS	Meningitis (in neonates)		PANDAS (see below)
General	Septicaemia		Sydenham's chorea
Cardiac	Infective endocarditis	Streptococcal	Rheumatic fever (p. 164)
Renal		TSS (see below)	Glomerulonephritis (p. 235)

Scarlet fever

This is due to a strain of Group A β–haemolytic streptococci producing an **erythrogenic exotoxin** in individuals who have no neutralizing antibodies. The entry site is usually the pharynx (after tonsillitis).

Transmission	Contact, droplet
Incubation	2–4 days

Clinical features

- Sudden onset of fever, rigors, headache, vomiting, sore throat, anorexia
- White strawberry tongue (white tongue with red papillae), then strawberry tongue (bright red tongue)
- Flushed cheeks and pale around the lips, and a coarse (feels like sandpaper) red rash over the body that desquamates after a few days

Management

Diagnosis	Confirmed with throat swab, and detection of ASOT and anti-DNAse B in the serum
Treatment	Oral penicillin

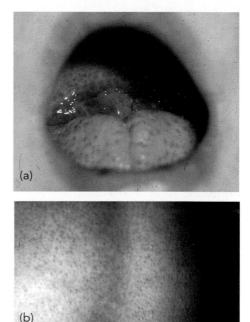

(a)

(b)

Figure 5.11 Scarlet fever. (a) White strawberry tongue. (b) Rash on the trunk

Streptococcal toxic shock syndrome

This is similar to staphylococcal TSS but often due to a deep-seated streptococcal infection.

PANDAS (paediatric autoimmune neuropsychiatric disorders associated with streptococcal infections)

These are children with childhood–onset obsessive-compulsive disorder and/or tic disorders in whom there is an onset or symptom exacerbation following GAS infection (scarlet fever or streptococcal throat infection), and symptoms are episodic.

CAT SCRATCH DISEASE

This common worldwide childhood infection is caused by the Gram-negative bacillus *Bartonella henselae*.

Transmission	Scratch or contact from a cat (especially kittens); sometimes a dog (but in half of cases no history of scratch is obtained)
	Mostly September–February
Incubation	3–30 days

Clinical features

- 50% have an inoculation pustule or papule (lasts days–months) or conjunctivitis
- Regional lymphadenopathy (2–4 months)
- Well child (50%)
- Malaise, low grade fever (50%)
- Other features unusual – conjunctivitis, maculopapular rash, neuroretinitis, thrombocytopaenia, hepatitis, splenomegaly, encephalopathy + convulsions (usually recover well)

Diagnosis

- History and primary innoculation lesion found
- Serology for *B. henselae*

Treatment

- Spontaneous recovery is common
- Antibiotics (azithromycin) effective for severe disease

LYME DISEASE

Lyme disease is due to infection with the spirochaete *Borrelia burgdorferi*.

| Transmission | From the bite of an ixodid tick from deer (or sheep, cattle, dogs or squirrels) in Europe, Asia, North America and Australia |
| Incubation | 7–30 days |

Clinical features

Within days	**Erythema chronicum migrans** (a painless annular rash slowly enlarging) develops from the site of the tick inoculation
	Malaise, conjunctivitis, headache, fever, arthralgia, myalgia, lymphadenopathy
Weeks to months	CNS – meningoencephalitis, cranial neuropathy (especially VII nerve palsy)
	Cardiac – myocarditis, heart block
	Arthritis – episodic oligoarthritis (often the knee)
	Other – hepatosplenomegaly, conjunctivitis
	Recurrent arthritis with erosion of bone and cartilage

Diagnosis

- Primarily a clinical diagnosis as confirmation is difficult
- Serology (may be positive after 3–6 weeks, false positives seen)
- Organism isolation (from serum, skin biopsy or CSF)

Treatment

This is dependent on the clinical features:

- For *early general symptoms*, oral antibiotics are given (amoxicillin or erythromycin if < 8 years old, doxycycline if > 8 years old)
- If *CNS or articular disease*, use ceftriaxone instead
- NB: when removing a tick ensure that the head is also removed. If simply pulled off, head will remain embedded and tick's stomach contents including the bacteria will be disgorged into the human host

MYCOPLASMA

Mycoplasma pneumoniae is the smallest organism that can survive outside a host cell and has no cell wall. It can produce a range of clinical features, the most common being a bronchopneumonia in school-age children and adolescents (see below).

Transmission	Droplet
Incubation	10–14 days

Clinical features

Bronchopneumonia	Gradual onset of mild URTI and then a persistent cough with fever, malaise, wheeze and headache
Other	Skin rashes are common (red maculopapular or vesicular)
	Vomiting, diarrhoea, arthralgia and myalgia (common)
	Bullous myringitis, haemolytic anaemia, Stevens–Johnson syndrome (p. 301)
	Hepatitis, pancreatitis, splenomegaly
	Aseptic meningitis, encephalitis, cerebellar ataxia, Guillain–Barré syndrome

Diagnosis

- Chest X-ray shows diffuse patchy shadowing and is often unexpectedly severe in appearance
- Mycoplasma infection can be identified by serology (specific IgM antibody) which is positive in around 50% of cases

Treatment

It is treated with erythromycin for 2 weeks.

TUBERCULOSIS

- Caused by infection with mycobacteria, usually *Mycobacterium tuberculosis* (an acid- and alcohol-fast bacillus)
- On the increase in the UK, particularly London, as a result of the widespread migration of people from Asia, Africa and central Europe
- Clinical features depend greatly on the host reaction. If there is a good immune response, the infection is locally contained and can become dormant. Small numbers of organisms may spread via the bloodstream and infect other organs. If there is a poor immune response, the infection becomes overwhelming and disseminated
- In children, tuberculosis is usually a *primary* infection (rarely becoming disseminated), whereas in adults it is usually a *reactivation* of previous pulmonary infection
- Amount of TB organisms in primary TB in children is *very* small
- Lung manifestations are mostly due to a marked **delayed hypersensitivity reaction**
- Children are usually infected from an adult with active pulmonary TB
- Children with primary TB are generally *not* infectious

Primary infection

Asymptomatic primary pulmonary tuberculosis

- A **primary asymptomatic complex** develops – a small local lung parenchymal area of TB infection and regional lymph node involvement
- On CXR the lymph nodes are usually visible but not the TB focus
- Mantoux/Heaf test may become positive (in which case anti-TB medication should be given)
- Becomes dormant and goes fibrotic. The lung focus may calcify over a couple of years and may then be visible on the CXR

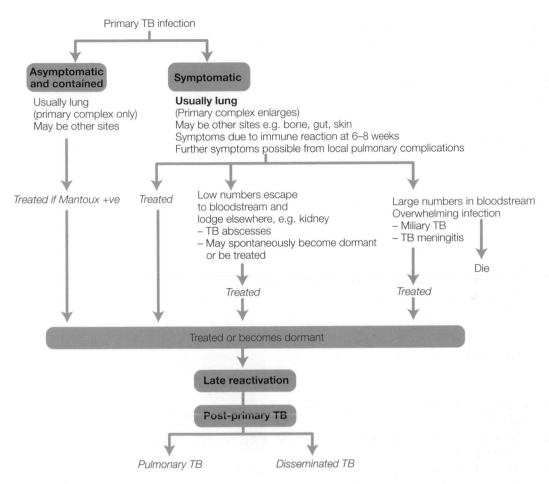

Figure 5.12 TB infection

> ❗ **NB: Asymptomatic primary pulmonary TB can reactivate later in life and develop into highly infectious 'open' pulmonary TB, and should therefore be treated.**

Symptomatic primary pulmonary tuberculosis

■ Enlargement of the **primary complex** (in around 50% of children), i.e. local lung reaction + regional lymph nodes, visible on CXR (the lymph nodes but not the lung TB focus)

■ Child becomes *symptomatic* after 4–8 weeks when the immune system responds – wheeze, cough, dyspnoea, fever, anorexia, weight loss

■ Local pulmonary complications can occur from:
  – Obstruction of a bronchus (due to lymph nodes) – cough, localized wheeze
  – Rupture into a bronchus – bronchopneumonia, bronchitis
  – Rupture into pleural cavity – pleural effusion

■ Treated with anti-TB medication

■ May become dormant (and may reactivate later), fibrotic and calcifying over a couple of years when the lung focus is visible on the CXR (see Figure 5.13a)

- Small numbers of bacilli may escape into the bloodstream and lodge in other sites where they can cause abscesses or spontaneously become dormant, e.g. the kidney
- Sometimes this primary infection is not contained by the immune system and spreads (see below)

> **!** **NB: It is the *immune response* mounted by the child that is primarily responsible for the lung manifestations. Only a few organisms may be present, but release of organisms with rupture causes a marked hypersensitivity reaction, as delayed hypersensitivity to TB has developed by this time (4–8 weeks post-infection).**

Sites of primary tuberculosis infection other than the lung

The site of the primary TB infection is usually the lung, but may be in other organs (and is sometimes in multiple sites):

Skin	Primary inoculation TB
Superficial lymph nodes	Tender lymphadenopathy in neck (from the mouth)
Gut	Mesenteric lymphadenopathy, abdominal pain, fever and weight loss

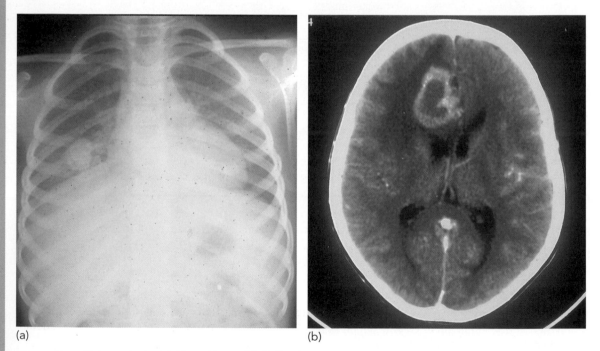

(a) (b)

Figure 5.13 Tuberculosis. (a) Chest X-ray. (b) CT brain

Massive tuberculosis spread (acute miliary tuberculosis)

- TB will rarely enter the bloodstream (from the primary infection – lung or other, or from reactivation of dormant TB)
- Can result in a few tubercles that can lodge in other organs, e.g. kidney, and spontaneously become dormant, or form a local abscess

- Or can result in disseminated TB, which has a high mortality if untreated
- Disseminated infection is more likely in children < 4 years, with malnutrition and immunosuppression

Clinical features of disseminated tuberculosis

Acute miliary TB   Acutely unwell, fever, weight loss, hepatosplenomegaly, lymphadenopathy, widespread internal organ infection including:
- TB pericarditis – a constrictive pericarditis
- Renal TB
- Bones and joints – osteomyelitis, infective arthritis
- 'Miliary' picture on CXR, i.e. scattered white dots throughout the lung fields

TB meningitis   A slow, insidious onset of meningitis:
- Night sweats, weight loss, malaise
- Symptoms of meningeal irritation occur later

Skin features of tuberculosis

Primary TB infection	Inoculation TB developing at skin site of inoculation
Lupus vulgaris	Red plaque(s), usually on head and neck
Metastatic TB abscess	Subcutaneous TB abscess from endogenous spread
Scrofuloderma	TB lymphadenitis which ulcerates. Often on neck from endogenous spread
Acute miliary TB	Scattered macules and papules may occur
Erythema nodosum (see p. 288)	Hypersensitivity reaction

Late reactivation

Dormant TB (post-asymptomatic or symptomatic) can reactivate any time, usually during intercurrent illness or immunosuppresion, causing **post-primary TB**. This can be:

- Disseminated TB (as above)
- Open 'pulmonary' TB which is very infectious. This generally occurs in adults, with an approximate life-long risk of 5–10%

Diagnosis

TB is an elusive disease. There are two main forms of investigation:

- Direct detection of bacilli (microscopy, PCR)
- Assessment of host immunity

Ideally, all TB would be diagnosed by visualization of the bacteria; however, this is rarely the case. More frequently diagnosis is made through a combination of radiological findings and evidence of host immunity to the organism.

Immunological tests

The immunological test is the Mantoux test.

- Test of delayed hypersensitivity to tuberculin using an intradermal injection of purified protein derivative (PPD) of tuberculin on the forearm
- Presence of induration is measured at 48–72 h
- A positive Mantoux is > 10 mm induration (indicating active infection)
- Interpretation is variable depending on the individual estimated risk of TB

Elispot (enzyme-linked immunosorbent spot) assay is a blood test which identifies interferon-gamma (IFN-γ) release from T cells in response to mycobacterial antigens.

Direct detection of organisms

Places to look for TB organisms:

- Early morning urine
- Sputum: early morning gastric aspirate
  - Bronchoscopy washings
  - Coughed up sputum (older child)
- Biopsies (of lymph nodes, pleura, skin, gut, tuberculoma)

} Samples for PCR and microscopy (Ziehl–Neilson stain) and culture (4–8 weeks)

Management

- Mantoux positive but no other evidence of disease:
  - Isoniazid (or rifampicin + pyrazinamide) for 3–6 months. (Two agents given if concern about multiresistance)
- Evidence of infection in addition to a positive Mantoux test:
  - For pulmonary disease: 6 months combination therapy
  - For disseminated disease: 12 months therapy

Combination therapy is used with various combinations of isoniazid, rifampicin, pyrazinamide and ethambutol.

Prevention

- Vaccination with the **BCG** (Bacille–Calmette–Guérin, a live attenuated strain) gives up to 75% protection
- This is now recommended for neonates in high-risk groups, i.e. most infants in London, and Asian and African populations, and at 10–14 years to tuberculin test-negative children

TROPICAL INFECTIONS

TYPHOID FEVER

Typhoid fever is due to the bacillus *Salmonella typhi*.

Transmission	Ingestion of food contaminated from faeces (humans are the only reservoir)
	Common in Asia, Africa and South America
Incubation	10–14 days

Clinical features

Week 1	Fever, malaise, sore throat, headache, abdominal pain
	Toxic child (tachycardic, tachypnoeic), often confused
	NB: Up to 80% of infections are subclinical
Week 2	Pink macules ('**rose spots**') on chest and abdomen
	Hepatosplenomegaly, toxic, confused
Week 3	Complications – pneumonia, myocarditis, heart failure, renal failure, glomerulonephritis, hepatitis, gastrointestinal haemorrhage and perforation
Week 4	Recovery

Diagnosis

- Blood cultures (80% positive in first week, 30% positive by week 3)
- Stool cultures (more positives after second week)

- Urine cultures (positive with bacteraemia)
- Widal test (high titre of O antigens)
- Anaemia and leucopaenia

Treatment

This depends on the age of the child and clinical severity. If unwell, IV antibiotics are given.

Carrier state

Rarely, children may become chronic carriers (sometimes secondary to defective cell-mediated immunity) and are treated with antibiotics (ciprofloxacin).

Paratyphoid fever is a similar but milder illness caused by *S. paratyphi* A, B or C.

MALARIA

Malaria is found in all countries between latitude 40 °N and 30 °S. It is increasing in incidence with resistance to treatment developing, and becoming the major infective cause of morbidity and mortality worldwide. It should be considered in any febrile child who has returned from a malaria-endemic area.

Life cycle of the malaria parasite

The malaria parasite lives in the female *Anopheles* mosquito as a **sporozoite**, and this is injected into the human bloodstream when the mosquito bites. These multiply in the liver as **schizonts** (and some remain latent here as **hypnozoites** in all forms except *Plasmodium falciparum*), and then re-enter the bloodstream as **merozoites**. These merozoites invade the red blood cells, become **schizonts** again and eventually cause rupture of the RBC with release of **merozoites** resulting in the fever.

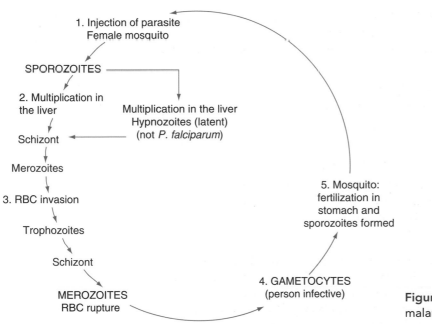

Figure 5.14 Life cycle of the malaria parasite

There are four species of malaria parasite, each causing different clinical features:

- *Plasmodium vivax*
- *P. ovale*
- *P. malariae*
- *P. falciparum*

Clinical features

Fevers	**Cold stage** 1–1½ h (rapid temperature rise but the patient feels cold), and then:
	Hot stage (2–6 h, patient feels hot and is delirious)
	Sweating stage (profuse sweating, patient sleeps)
Other features	Anaemia, splenomegaly, hepatomegaly

Malaria species-specific symptoms

P. vivax } *P. ovale* }	Mild disease, young RBC only affected, difficult to eradicate due to latent phase
P. malariae	Only old RBCs affected. Mild chronic disease with massive splenomegaly and growth retardation
	Nephrotic syndrome may occur
P. falciparum	Most severe form. All RBCs affected and become sticky to endothelium causing vascular occlusion with ischaemic organ damage, e.g. brain, kidneys, liver. Complications may occur:

- Cerebral malaria, fits
- Severe anaemia
- Acute renal failure (Blackwater fever)
- Shock, metabolic acidosis, DIC
- Hypoglycaemia

Management

- Both *thick* (for initial diagnosis) and *thin* (for sub-typing) **peripheral blood smears** are taken, where the parasite is seen with staining
- Three negative smears on three consecutive days are required to declare the child malaria free
- Disease type-specific medication is given, and because resistance is increasing, up-to-date advice for therapy should be obtained from the malaria reference laboratory
- If the infective species is not known or is mixed, the initial treatment is as for **falciparum malaria** with IV quinine and intensive care as necessary
- Primaquine is given for 2–3 weeks after the acute treatment for eradication of latent parasites in *P. vivax* and *P. ovale*

Prophylaxis   The appropriate area-specific anti-malarial drugs should be taken.

ROUNDWORM (NEMATODE)

Many different roundworms infect humans worldwide. In the UK threadworm infection is very common in children.

Threadworm (*Enterobius vermicularis*)

- Common intestinal infection with these small worms is often asymptomatic
- Host – humans
- It can result in an itchy bottom (**pruritis ani**), particularly at night when the worms come out to lay their eggs perianally
- The **sticky tape test** is used to identify the organisms (briefly attach selotape perianally and send eggs and worms that stick to it to the lab for microscopic examination)
- Easily treated with oral mebendazole, treat all family members simultaneously, and change all bed linen on the same day

Hookworm

- A quarter of the world's population is supposedly infected with hookworms
- Host – dogs
- The worms are:
  - *Ankylostoma duodenale* (around the Mediterranean – Europe, Middle East, N. Africa)
  - *Necator americanus* (South America, South and Central Africa)
- Worms penetrate the skin and migrate to attach to the jejunal intestinal lining, and cause **gastrointestinal bleeding**
- Infection is asymptomatic or results in **anaemia** (up to 150 mL/day blood loss) and intestinal ulcer-like symptoms
- Eggs can be detected in the stool
- Treatment is with mebendazole or albendezole

Tapeworm

Taenia solium (pork)
Taenia saginata (beef)
- from poorly cooked meat
- rare in UK
- mebendazole treatment

VACCINATION SCHEDULES

Birth	BCG (in at-risk individuals)
2 months	DTP, Polio, Hib, Men C
3 months	DTP, Polio, Hib, Men C
4 months	DTP, Polio, Hib, Men C
Infancy	BCG for 'at-risk' infants
12 months	MMR, Hib
3–5 years	DTaP, Polio, MMR
15 years	dT, Polio

Key: D = diphtheria, d = low concentration diphtheria, P = pertussis, aP = acellular pertussis, T = tetanus, MMR = measles, mumps and rubella, Men C = meningococcal C conjugate, Hib = *Haemophilus influenzae* type b conjugate, BCG = Bacille–Calmette–Guerin.

> **!** **NB: Premature infants have their vaccines for age since *birth* (i.e. chronological age), irrespective of their prematurity (post-conceptional age).**

Clinical scenario

An 11-month-old child is brought to the Emergency Department non-specifically unwell and is seen by one of the on call paediatric team. He displays a fever of 38.5°C, is lethargic and irritable, feeding poorly, vomiting, and on examination has a bulging fontanelle, and rapidly develops a non-blanching rash over his limbs and trunk.

1. What would you do first?

The stabilization occurs and he is treated with appropriate antibiotics and is sent home 5 days later.

He is readmitted 6 months later with an abscess under his left arm and it is diagnosed as a staphylococcal infection.

2. What antibiotic would be most effective?
3. Given two significant infections would immunological investigations be useful, and if so which one/s?

ANSWERS

1. ABC and resuscitate. If more than 40 ml/kg of IV fluid are needed then intubate and call the nearest PICU. Simultaneously administer parenteral antibiotic such as benzylpenicillin or third generation cephalosporin (cefotaxime or ceftriaxone are good examples)
2. Flucloxacillin
3. Ask for an immunology opinion first. Relevant investigations might include: FBC; immunoglobulins and IgG subclasses; T cell subsets; NBT test for chronic granulomatous disease; memory phenotypes of lymphocytes for previous immunizations such as tetanus; neutrophil function tests etc.

FURTHER READING

Department of Health. *Immunisation against infective diseases*. London: HMSO, 2006.

Shingadia D (ed.). *Manual of Childhood infection*, 3rd edn. Oxford: Oxford University Press, 2011.

Feigin R, Cherry J, Demmler-Harrison G, Kaplan S (eds.). *Feigin and Cherry's Textbook of Pediatric Infectious diseases*, 6th edn. London: Elsevier, 2009.

Nelson's Textboook of Paediatrics, Berhman, Klegman, Arvin, Elsevier, 1995.

6 Immunodeficiency disorders

- Clinical features of immunodeficiency
- Components and development of the immune system
- Investigations
- Treatment modalities
- Inherited immunodeficiencies
- Acquired immunodeficiencies
- Further reading

CLINICAL FEATURES OF IMMUNODEFICIENCY

Immunodeficiency may be *inherited* or *acquired*, and the latter may be *temporary* or *permanent*. The features of immunodeficiency can be related to the specific deficiency present, but there are also general features that help with recognition of an immune problem.

Important points in the history

Infections	*Frequent?*
	Age of onset? (? since birth)
	Unusual organisms, opportunistic infections?
	Atypical infections, i.e. unusually severe and widespread, involving unusual sites?
	Recurrent skin infections, periodontitis, abscesses, sinopulmonary infections, chronic candidiasis
Family history	Consanguineous parents?
	Parents unwell?
	Previous unexplained neonatal deaths?
	Immunodeficiency?
Medications	Immunosuppressive therapy?
Underlying	Leukaemia?
Illness	Organ transplant patient?
Other	Diarrhoea, failure to thrive
	Prolonged wound healing, rashes

Features of the examination

Appearance	Dysmorphism? (some syndromes are associated with immunodeficiency)
General	Failure to thrive?
Skin	Rash? Eczema? Infections? Telangiectasiae? Granulomas?
Lymphoid tissue	Lymphadenopathy? Tonsils present?
Eyes	Conjunctival telangiectasiae? Retinal abnormalities?
CNS	Ataxia? (ataxia telangiectasia)

COMPONENTS AND DEVELOPMENT OF THE IMMUNE SYSTEM

The immune system is extremely complex and contains many components. A basic knowledge of these components and the development of the immune system helps in understanding these immunodeficiency disorders and the effects that they have.

IgG	Crosses placenta. Secondary response to infection. Adult levels 6/7 yrs
IgM	Primary response to infection (appears immediately). Adult levels 4/5 yrs
IgA	In breast milk. Secretory (sIgA) is important in protection of mucosal surfaces. Adult levels > puberty
IgE	Involved in type I hypersensitivity reaction. Adult levels > puberty
IgD	Precise function unknown

The immune response involves an initial *generalized* reaction (**innate immunity**), then a *specific* reaction to the foreign material. The response is complex and the mechanisms of activation and interaction are integral.

Innate immunity

Phagocytes	Mononuclear phagocytes – monocytes (blood), macrophages (tissues), dendritic cells, Kuppfer cells (liver)
	Polymorphonuclear granulocytes – neutrophils, eosinophils
Complement	
c-type lectins	e.g. mannose-binding lectin
Soluble mediators	Cytokines
	Antibodies (for non-specific response)
	Acute phase proteins
Other cells	Basophils and mast cells
	Antigen presenting cells, platelets, endothelial cells

Specific immunity

Leukocytes have molecules on their surfaces known as **clusters of differentiation (CD)**, identified using monoclonal antibodies, which are used to differentiate subpopulations.

T lymphocytes (CD3)	T-helper cells (CD4):
	■ Th1 subset
	■ Th2 subset
	T-cytotoxic cells (CD8)
B lymphocytes	When active become plasma cells and make antibodies – IgG, IgM, IgA, IgE, IgD
Natural killer cells	CD56 and CD16
	Eliminate tumour and virus-infected cells using cytotoxic means.

INVESTIGATIONS

Investigations to identify the immunodeficiency include initial screening tests of the immune system and then relevant more specialized tests (see below). Finally, gene analysis can be performed for some disorders for which the genetic defect has been identified, e.g. X-linked agammaglobulinaemia.

General initial immunological investigations

Blood tests	FBC with film (count and appearance of neutrophils, lymphocytes, monocytes, eosinophils, basophils and platelets)
	Immunoglobulins (IgA, IgM, IgG, IgD, IgE)
	Complement tests (C3, C4, CH100)
	HIV testing (if appropriate and following counselling)
Ultrasound scan	Thymus (or by CXR), liver and spleen (as indicated)

Specific investigations

Cell-mediated immunity	Quantitative:
	■ T cell subsets (CD3, CD4, CD8, CD4:CD8 ratio)
	■ NK cells (CD16 and CD56)
	■ Monocytes (CD14)
	Functional:
	■ *General* – mitogen stimulation of T cell function, e.g. PHA (phytohaemagglutinin) anti-CD3
	■ *Specific* – antigen specific assays, e.g. PPD, candida killing test
Humoral immunity	Quantitative:
	■ B cell numbers (CD19, CD20)
	■ Immunoglobulins (IgA, IgG, IgM, IgE, IgG subclasses 1–4)
	Functional:
	■ Antibody response to vaccines, e.g. diphtheria, Hib, polio
Phagocytes	Neutrophil function tests (nitroblue tetrazolium test)
	Adhesion molecule expression – CD18 (LAD1), CD15s (LAD2)

Infections associated with specific immunodeficiencies

Deficiency	Organisms
Humoral (B cells/antibodies)	Bacteria – staphylococci, streptococci, *Haemophilus influenzae*, mycoplasma, campylobacter Enteroviral infections, giardia
Cellular (T cells)	Viruses – herpes viruses, measles Intracellular bacteria – TB Protozoa – *Pneumocystis jejunii* (formerly *carinii*), toxoplasmosis Fungi – candida, aspergillus
Combined (B and T cells)	Both of above groups
Neutrophils	Bacteria – Gram-positive and -negative (especially staphylococcal infections and abscesses) Fungi – candida and aspergillus infections

TREATMENT MODALITIES

Infection treatment	Treat individual infections
	Prophylactic long term antibiotics and antivirals
	In addition, monoclonal antibodies against organism and target cell, e.g.
	B cells in EBV infections
Immune component replacement	Immunoglobulin infusions
Cure	Stem cell transplant
	Gene therapy, e.g. γ chain–deficient severe combined immunodeficiency and X-linked chronic granulomatous disease (limited use currently)

INHERITED IMMUNODEFICIENCIES

Transient hypogammaglobulinaemia of infancy

- Common transient deficiency of IgG and also sometimes IgA during the first few months of life
- Consequence of the gradual loss of maternally derived IgG (transplacentally acquired), but the infant's own production of IgG is not being fully developed (see Fig. 6.1). IgA is derived from breast milk in addition to the infant's own production, so a bottle-fed baby will have low levels of IgA until his/her own production is established
- More common in preterm babies as they have received less placental IgG
- Manifests as recurrent respiratory tract infections and will *spontaneously* improve with age
- Some cow's milk protein allergic infants are known to have low IgA and IgG subclass abnormalities

Selective IgA deficiency

- Common condition affecting 1 in 500 Caucasians
- Low or absent IgA (and sometimes also IgG2 and IgG4)
- Can result in recurrent respiratory infections (URTIs, sinusitis, wheeze) and sometimes chronic diarrhoea

X-linked agammaglobulinaemia (Bruton XLA)

This X-linked recessive disorder of boys is caused by very low or absent B cells due to a mutation in the Bruton tyrosine kinase (*btk*) gene at Xq22.3–22. It presents after 6 months of age when the maternally derived immunoglobulins are gone.

Clinical features

- Recurrent bacterial infections
- Unusual enteroviral infections, e.g. chronic meningoencephalitis
- Absent or small tonsils, adenoids and lymph nodes

Treatment

Regular 3–4 weekly infusions of intravenous or subcutaneous immunoglobulin replacement.

DiGeorge anomaly

This autosomal dominant condition is predominantly a T-cell disorder and is a result of a microdeletion of chromosome 22q. There are decreased malfunctioning *T cells* and specific *antibody* deficiencies causing:

- Respiratory infections
- Chronic diarrhoea

There is also malformation of the **4th branchial arch**, resulting in:

- Thymus aplasia or hypoplasia
- Facial dysmorphism (micrognathia, bifid uvula, low-set notched ears, short philtrum)
- Hypoparathyroidism (causing hypocalcaemia, neonatal seizures and cataracts)
- Cardiac defects (right-sided aortic arch defects, truncus arteriosus)

Treatment

The condition can be managed with a thymus transplant and, if necessary, a bone marrow transplant.

Severe combined immunodeficiency (SCID)

This term encompasses various disorders with absent or impaired function of both T and B cells, and which share the following basic characteristics. The features are similar to those of AIDS, from which it must be differentiated.

Clinical features

- Severe failure to thrive
- Absent lymphoid tissue
- Diarrhoea
- Infections (pneumonia, otitis media, sepsis, cutaneous infections, opportunistic infections)

These children will die in infancy unless they are given a successful bone marrow transplant or gene therapy.

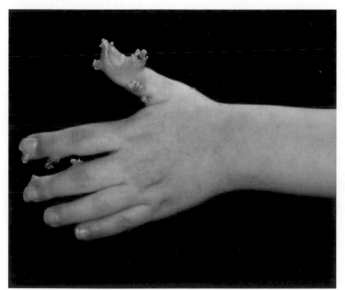
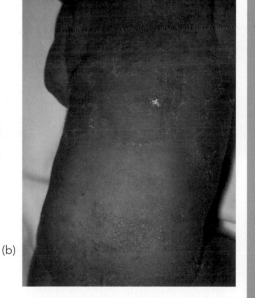

(a)　　　　　　　　　　　　　　　　　　　　　　(b)

Figure 6.1 Severe combined immunodeficiency.
(a) Multiple viral warts in a child.
(b) Widespread cutaneous candidiasis in an infant

Wiskott–Aldrich syndrome

An X-linked recessive disorder of boys with progressive T-cell depletion, and impaired antibody production, due to mutation of the *WASP* gene on Xp11. These children are distinguished by severe eczema and purpura due to thrombocytopaenia.

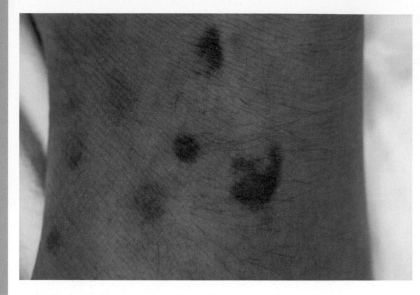

Figure 6.2 Petechiae and eczema in a child with Wiskott–Aldrich syndrome

Clinical features

- Severe eczema
- Thrombocytopaenic purpura
- Infections (pneumonia, otitis media, meningitis, HSV, VZV)
- Increased incidence of lymphoma
- Autoimmune disorders, e.g. juvenile chronic arthritis, haemolytic anaemia

Treatment

Treatment is with a bone marrow transplant.

Ataxia telangiectasia

In this autosomal recessive condition there is both impaired cell-mediated immunity and antibody production. There is abnormal DNA repair, leading to an extreme sensitivity to ionizing radiation and increased incidence of lymphoma and adenocarcinoma. Mutations in the *ATM* gene on chromosome 11q23.1 have been found.

Clinical features

- Progressive cerebellar ataxia
- Oculocutaneous telangiectasiae
- Chronic sinopulmonary infections
- Lymphomas and adenocarcinomas

Treatment

Treatment is supportive only.

Chronic granulomatous disease

This is a disorder of defective neutrophils which cannot kill organisms due to a failure of superoxide production. This is due to a defect in cytochrome b558 (the enzymatic unit of NADPH oxidase). These children suffer from:

- Recurrent abscesses (bone, gut, liver, gastrointestinal tract)
- Granulomas (bone, lung, liver, skin, gastrointestinal tract)

Diagnosis is confirmed with the nitroblue tetrazolium (NBT) test of neutrophil function (there is a failure of their lymphocytes to reduce NBT). *Management* is to treat the infections and give long term γ-interferon and prophylactic antibiotics.

Summary of inherited immunodeficiencies and their management

Disorder	Immune defect	Genetics	Clinical features	Treatment
Transient hypogamma-globulinaemia of infancy	Low IgG ± low IgA	None	Recurrent respiratory infections	None specific
Selective IgA deficiency	Low or absent IgA	Variable	Recurrent respiratory infections ± chronic diarrhoea	None specific
XLA	Low or absent B cells (+ low or absent immunoglobulins)	*btk* gene Ch Xq22.3–22 XLR (boys)	Absent or small tonsils, adenoids and lymph nodes Recurrent bacterial infections	3–4 weekly immunoglobulin infusions
Common variable immuno-deficiency (CVID)	Abnormal B-cell function and abnormal T-cell function	Unknown	Recurrent sinopulmonary infections Lymphoma and GI malignancies	Regular immunoglobulin infusions
DiGeorge anomaly	Low malfunctioning T cells and antibody deficiencies	Ch 22q microdeletion AD	Thymus small or absent Hypoparathyroidism Cardiac defects Dysmorphism Chronic diarrhoea Respiratory infections	Thymus transplant Bone marrow transplant
SCID	Absent or impaired T cells Impaired or absent B cells	Various	Severe failure to thrive Absent lymphoid tissue Diarrhoea Infections	Bone marrow transplant
Wiskott–Aldrich syndrome	Progressive T-cell depletion Impaired antibody production	*WASP* gene mutation Ch Xp11 XLR (boys)	Thrombocytopaenic purpura Severe eczema Infections (see text) Lymphoma Autoimmune disorders	Bone marrow transplant
Ataxia telangiectasia	Reduced malfunctioning T cells Impaired antibody production Impaired DNA repair	*ATM* gene mutations Ch 11q23.1 AR	Progressive cerebellar ataxia Telangiectasiae Sensitivity to ionizing radiation Malignancies Sinopulmonary infections	Supportive only
Chronic granulomatous disease (CGD)	Neutrophil killing failure (NADPH oxidase defective)	Absent *gp91 phox* or absent *p22 phox* XLR or AR	Abscesses Granulomas	γ-interferon Antibiotic prophylaxis

AR = autosomal recessive; XLR = X-linked recessive

ACQUIRED IMMUNODEFICIENCIES

Many of the causes of acquired immunodeficiency are temporary, with HIV infection being the notable exception.

Causes

Immunoglobulin deficiency	Lymphoproliferative diseases, e.g. leukaemia
	Bone marrow aplasia
	Hypersplenism
	Protein loss, e.g. malnutrition states, burns, nephrotic syndrome
Cell-mediated deficiency	Drugs – cytotoxic, e.g. cyclosporin, azathioprine (transplant and cancer patients), high-dose steroids
	Lymphoproliferative disease, e.g. lymphoma
	Bone marrow aplasia
	Hypersplenism
	HIV infection

HIV AND AIDS

Human immunodeficiency virus (HIV) is a retrovirus. Retroviruses contain the enzyme reverse transcriptase which enables viral RNA to be incorporated into host cell DNA. The HIV cellular receptor is the CD4 molecule found on T helper cells (Th1 subset), which are the cells most affected by the disease. The CD4 cell numbers gradually decline and a profound immunodeficiency develops with resultant multiple and often opportunistic infections. The virus also has a direct effect on organs, e.g. gut, brain.

Transmission

This is via bodily fluids:

- Vertical transmission (mother to child, the majority of childhood HIV)
- Mucous membranes during sexual intercourse (NB: sexual abuse)
- Direct blood inoculation, e.g. IV drug abusers

Vertical transmission can occur:

- Prenatally (placental)
- Intrapartum
- Postnatally (via breast feeding)

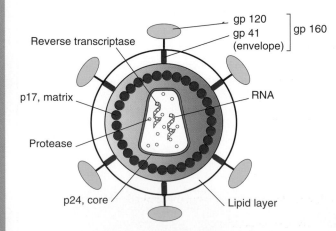

Figure 6.3 HIV virus

Reduction of vertical transmission

Pregnant women with HIV have a transmission risk (untreated) of approximately 15–30%. Measures to reduce transmission to < 5% are:

- Antiretroviral therapy during pregnancy and delivery
- Antiretroviral therapy during delivery only if unable to administer during pregnancy
- Oral AZT to the infant for the first 4–6 weeks
- Elective Caesarean section
- Avoid invasive fetal procedures, e.g. fetal scalp electrodes
- Avoid breast feeding (the WHO advises breast feeding continues in developing countries to avoid malnutrition)

Clinical manifestations

- Infants are generally asymptomatic during the neonatal period
- Disease develops more rapidly in children than adults
- Initially, lymphadenopathy and prominent parotitis develop, then moderate infections, e.g. recurrent otitis media and bacterial pneumonia, and finally severe conditions, e.g. PCP, encephalopathy
- In addition to multiple and opportunistic infections, particular clinical presentations include failure to thrive, lymphocytic interstitial pneumonitis (LIP) and HIV encephalopathy

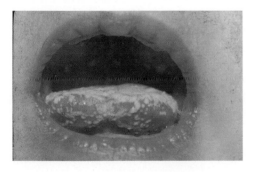

Figure 6.4 Widespread oral candidiasis in a child with AIDS

Two patterns of infection are seen:

Early-onset (25%)   AIDS-defining symptoms (within a few months)
Late-onset (75%)   AIDS-defining symptoms (around 8 years)

Failure to thrive
This is due to:

- Reduced intake (poor appetite, HIV encephalopathy)
- Malabsorption (HIV enteropathy, GI infections)
- Increased metabolic requirements (recurrent infections)

Lymphocytic interstitial pneumonitis (LIP)
A chronic lung disease of uncertain aetiology seen in around half of infected children.

Clinical features are variable:

- Respiratory distress, dyspnoea, hypoxia
- May be asymptomatic
- CXR – diffuse interstitial reticulonodular infiltrate, hilar and mediastinal lymphadenopathy

Treatment is symptomatic only; steroids may reduce oxygen dependency.

Clinical categories of HIV infection in children

The CDC classification for HIV disease in children < 13 years was devised in 1994 and involves four clinical categories and three immunological categories based on the CD4 lymphocyte count.

Category	Clinical features
N Asymptomatic	
A Mildly symptomatic	> 2 of: lymphadenopathy, parotitis, hepatomegaly, splenomegaly, dermatitis, recurrent URTIs
B Moderately symptomatic	Moderate infections, e.g. oropharyngeal candidiasis, and LIP
C Severely symptomatic	Any condition listed in the 1987 surveillance case definition of AIDS (except LIP), e.g. PCP, severe failure to thrive, HIV encephalopathy

HIV encephalopathy
- Developmental delay of motor skills and language
- Acquired microcephaly
- MRI – cortical atrophy, basal ganglia calcification, ventricular enlargement

Pneumocystis jejunii (formerly *carinii*) pneumonia (PCP)
Pneumocystis jejunii is an extracellular protozoan which causes an opportunistic infection in the immunocompromised. In severely affected infants, it can present as early as 3 months of age.

Clinical features are:

- Persistent non–productive cough
- Dyspnoea
- High fever
- Hypoxia (often more severe than the CXR would suggest)

Treatment is with high-dose oral or IV co-trimoxazole (Septrin), or IV pentamidine, then prophylaxis with low-dose oral Septrin or monthly pentamidine nebulizers.

Diagnosis
Serologically to confirm HIV infection in infants:

- Virus can be detected by PCR (rapid, sensitive) or viral culture (slower)
- Detection of IgG antibody to viral envelope components

> **NB: Repeat testing for HIV should be done to ensure an infected infant is not missed and to confirm a positive test.**

> **NB: Viral antibodies are IgG and therefore they cross the placenta; therefore, *all* infants of HIV-positive mothers will possess antibodies whether they are infected or not. The antibody disappears by 18 months of age if the infant is not infected.**

Therapy

A multidisciplinary approach is necessary to manage both the physical and considerable emotional needs of these children and their families. A great deal of support is necessary to help deal with issues such as education and schooling, confidentiality, terminal illness in a child (many of these children now live well into their teens), complex drug regimens and side effects, parental illness and death.

Currently, Septrin prophylaxis is given until the child is shown to be HIV negative. If HIV positive, Septrin is continued until 12 months of age, and then treatment is given according to the CD4 count and viral load. Combinations of drugs are used; the specific treatment recommendations frequently changing due to rapid therapeutic developments. The CD4 count and viral load are used as monitors of therapy. The drugs have many side effects.

Types of antiretrovirals available

- Nucleoside analogues (reverse transcriptase inhibitors), e.g. AZT (3-azido-3-deoxythymidine)
- Non-nucleoside analogues (reverse transcriptase inhibitors), e.g. nevirapine
- Protease inhibitors (prevent viral maturation), e.g. Indinavir
- Entry (fusion) inhibitors

Clinical scenario

An infant presents with severe failure to thrive, chronic profuse diarrhoea and repeated bacterial infections.

1. Which components of the immune system are likely to be affected and what is the likely diagnosis?
2. What blood tests would you arrange?
3. If these blood tests were positive for the suspected condition what definitive treatment would you refer the child for?

ANSWERS

1. B cells, T cells. Subacute combined immunodeficiency (SCID)
2. Immunoglobulins; T cell stimulation; FBC with B and T cell subsets
3. Bone marrow transplant

FURTHER READING

Roitt I, Brostoff J, Male D. *Immunology*, 6th edn. London: Elsevier, 2001.

Ohls R, Yoder M. *Hematology, Immunology and Infectious disease: Neonatology Questions and Controversies*. London: Saunders, 2008.

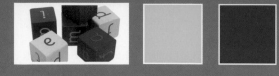

7 Ear, Nose and Throat

- The ear
- The nose
- The throat
- Further reading

THE EAR

HEARING TESTS

Mild hearing loss	25–35 dB
Moderate hearing loss	40–60 dB
Severe hearing loss	60–90 dB
Profound hearing loss	> 90 dB

Otoacoustic emission

- Simple and quick to perform, can be done at any age although *requires some cooperation*
- Routinely done on all infants either at birth or at their 6-week check in some health authorities. It is intended that this will soon be universal, as it currently is in the USA
- An ear-piece is inserted into the external auditory meatus which emits sounds and, if the hearing apparatus is normal, the inner ear makes a sound in response which can be detected. In neonates these responses are particularly large

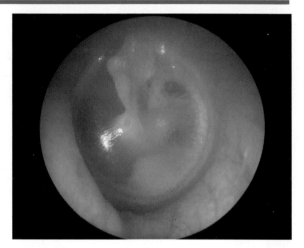

Figure 7.1 Normal ear drum

- *Disadvantages* – not very specific. If you get a normal result then you can be almost certain that hearing is normal. However, an abnormal result can be due to a number of different factors, some of which are artefactual. Any mild conductive hearing loss, such as fluid in the external auditory canal (EAC), wax or glue ear will give a failed response. Should this be the case, then the test is repeated and, if it is again negative, then further testing in the form of a brain-stem evoked response (BSER) is performed

Brain stem evoked responses

- Usually performed in a child who is asleep or sedated. Electrodes are placed on the scalp and clicks are made into the ear
- Multiple responses are averaged to give the brain-stem response, and the minimum threshold at which a response is obtained is a good guide to the true hearing thresholds of the child

Audiograms

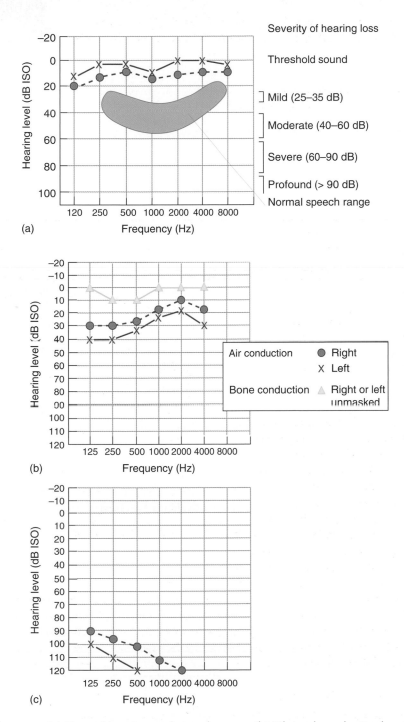

Figure 7.2 Audiograms. (a) Normal hearing and speech range. (b) Bilateral conductive hearing deafness. (c) Bilateral profound sensorineural hearing loss

Age-related hearing tests

Age	Objective hearing test	Use
Birth	*Otoacoustic emission* (OAE)	Neonatal screening
	Brain-stem evoked response (BSER) (gold standard)	When OAEs are failed
9–24 months	*Distraction test*/behavioural audiometry (baby turns towards sounds made)	Establish thresholds, more frequency specific
15 months–2½ years	*Cooperative testing* (whisper instructions with hand covering mouth)	Hearing assessment
2–3 years	*Performance testing* (conditioning, e.g. balls into bucket when sounds heard, and play audiometry)	Hearing assessment
2–4 years	*Speech discrimination tests* (similar words used, e.g. man, lamb)	Hearing assessment
> 3 years	*Impedance audiometry*	For conductive loss
	Pure tone audiometry	Formal hearing assessment

DEAFNESS

- Deafness can go unnoticed for some time in infants, particularly if mild. The parents are usually, but not always, the first to notice. Some children develop good lip reading skills and may elude detection for some time
- If deafness is not detected early the child will have problems with communication and socialization, and speech and language delay
- It is important to consider deafness developing later in an older child who may have new behavioural problems or poor school performance, such as may occur with glue ear
- Deafness may be conductive or sensorineural (see below)

Causes for concern in newborns regarding hearing

- Family history of deafness
- Craniofacial malformations
- Birthweight < 1500 g
- Neonatal meningitis
- Severe perinatal asphyxia
- Potentially toxic levels of ototoxic drugs, e.g. gentamicin
- Neonatal jaundice requiring exchange transfusion
- Congenital infection, e.g. rubella, CMV, toxoplasmosis
- Parental concern at 6-week check

Conductive and sensorineural deafness

	Conductive deafness	Sensorineural deafness
Site of lesion	Middle ear defects, e.g. Eustachian tube blockage	Cochlear or central neural damage

	Conductive deafness	Sensorineural deafness
Incidence	Common in children	Uncommon
Cause	Usually secretory otitis media (glue ear) Congenital middle ear defect (craniofacial malformations), e.g. Pierre–Robin sequence, cleft palate Foreign body, e.g. bean in ear, wax	Usually congenital or neonatal Genetic, e.g. familial deafness syndromes, Craniofacial malformations Ototoxic drugs, e.g. gentamicin Congenital infection, e.g. rubella, CMV, toxoplasmosis Meningitis (neonatal or later) Profound neonatal jaundice Perinatal asphyxia (intracranial haemorrhage)
Presentation	Poor school performance and behavioural problems	Developmental delay OAEs can detect very early
Severity	Usually mild or moderate	May be profound
Management	Watchful waiting, medical or surgical therapy	Hearing aids, cochlear implants (in the absence of hearing, i.e. a profound loss)

ACUTE OTITIS MEDIA

Acute otitis media is an infection of the middle ear and is common in children.

Causes

Viral	Respiratory syncytial virus (RSV), rhinovirus
Bacterial	*Streptococcus pneumoniae, Haemophilus influenzae, Moxarella catarrhalis,* Group A β–haemolytic streptococcus, *Streptococcus pyogenes*

❗ NB: The majority of cases of acute otitis media begin as a viral infection with bacterial secondary infection.

Clinical features

Symptoms	Severe earache (not present in about 20%) URTI symptoms Hearing loss Pre-verbal children will often pull at or scratch the involved ear
Signs	Injected tympanic membrane (TM), bulging TM, loss of light reflex Fever Perforated TM and discharge (late signs) Middle ear effusion post-infection in most children for at least 2–3 weeks

❗ NB: Ear pulling is not a reliable sign of otitis media, especially if no other features are present, e.g. fever, URTI, but can occasionally be instructive in the pre-verbal child.

Management

1. Analgesia and antipyretics for 24 h; if no improvement, commence oral antibiotics
2. Ear toilet in the presence of discharge
3. Oral antibiotics
4. Myringotomy and drainage very rarely required

GLUE EAR (OTITIS MEDIA WITH EFFUSION)

Glue ear follows acute otitis media when fluid persists in the middle ear for > 8 weeks without signs of inflammation. The initial infection may have gone unnoticed. Although glue ear is very common, most effusions resolve spontaneously.

Clinical features

- Conductive hearing loss
- Earache
- Speech and learning difficulties if long term
- Behavioural difficulties
- Signs:
  - Retracted TM, loss of light reflex, bubbles and fluid levels may be seen through the TM
  - There may be a normal looking drum
  - Tympanometry shows a flat response as TM is non-mobile
  - Pure tone audiometry, if the child is old enough, shows a conductive hearing loss

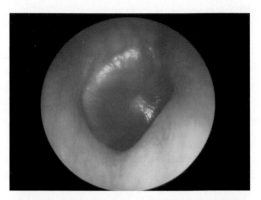

Figure 7.3 Tympanic membrane in glue ear

Management

1. Initial observation for spontaneous resolution, i.e. '*watchful waiting*' for 3 months
2. Trial of antibiotics may benefit some children, e.g. 6 weeks of low-dose augmentin or erythromycin, although the response rate is low
3. Grommet insertion
4. Adenoidectomy may be combined with grommets (leads to higher resolution rates, but higher morbidity)

CHRONIC OTITIS MEDIA

The term **chronic otitis media** applies to chronic disease of the middle ear, and is subdivided into different conditions depending on where the perforation lies and whether it is active:

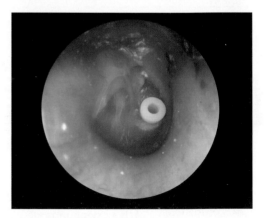

Figure 7.4 Grommet *in situ*

- Perforation of the *central TM* (pars tensa, mucosal) is a '*safe perforation*', and may be active (i.e. discharging) or inactive. There is a conductive deafness and if long-standing, a coexistent sensory loss. This can heal spontaneously leaving tympanosclerosis
- Perforation of the *margin of the TM* (squamous epithelial) or pars tensa that has retained squamous epithelium is an '*unsafe perforation*' which may become an active **cholesteatoma**

Cholesteatoma

This is a potentially serious condition in which squamous epithelial debris, granulation tissue and pus develop in the middle ear and progress to damage neighbouring structures. Treatment is nearly always surgical in children. The *complications* are:

| Extracranial | VIIth nerve palsy, perimastoid abscess, suppurative labyrinthitis |
| Intracranial | Extradural, subdural and intracerebral abscess, meningitis, sigmoid sinus thrombosis and hydrocephalus |

ACUTE MASTOIDITIS

This is an uncommon but serious condition.

Clinical features

- Symptoms of acute otitis media
- Swelling and tenderness in the postauricular region with the pinna being pushed forward

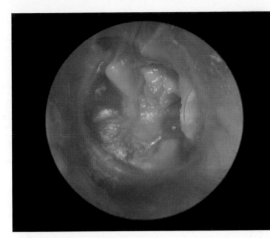

Figure 7.5 Cholesteatoma

Investigations

- CT scan is not mandatory but will show opacification of the mastoid air cell system and breakdown of the bony septa (the diagnostic finding)
- Blood tests – FBC (neutrophilia), blood cultures

Treatment

- Admit for IV antibiotics and analgesia
- Surgical exploration and mastoidectomy are performed in cases that fail to resolve on medical therapy or are advanced on presentation

Complications

- Sinus venosus thrombosis
- Intracerebral abscess (very rare)

THE NOSE

Causes of chronic nasal symptoms

- Allergic rhinitis
- Non-allergic rhinitis
- Foreign body
- Sinusitis
- Anatomical obstruction (deviated nasal septum, nasal polyps?)
- Trauma – cerebrospinal rhinorrhoea (cribriform plate sphenoid or frontal sinus fracture or suborbital ethmoid fracture). Check nasal discharge for glucose level if fracture suspected (CSF glucose > 60% plasma glucose)
- Rhinitis medicamentosa (over usage of decongestants causing blocked nose due to mucosal vasodilatation)
- Illicit drug use (sniffing glue or cocaine)

RHINITIS

Rhinitis can be divided into *allergic* rhinitis (where allergens trigger the symptoms) and *non-allergic* rhinitis.

Clinical features (similar in both types)

- Persistently runny nose, clear discharge occasionally becoming purulent
- Sneezing and itchy nose
- Nasal obstruction
- Mouth breather, hyponasal speech in extreme cases
- Family history of atopy (in allergic rhinitis)

! NB: Hay fever is allergic rhinitis triggered by pollen.

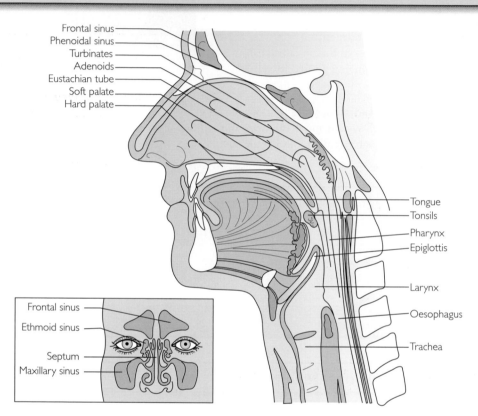

Figure 7.6 Anatomy of the nose and throat

Clinical signs and investigations

- Appearance of the nasal mucosa is unreliable. A good history of symptoms following allergen exposure is the most reliable factor
- Skin tests or serum IgE/RAST tests (see below) to identify specific allergens positive (allergic rhinitis)
- Post-nasal space X-ray is helpful in diagnosing/ruling out adenoidal hypertrophy

! NB: Check for nasal foreign body if unilateral discharge.

Management

- Avoidance of allergens (allergic rhinitis)
- Topical steroid nasal spray or drops (best for nasal blockage)

- Decongestants for short term use only (< 1 week) for acute exacerbations, e.g. ephedrine
- Antihistamines (nasal or oral) (best for itching and sneezing)

The RAST test

RAST (radioallergosorbent assay) is a blood test in which the amount of IgE to specific allergens is measured, e.g. RAST to tree pollens = amount of IgE mediated towards tree pollens present. The result is given as a level (1–6) that indicates how much IgE is present. If an individual is allergic to a substance, he/she will normally have a high RAST level to it (i.e. 3–6).

Neonatal rhinitis

This is a common cause of neonatal nasal blockage, which leads to difficulty feeding etc. The management involves the use of saline nasal drops as well as judicious use of a decongestant such as ephedrine.

COMMON COLD (NASOPHARYNGITIS)

The common cold is a very common viral infection. Children have 5–8 colds/year.

Causes

Rhinoviruses, coronaviruses, RSV.

Clinical features
- Snuffles, nasal discharge, sneezing
- Nasal obstruction with mouth breathing
- Headache
- Fever, malaise, anorexia
- Congested ear drums
- Sore throat

Management
- Rest, oral fluids and simple analgesics as required
- Infants benefit from saline nasal drops to help clear the nose

EPISTAXIS

Epistaxis is a common problem in childhood, usually involving bleeding from Little's area of the nasal mucosa.

Management

Immediate	Apply pressure to soft part of nose
	Vasoconstrictors, e.g. otrivine spray, to the area if pressure alone fails
	Admit and insert a nasal pack if above fails
Recurrent nose bleeds	Check for:

- Underlying defect of coagulation ⎫
- Hypertension ⎬ All exceedingly rare
- Nasal neoplasm ⎭

Cauterization to Little's area if necessary

SINUSITIS, FACIAL PAIN AND HEADACHES

Infection of the sinuses in children usually involves the maxillary and ethmoid sinuses as the frontal sinuses are not fully developed.

Clinical features

- Purulent nasal discharge, fever, general malaise
- Local tenderness, facial pain and headaches
- Post-nasal drip and chronic cough (in chronic sinusitis)

Sinusitis in children may present with the serious complications of **orbital cellulitis**, **subperiosteal** or **orbital abscess** (see p. 417 [orbital cellulitis]). If orbital cellulitis is present, both an ophthalmologist and an ENT surgeon must be involved.

Investigations

CT scan sinuses	Investigation of choice if complications are suspected. This will show both sinus involvement and intraorbital complications and allow the need for surgical intervention to be assessed
Sinus X-rays	Less frequently requested. They may be useful to exclude obvious intrasinus infection, and may show opaque maxillary sinuses + air–fluid level
Blood tests	FBC, blood cultures

Management

- Broad-spectrum antibiotics (IV if acutely unwell)
- Nasal decongestion (ephedrine or otrivine)
- Intranasal steroids (betnesol drops)
- Steam inhalations

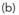 **NB: Sinusitis is a rare cause of facial pain and symptoms in children.**

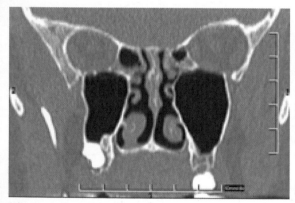

(a)

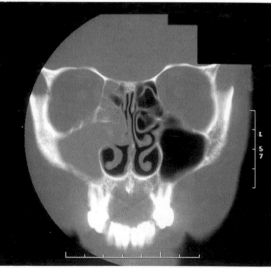

(b)

Figure 7.7 Sinusitis. (a) Coronal CT through the maxillary sinuses (normal). (b) CT sinuses showing an opaque antrum and patchy ethmoid opacification in sinusitis

THE THROAT

CLEFT LIP AND PALATE

These are inherited in a polygenic fashion. Incidence 1 in 1000. The subsequent pregnancy risk is 5%. They may be unilateral, bilateral or combined.

Associations

- Older mothers
- Syndromes, e.g. Patau syndrome
- Drugs, e.g. maternal anticonvulsant therapy

Problems

- Inability to feed
- Choking episodes
- Otitis media (acute/chronic)
- Speech problems

A multidisciplinary approach is needed with input from ENT surgeons, plastic surgeons, geneticists, paediatricians, speech therapists, audiologists and orthodontists. Most children are now managed in one of a small number of specialist centres.

Treatment

- Special feeding teats
- Speech therapy
- Surgical repair (lips are generally repaired at 3 months of age, palates – variable)

Pièrre–Robin sequence

These children have feeding and speech difficulties, and upper airway obstruction. They are managed with a special feeding teat, a nasopharyngeal airway initially, and surgical repair of the palate. Rarely, they may require a tracheostomy.

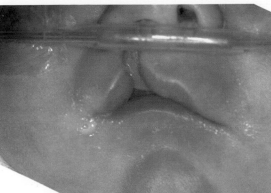

Figure 7.8 Cleft lip in an infant. Note the nasogastric tube necessary for feeding as the infant also had a cleft palate

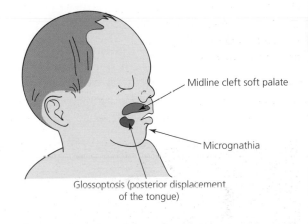

Midline cleft soft palate

Micrognathia

Glossoptosis (posterior displacement of the tongue)

Figure 7.9 Pièrre–Robin sequence

Causes of upper respiratory tract infection (URTI)

URTI is a widely used general term covering infections of the ears, nose or throat:

- Acute otitis media
- Common cold (coryza)
- Croup, epiglottitis
- Pharyngitis
- Tonsillitis + adenoiditis
- Sinusitis

STRIDOR

Stridor is a harsh sound caused by upper airway obstruction. *Inspiratory* stridor is caused by an upper airway (supralaryngeal) obstruction, *expiratory* stridor is caused by a sublaryngeal obstruction. Stridor arising from the subglottis and trachea is often *biphasic*.

Causes of cervical lymphadenopathy

Acute

Reactive:
- URTI
- Tonsillitis
- Dental abscess
- Cellulitis

Viral infection – EBV, CMV

Lymphadenitis (tender enlarged lymph nodes)

Bacterial infection, e.g. *Staphylococcus aureus*, TB (atypical)

Kawasaki disease

Acute leukaemia

Chronic

Viral infection: EBV, CMV, HIV

TB (usually atypical)

Lymphoma

NB: Children have very small airways, and the trachea is a few millimetres in diameter only; therefore, any swelling of the tracheal wall, pressure on it resulting in distortion, or object in the trachea will easily cause an obstruction and result in stridor.

Area of a circle = πr^2: 3 mm diameter = 29 mm^2 area
2 mm diameter = 13 mm^2 area
1 mm diameter = 3.14 mm^2 area

Associated findings

- Hoarse cry/voice
- Barking rough cough
- Tracheal tug
- Sternal recession
- Dyspnoea
- Tachycardia and tachypnoea
- Cyanosis (if severe)
- Agitation then drowsiness

Causes of stridor

Intraluminal	Intramural	Extramural
Foreign body (acute)	Infection (e.g. croup, epiglottis, diphtheria) (acute)	Goitre (chronic)
Haemangioma (acute or chronic)	Laryngomalacia (chronic)	Haemangioma (acute or chronic)
Tumour (acute or chronic)	Subglottic stenosis (chronic)	Cystic hygroma (chronic)
Papilloma (chronic)	Haemangioma (chronic)	Mediastinal tumour (acute or chronic)
Diphtheria (acute)	Vocal cord paralysis or prolapse (chronic)	Retropharyngeal abscess (acute)

LARYNGOMALACIA

- A common condition also known as a 'floppy larynx'; soft cartilage collapses on inspiration or an elongated epiglottis flops into the larynx, resulting in stridor
- Stridor becomes worse (or may only be present) on crying, agitation or lying supine
- Diagnosis is clinical or by direct laryngoscopy
- It comes on in first few days of life and resolves spontaneously, usually within a year but occasionally up to 2 years of age
- Gastro-oesophageal laryngo-respiratory reflux (GOLR) may prolong or exacerbate it

CROUP (ACUTE LARYNGOTRACHEOBRONCHITIS)

- **Commonest cause of acute stridor in children**
- Caused by a viral infection (parainfluenza virus, occasionally RSV or rhinovirus)
- Oedema and secretions narrow the child's already small airway

Clinical features

- Usual age 1–2 years
- Mild fever, hoarse voice, barking cough, stridor
- Worse in the evening and overnight
- Little constitutional disturbance
- Watch carefully for cyanosis developing (is the child becoming dusky? Attach an oxygen saturation monitor)
- Sometimes a viral croup can deteriorate into a much more severe condition, especially in the very young (narrower airway) or if a predisposing pathology

Management

1. Give humidified oxygen to keep oxygen saturation > 92% (by head box, face mask, or nasal prongs)
2. Steroid given as steroid nebulizer (budesonide 12 hourly) or oral dexamethasone (12 hourly)
3. Racemic adrenaline nebulizer if child rapidly deteriorating. (NB: Transient improvement. Close monitoring with ECG and oxygen saturation necessary. A rebound increased stridor is common 30–45 min after adrenaline)
4. Intubation and ventilation is necessary in < 1% of children. Consider alternative diagnosis: epiglottitis, tracheitis, foreign body (although very rare now since *H. influenzae* vaccination)

Indications for intubation and ventilation

- Drowsiness due to hypoxia, not controlled with additional oxygen
- Child tiring
- Rapid deterioration

NB: Call an experienced anaesthetist if epiglottitis is suspected.

Recurrent (spasmodic) croup

- Sudden onset at night of inspiratory stridor and croupy cough
- Most common in infants aged 1–3 years
- Recurrent episodes
- Responds to inhaled corticosteroids in acute phase
- Thought to be related to bronchial hyperreactivity/reflux (GOLR)

Bacterial tracheitis (pseudomembranous croup)

This is an uncommon condition of bacterial croup, usually caused by *Staphylococcus aureus*. The child is usually severely unwell and toxic on presentation, with a history of being unwell for 2–3 days. Very soft, hoarse voice, quiet cough, soft stridor. Intubation and ventilation for several days is often required, together with antibiotic therapy.

EPIGLOTTITIS

Epiglottitis is an infection of the epiglottis, usually caused by *Haemophilus influenzae* type b. It has become rare since the introduction of the Hib vaccination. It presents between 1 and 7 years (peak incidence 2–3 years).

Clinical features

- Toxic, unwell child, short history
- Drooling, stridor, high fever, no cough, tachypnoea and tracheal tug
- Sits upright with mouth open and extended neck
- Muffled voice, pain in throat

Management

- Immediate involvement of a senior anaesthetist and ENT surgeon
- Calm environment, do *not* examine mouth or X-ray neck
- Transfer to intensive care or a high-dependency setting with intubation equipment and anaesthetist, paediatrician and ENT surgeon
- Intubation and ventilation for 1–3 days electively or in response to hypoxia
- IV antibiotic therapy
- Rifampicin prophylaxis for close contacts

! **NB: Children with epiglottitis deteriorate rapidly and can be difficult to intubate due to the extreme narrowing of the airway caused by oedema.**

Differences between viral croup and epiglottitis

	Viral croup	Epiglottitis
General state	Child mildly unwell	Very unwell, toxic child
Fever	Low-grade fever	High fever
Length of history	Unwell few days	Rapid, unwell few hours
Drooling	No drool	Drooling
Cough	Barking cough	No cough
Voice	Hoarse voice	Muffled voice
Incidence	Common	Rare
Age	Infants (1–3 years)	Older (2–7 years)

PHARYNGITIS

A common infection usually caused by a virus (adenovirus or parainfluenza virus) and rarely by a bacterium (Group A streptococcus).

Clinical features

■ Sore throat, fever, nasal congestion
■ Oropharyngeal inflammation (red pharynx)

Treatment

■ Symptomatic treatment with antipyretics and plenty of fluids
■ Antibiotics given if a bacterial cause is suspected/established

TONSILLITIS

Acute tonsillitis may be bacterial (usually *Streptococcus pneumoniae*) or viral. It can be difficult to distinguish the two clinically.

Clinical features

■ Sore throat, fever, malaise
■ Red tonsils + pus
■ Cervical lymphadenopathy

Infectious mononucleosis (Epstein–Barr virus [EBV]) must be differentiated. This may present with similar features, although malaise is more generalized, often with tender splenomegaly. Hepatitis and blood abnormalities may also be present. An impressive red generalized rash develops if ampicillin is given to children with EBV infection in 90% of cases.

Investigations

■ Throat swab
■ FBC and monospot
■ EBV IgM

Management

■ Analgesics, antipyretics and plenty of fluids
■ Antibiotics are required if bacterial infection is suspected (penicillin V as first-line therapy)

Complications

■ Quinsy (a peritonsillar abscess) – surgical drainage required under local or general anaesthesia
■ Post-streptococcal complications (see p. 89)
■ Obstructive sleep apnoea syndrome

Indications for tonsillectomy

■ Six attacks of tonsillitis/year for 2 years
■ Three attacks/year over a number of years for the older child
■ Obstructive sleep apnoea syndrome

OBSTRUCTIVE SLEEP APNOEA SYNDROME

This is upper airway obstruction with periods of desaturation. It can theoretically lead to complications secondary to the prolonged periods of hypoxia and hypercapnoea of:

■ Right ventricular hypertrophy, hypertension, polycythaemia
■ Eventually cor pulmonale

It is one end of a spectrum of (usually) adenotonsillar hypertrophy that begins with snoring and milder sleep disordered breathing. Children with certain craniofacial abnormalities are more likely to be affected, as are children with sickle cell disease due to a lower resting oxygen saturation and a propensity for precipitating sickle cell crises.

Failure to thrive may occur.

Adenoids

These enlarge until age 7 years. If very large they may:

- Cause obstructive sleep apnoea syndrome (usually in association with tonsillar hypertrophy)
- Contribute to nasal blockage, snoring, chronic ear disease

Clinical features

During sleep	Snoring with apnoeas for > 10 s as the child struggles for breath
	Mouth breathing
	Intercostal and subcostal recession during the apnoeas
	Frequent awakenings
	Unusual sleeping postures
Tiredness	Daytime somnolence
	Learning problems and behavioural change
	Morning headache

Investigations

ENT examination	Large tonsils ± adenoids
X-ray post-nasal space	
Sleep studies	If the diagnosis is in doubt or child at high risk (overnight pulse oximetry may have some role in identifying severe cases that need HDU support postoperatively)

Treatment

Adenotonsillectomy is usually curative.

Clinical scenario

An 18-month-old infant girl is seen by her GP. A mild fever of 38.0°C, hoarseness, a barking cough, and symptoms over the last 48 h, which are worse at night, have been noted.

1. What is the diagnosis?
2. What three organisms are most likely to be responsible?
3. What are you immediate actions in the Emergency Department?
4. What three drugs may be useful in treatment?

ANSWERS

1. Croup (laryngo-tracheo-bronchitis)
2. Adenovirus; parainfluenza; influenza
3. ABC
4. Nebulized racemic adrenaline; nebulised beclomethasone; oral steroids

---

FURTHER READING

Graham J, Scadding G, Bull P (eds.). *Pediatric ENT*. Berlin: Springer-Verlag, 2008.

8 Respiratory Medicine

- Bronchiolitis
- Inhalation of foreign body
- Aspiration (acute and recurrent)
- Wheeze
- Asthma
- Pneumonia (chest infection)
- Pertussis (whooping cough)
- Bronchiectasis
- Cystic fibrosis
- Further reading

Symptoms and signs of respiratory distress

Symptoms	Signs
Breathlessness	Tachypnoea
Difficulty feeding or talking	Tachycardia
Wheeziness	Dyspnoea
Sweatiness	Recession – intercostal, subcostal and suprasternal
	Nasal flaring
	Use of accessory muscles of respiration (shoulders up, leaning forward, head bob in infants)
	Expiratory grunting
	Wheeze
	Crackles
	Cyanosis
	Downward displacement of liver (hyperinflation of lungs)

Causes of wheeze

Common	Rare
Infection – bronchiolitis, viral-induced wheeze, pneumonia	Cystic fibrosis
	Immunodeficiency
Asthma	Whooping cough
Recurrent aspiration	External compression of airway: congenital vascular ring, mediastinal mass (glands, tumour, cysts): stridor more than wheeze
Foreign body inhalation	
Gastro-oesophageal reflux	
	Heart failure
	Fibrosing alveolitis

Causes of chronic cough

- Asthma
- Recurrent aspiration
- Inhaled foreign body
- Prolonged infection, e.g. pertussis, mycoplasma, RSV, TB
- Habit cough (after an acute chest infection; these children do not cough while asleep)
- Post-nasal drip
- Lung disease, e.g. cystic fibrosis, bronchiectasis
- Immunodeficiency, e.g. cancer therapy, HIV

BRONCHIOLITIS

This is a common condition in young children (usually between 1 and 12 months old) caused by a viral infection of the bronchioles. Most cases (80%) are due to respiratory syncytial virus (RSV), and the remainder to adenovirus types 3, 7 and 21, parainfluenza viruses, rhinovirus or influenza viruses.

Clinical features

- Coryza, snuffles, chesty cough, tachypnoea, dyspnoea, sometimes wheeze
- Worsening over first 5–6 days, then plateau for 1–2 days, then resolution over next 2 weeks
- Feeding difficulties (secondary to breathing difficulties), poor intake and vomiting
- Apnoea in small babies
- Secondary bacterial chest infection can develop, making the child more unwell

Signs

- Tachypnoea, tachycardia
- Intercostal, subcostal and suprasternal recession
- Inspiratory crackles, occasionally wheeze
- Low grade fever, and if severe, cyanosis
- Respiratory distress preventing feeding

Investigations

Nasopharyngeal aspirate — Sent for immunofluorescent antibody test looking for RSV + other viruses
Bedside rapid diagnostic kits are available

CXR — Only if severe or bacterial superinfection suspected:
- Hyperinflation (horizontal ribs and flattened diaphragm)
- Patchy atelectasis (often RUL)
- *Peribronchial thickening*

Treatment

- Oxygen via nasal prongs or a head box
- IV fluids as necessary; nasogastric in recovery phase
- CPAP via nasal prongs or intubation and ventilation if deterioration with exhaustion or persistent apnoeas
- Bronchodilators, including nebulized adrenaline, are advocated in some centres. These cause short term improvement in clinical signs in a minority of patients and must be carefully monitored for efficacy
- Antibiotic therapy only if secondary bacterial infection is suspected
- Ribavirin via SPAG aerosol generator machine for infants who are very unwell or at risk of severe disease, e.g. CHD, CF

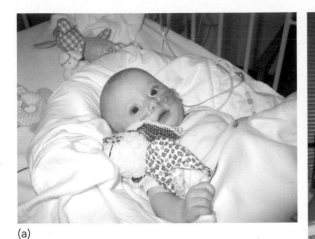

(a)

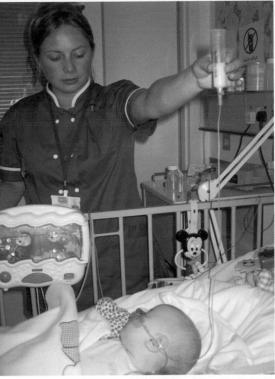

(b)

Figure 8.1 (a) Five-month-old girl in respiratory distress. Note the nasal prong oxygen, IV infusion and nursing at 30° head elevation. (b) Same child 24 h later and now requiring regular 2-hourly nasogastric milk feeds, as not able to cope with small volume oral feeds, but unable yet to breast feed

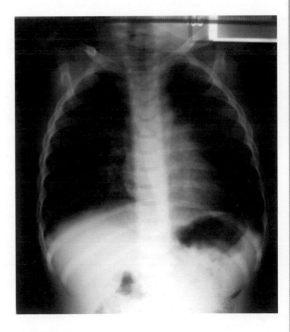

Figure 8.2 Chest X-ray of a 1-year-old infant with bronchiolitis showing horizontal position of the ribs secondary to chest hyperinflation, and diffuse patchy pulmonary infiltration

INHALATION OF FOREIGN BODY

- Children may accidentally inhale foreign bodies
- Classic history is of a coughing/choking episode whilst eating (often peanuts)
- Inhaled foreign body will usually go down the *right* main bronchus, because this is more vertical than the left
- Clinical features depend on the level the object lodges at
- May present acutely or chronically

Clinical features

Acute episode — Acute coughing or choking episode followed by stridor (in upper airway) or wheeze (in lungs) – often localized

Positive history of small object inhaled

Chronic symptoms — Respiratory infection not resolving

Recurrent lobar pneumonias involving the same lobe

Persistent wheeze

Investigations

Chest X-ray — Foreign body only radio-opaque in 10–15% of cases

Lobar pneumonia may be visible

If possible, do inspiratory film (both sides appear equally inflated) and expiratory film (foreign body side may be *hyperinflated* due to foreign body acting as a ball valve)

Management

Removal of the foreign body using **rigid bronchoscopy** under general anaesthetic.

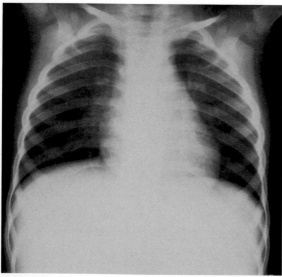
(a)

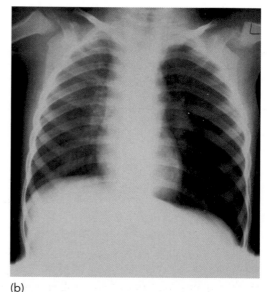
(b)

Figure 8.3 Chest X-rays of a 36-month-old child with obstructive emphysema due to an inhaled walnut. (a) Peak inspiration – both lungs appear equally aerated and the mediastinal structures are in the midline. (b) Deep expiration – there is marked hyperlucency of the left lung. The right lung has de-aerated normally. At bronchoscopy a walnut piece was retrieved from the left bronchus (courtesy of Dr Kapila Jain and Dr Simon Padley)

ASPIRATION (ACUTE AND RECURRENT)

Causes

There are many causes of aspiration, which may be *acute* or *recurrent*.

Acute	Recurrent
Depressed gag reflex	Neurological swallowing disorder, e.g.
Depressed state of consciousness, e.g.	cerebral palsy
post anaesthetic	GOR
Infants with acute viral illness exacerbating	Oesophageal incoordination
existing gastro-oesophageal reflux (GOR)	Structural anomaly, e.g. tracheosophageal fistula

Clinical features
- Cough, stridor and wheeze (acute or recurrent)
- Signs of pneumonia (acute or recurrent)

Investigations

CXR   Consolidation (often RLL in older children, RUL in infants)
   In chronic aspiration more than one lobe may be involved; there may be collapse with features of hyperinflation and hilar shadowing

Other   Depend on the suspected cause of the aspiration – GOR reflux studies (24-h pH study) and contrast studies; broncho–alveolar lavage by bronchoscopy

Management

Treat the acute infection, and then identify and treat the underlying cause.

WHEEZE

Viral-induced wheeze

Usually found in pre-school children. Individuals are often non–atopic and the symptoms resolve by school age.

Management
- As for any acute asthma attack (see below), dependent upon severity
- Acute relievers (bronchodilators) in the presence of symptoms
- Short course oral prednisolone (1–2 mg/kg)

Persistent wheeze in infancy

- Recurrent episodes of wheeze in infants, often with multiple admissions, sometimes following admissions with viral infections such as bronchiolitis
- Usually these children have small airways (boys, child of smoking mother)
- Divide into those who go on to wheeze in later life, often from atopic families, and those who resolve in first few years

Management
- Acute relievers (nebulized/nebuhaled ipratroprium bromide or β–agonists)
- If family history of atopy, consider inhaled steroids
- Exclude other diagnoses – tracheomalacia, cystic fibrosis, immune deficiency, foreign body

ASTHMA

Asthma is a common condition affecting up to 1 in 10. It is a chronic inflammatory condition of the airways, diagnosed essentially clinically and characterized by:

- Reversible bronchoconstriction
- Mucosal oedema
- Excessive mucous production

! NB: Asthma leads to a difficulty breathing *out*.

Asthma is an atopic condition and other atopic conditions are often coexistent, e.g. eczema and allergic rhinitis.

Features of atopy

- Asthma
- Eczema
- Allergic rhinitis
- Allergic conjunctivitis
- Raised serum IgE level
- Skin prick test positivity to various allergens, e.g. house dust mite
- Family history of atopy

Clinical features

The features can be *chronic* with frequent wheeze and cough (usually present if asthma is being undertreated), or *acute* with fast onset often associated with URTI. The disease varies from being extremely mild to very severe, with frequent and even life-threatening exacerbations, and interrupting daily life considerably.

Chronic features	Recurrent wheeze ⎱ Both often with exercise
	Difficulty in breathing ⎰
	If longstanding:
	■ Chest hyperinflation
	■ Harrison sulci (a permanent groove in the chest wall just above the costal margins at the insertion of the diaphragm)
	■ Faltering growth
	Nocturnal wheeze with cough
Exacerbation	Dyspnoea
	Expiratory wheeze (NB: Babies have crackles with bronchiolitis, not infant wheeze)
	Respiratory distress (tachypnoea, tachycardia, recession, cyanosis)
Life-threatening attack	Unable to speak or feed
	Central cyanosis
	Exhaustion/confusion/decreasing level of consciousness
	Silent chest on auscultation (due to minimal air entry)
	Peak flow < 30% of predicted
	Pulsus paradoxus (fall of inspiratory systolic BP greater than 10 mmHg from expiratory systolic BP)

Peak expiratory flow (PEF)

- Useful and simple lung function test. Performed much less nowadays due to relative lack of reproductibility
- Used to assess asthma severity, comparing the child's peak flow to his/her normal peak flow (charts of normal flow are available but should be used with caution)
- Varies with height, gender and ethnic group (no use if baseline not known)
- Varies during the day (lowest in the early morning)
- Varies with exercise (increases in normal individuals, drops in exercise-induced asthma by > 15%)

Important questions to ask in an asthma history

1. What triggers the asthma?
2. How often and how severe are the attacks?
3. Does the asthma affect daily living, e.g. sport, school, sleep?
4. Can they measure their peak flow properly to monitor their asthma?
5. Can they use their device properly (get them to demonstrate this)?
6. Do they understand the difference between quick relief and preventative medications?
7. Do they recognize a deterioration, and have a good management plan for this?
8. Do they recognize a severe attack and know to seek prompt medical attention?

Management

Acute attack Oxygen

β–agonist, e.g. salbutamol: either 10 puffs from a metered dose inhaler (MDI) via spacer device or nebulized as frequently as necessary (initially every 15 min)

Ipatropium bromide 6 hourly can be helpful, more in younger children

Systemic steroids (oral prednisolone 1–2 mg/kg [max. dose 40 mg] or IV hydrocortisone)

If severe attack, then may need:

- IV infusion or bolus of salbutamol or aminophylline infusion (if on oral theophylline, no loading dose)
- Intubation and ventilation if deterioration in general condition, i.e. peak flow, blood gases, drowsiness, tiring, despite above measures

Long term Essentially divided into:

- **Immediate relief** medications, e.g. salbutamol inhaler (to take whenever necessary [prn])
- **Long term preventative** medications, e.g. beclomethasone inhaler (to take regularly each day)

A stepwise progression of long term therapy has been devised by the British Thoracic Society, outlined in the British Guidelines on Asthma Management (see Table 8.1):

- Lowest step necessary to control the asthma is used
- Child should be regularly reviewed (every 3–6 months) and a step down is usually possible if control has been adequate for > 3 months
- β–agonists are used as relievers on all of the steps

> **!** **NB: A short course of oral steroids is often required to treat an acute exacerbation of asthma.**

Table 8.1 Stepwise progression of long term asthma therapy. (a) School children (5–12 years). (b) Children under 5 years (from the British Guidelines on Asthma Management)

(a)

Step 1	Step 2	Step 3	Step 4	Step 5
Mild intermittent asthma	*Regular preventer therapy*	*Add-on therapy*	*Persistent poor control*	*Frequent or continuous use of oral steroids*
Occasional β-agonist inhaled	Add inhaled steroids (200–400 μg/day*)	Add long acting β-agonist (LABA) Assess control: 1. LABA benefit, but still poor control, ensure 400 μg/day* inhaled steroids 2. LABA no response, stop LABA, ensure 400 μg/day* inhaled steroids. Trial other therapies, e.g. theophylline SR, leukotriene antagonist	Increase inhaled steroids to 800 μg/day*	Use daily steroid tablet in lowest dose to maintain control
If used > twice per week, go to Step 2				Ensure high-dose inhaled steroids maintained 800 μg/day*
				Refer to respiratory paediatrician

(b)

Step 1	Step 2	Step 3	Step 4
Mild intermittent	*Regular preventer*	*Add-on therapy*	*Persistent poor control*
Occasional inhaled β-agonist	Add inhaled steroid 200–400 μg/day*	2–5 years: consider leukotriene receptor antagonist	Refer to respiratory paediatrician
If used > twice per week, go to Step 2		< 2 years: consider Step 4	

*Beclamethasone equivalent

Asthma medications

Immediate relief bronchodilators

- **β-2 agonists:**
  - Bronchodilators acting directly on the β-2 receptors in the bronchi:
  - Side effects due to stimulation of β-receptors: tachycardia and arrhythmias, peripheral vasodilatation, headache, fine tremor, excitement, hypokalaemia if used frequently
- *Anticholinergics:*
  - Antimuscarinic bronchodilators,
  - Slower onset (30–60 min), last up to 6 h
  - Rarely used in children unless < 1 year old
  - Sometimes used in acute attacks

Example

- *Short acting*, e.g. salbutamol, terbutaline – used as acute relievers of symptoms
- *Longer acting*, e.g. salmeterol, eformoterol – used to prevent daily symptoms, e.g. exercise induced wheeze

e.g. frequent nebulizers in acute attack
e.g. ipatropium bromide, oxitropin

Long term preventative medications

- *Inhaled steroids:*
  - Anti-inflammatory effect on airways
  - Steroid side effects minimal unless high-dose inhaled or oral steroids given regularly
- *Mast cell stabilizers:*
  - Prevent mast cell degranulation
- *Methylxanthines:*
  - Bronchodilators, smooth muscle relaxer
  - Narrow margin between toxicity (arrhythmias, convulsions) and therapeutic dose
- Leukotriene receptor antagonists:
  - Selectively block the action of cysteinyl leukotrienes preventing bronchoconstriction, mucus secretion and oedema

Example

e.g. beclomethasone, budesonide, fluticasone

e.g. sodium chromoglycate, necrodomil

e.g. aminophylline, theophylline

e.g. *montelukast*

Delivery devices

There are many different asthma medications but essentially just three methods of delivery directly to the lungs:

1. Metered dose inhaler (MDI) + spacer
2. Dry powder devices
3. Nebulizer

- Most convenient and appropriate device is selected for each child
- Best devise to use for *all* children and adults is a pressurized **metered dose inhaler (MDI) with spacer**
- Some older children prefer to use smaller devices. Dry powder inhalers or automated firing MDIs may then be used, e.g. Turbohaler and Accuhaler
- Nebulizer: for acute severe asthma, give over 5–10 min; driven by oxygen in hospital

> **NB:** It is very important that the parents and child are taught how to use the equipment properly, as poor technique is very common, and results in most of the medication never reaching the lungs as it should.

Spacer devices

These increase the amount of small respirable particles, trap larger non-respirable particles and remove the need for coordination between inhalation and drug release. There are two main spacer devices which connect with different medications:

Nebuhaler   Terbutaline, budesonide
Volumatic   Salbutamol, beclomethasone, fluticasone, ipratropium bromide

There are other non-generic devices on the market.

PNEUMONIA (CHEST INFECTION)

Pneumonia may be viral (particularly in young children – up to 40% of pneumonias) or bacterial. As it is not possible to distinguish between the two clinically or on CXR, pneumonia is *always* treated with antibiotics.

Infections causing pneumonia

Newborn	Infants	Children	Immunocompromised
Group B β-haemolytic streptococcus	RSV	*Strep. pneumoniae*	As for children
Escherichia coli	Adenovirus	*Mycoplasma*	*Pneumocystis jejunii*
Listeria monocytogenes	Influenza virus	*pneumoniae*	*(carinii)*
Chlamydia trachomatis	Parainfluenza	*Haem. influenzae*	Atypical TB
Staphylococcus aureus	*Strep. pneumoniae*	TB	
CMV	*Staph. aureus*	*Staph. aureus*	
	Haemophilus influenzae		
	C. trachomatis		

Clinical features

- Respiratory distress symptoms and signs, RR > 50 (> 70 in infants)
- Febrile and unwell, temperature > 38.5°C

Investigations

Pneumonia is a *clinical* diagnosis.

Pulse oximetry
CXR   **Lobar pneumonia** (dense, localized consolidation) or **bronchopneumonia** (patchy consolidation)
                    Unnecessary in mild uncomplicated LRTI
Blood tests   Blood cultures
                    Blood gas to assess respiratory function if child unwell
Microbiology/virology Nasopharyngeal suction specimen for viral immunoflourescence and microscopy, culture and sensitivities
                    Sputum for microscopy, culture and sensitivities

Radiographic patterns of lobar consolidation and collapse on chest X-ray

It is very useful to understand the patterns of the CXR silhouette:

Consolidation Increased shadowing, may have air bronchogram but no loss of volume or shift of mediastinum or other lobes

Collapse Dense increased shadowing, but contracted, loss of lung volume, no bronchogram, shift of fissures and mediastinal structures

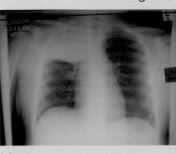
(a)

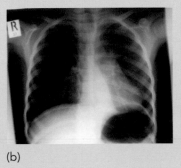
(b)

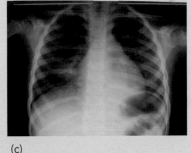
(c)

Figure 8.4 Pneumonia. (a) Right upper lobe consolidation. (b) Left lower lobe (LLL) collapse consolidation. Note the left hilar is displaced downwards and the LLL is contracted, indicating collapse in addition to consolidation. (c) Right middle lobe consolidation

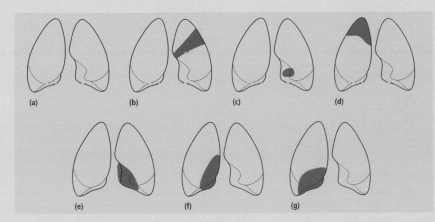

(a) (b) (c) (d)

(e) (f) (g)

Figure 8.5 Pneumonia shadowing patterns seen on chest X-ray. (a) Normal chest X-ray. (b) Left upper lobe segmental consolidation. (c) Lingular consolidation. (d) Right upper lobe consolidation with collapse (horizontal fissure and right hilar pulled up). (e) Left lower lobe collapse and consolidation (left hilar pulled down). (f) Loss of distinct right cardiac border (right middle lobe consolidation). (g) Right cardiac border still distinct. Right hemidiaphragm may be raised (right lower lobe consolidation)

Management

- Admit if toxic, hypoxic or dyspnoeic
- Humidified oxygen as needed to keep oxygen saturations > 92%
- Appropriate antibiotic treatment (intravenous if unwell)

Complications

- Pneumococcal pneumonia – meningitis, pleural effusion
- Staphylococcal pneumonia – empyema, lung abscess, pneumothorax
- Severe infection (esp. TB, whooping cough) – bronchiectasis (do CXR 4–6 weeks after pneumonia if persistent cough or original CXR showed collapse)

Causes of chronic or recurrent pneumonia

- Inhaled foreign body
- Bronchiectasis (post-infectious)
- Aspiration pneumonia
- TB infection
- Immunodeficiency
- Cystic fibrosis
- Tracheo-oesophageal fistula
- Congenital abnormality of the lung
- Ciliary dyskinesia (e.g. Kartagener's syndrome)

PERTUSSIS (WHOOPING COUGH)

This infection of young children is caused by the Gram-negative coccobacillus, *Bordetella pertussis*. It is a notifiable disease. The incidence is low due to vaccination at 2, 3 and 4 months.

Transmission	Droplet
Incubation	7–14 days

Clinical features

Catarrhal stage	1–2 weeks
	Runny nose, conjunctivitis, malaise
Paroxysmal stage	Up to 3 months (the 100 day cough)
	Paroxysms of coughing occur causing an inspiratory '**whoop**' and vomiting
	Coughing can be so intense that it causes conjunctival petechiae/sub-conjunctival haemorrhage and epistaxis
	Infants may not have the 'whoop' but often have **apnoeas** following coughing spasm
Convalescence	1–2 weeks
	Resolution of the symptoms

Management

- Diagnosis is confirmed by PCR and culture from a *per nasal swab*
- Child treated with antibiotics (erythromycin) as well as close contacts to prevent spread. (This does not change the severity or duration of the disease)
- Supportive care during paroxysms

Complications

- Lobar pneumonia (mostly secondary bacterial infection) – causes 90% of the deaths
- Atelectasis, bronchiectasis (late)
- Apnoea, cerebral anoxia with convulsions in young infants.
- Rectal prolapse, inguinal hernia, frenulum tear, periorbital petechiae ⎫ Due to prolonged coughing
- Subconjunctival haemorrhage ⎬ fits

BRONCHIECTASIS

Bronchiectasis is permanently *dilated bronchi* and may be localized or diffuse. There are inflamed bronchial walls, decreased mucociliary transport and recurrent bacterial infections.

Causes

It occurs secondary to damage of the lung due to:

- Severe pneumonia
- Post whooping cough, measles and TB
- Inhaled foreign body
- Cystic fibrosis
- Primary ciliary dyskinesia

Clinical features

- Chronic productive cough, sometimes haemoptysis
- Dyspnoea and clubbing after time
- CXR:
  - Hyperinflation
  - Peribronchial thickening of the affected area
  - Tram tracking
- CT thorax demonstrates dilated bronchi with thickened walls

Management

- Antibiotics for acute infections and long term antibiotic prophylaxis if necessary
- Physiotherapy and bronchodilators as appropriate
- If an isolated lobe is affected it can be resected

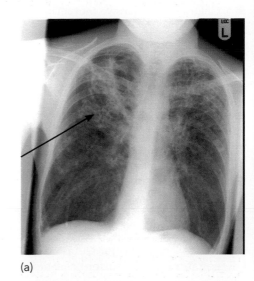

(a)

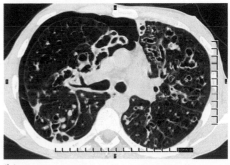

(b)

Figure 8.6 (a) Chest X-ray demonstrating widespread bronchiectasis, aetiology unknown. Note the bronchial wall thickening and tram tracking (non-tapering thick walled bronchi – arrow). (b) CT scan demonstrating severe bronchiectasis and right-sided pneumothorax (courtesy of Dr Kapila Jain and Dr Simon Padley)

Immotile cilia syndrome

- Several conditions with either absent or severely reduced ciliary motility
- Primary ciliary dyskinesia – 50% of cases, autosomal recessive condition
- Defective ciliary action in lungs, ears, nose and sperm ducts
- Features – chronic productive cough, chronic sinusitis, otitis media and wheeze
- Males are infertile

Kartagener syndrome is the triad of immotile cilia, situs inversus (dextrocardia and visceral inversion) and chronic sinusitis

CYSTIC FIBROSIS

- *Commonest* inherited autosomal recessive disorder in the UK: ~ 1 in 2500 births
- Due to a defect in CFTR (cystic fibrosis transmembrane regulator) protein, which is a **chloride channel**
- Chloride (with passive movement of sodium and water) is poorly secreted, causing secretions that are dehydrated and thick
- Two main problems:
  - Recurrent chest infections causing chronic lung damage (bronchiectasis)
  - Malabsorption (due to reduced pancreatic enzymes) causing failure to thrive
- Life limiting, with a median survival of 32 years in 2000

Genetics

- CFTR protein is located on chromosome 7
- > 1000 different gene mutations have been found
- Loss of phenylalanine at position 508 (Δ508) on at least one chromosome is present in 75% of UK cases
- Carrier rate in Northern Europeans is about 1 in 25

Clinical features

General	Failure to thrive Finger clubbing
Respiratory	Recurrent chest infections (*Staphylococcus aureus*, *Haemophilus influenzae*, *Pseudomonas aeruginosa*) Restrictive (and obstructive in one-third) lung disorder Chronic lung damage (bronchiectasis, lobar collapse, pneumothorax, respiratory failure) Hyperinflation, scoliosis Chest scars (portacath)
ENT	Nasal polyps Sinusitis
Cardiovascular	Right heart failure (late feature, secondary to severe lung disease)
Pancreas	85% have decreased pancreatic enzyme production (lipase, amylase, proteases), this causes loose fatty stool CFRD (CF-related diabetes) – increasing incidence with age (one-third of adults)
Liver	Fatty infiltrate, cholesterol gallstones, cirrhosis, pericholangitis, portal hypertension
Abdominal	Meconium ileus: this presents soon after birth with delayed passage of meconium and bowel obstruction (relieved either surgically or with Gastrografin enema) (NB: it can present antenatally with bowel damage) Rectal prolapse (> 18 months): resolves quickly on starting enzyme replacement Hepato(spleno)megaly, pubertal delay Surgical scars, e.g. meconium ileus, gastrostomy, liver transplant Intussusception, constipation
Joints	Cystic fibrosis-related arthropathy
Reproductive	Males are infertile (as the vas deferentia are absent) Delayed puberty

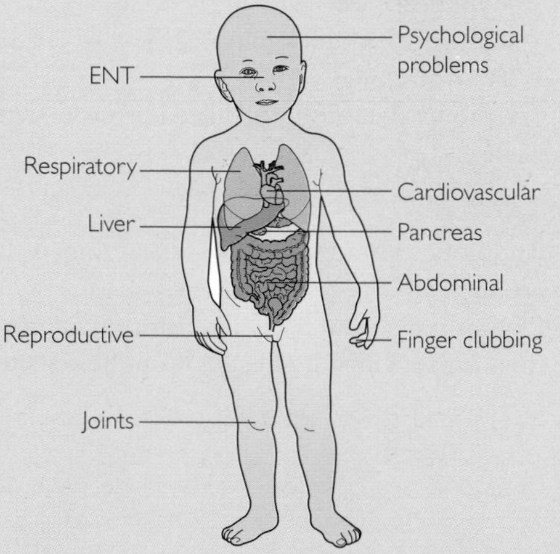

Figure 8.7 Clinical features of cystic fibrosis

Neonatal presentations of cystic fibrosis

- Meconium ileus
- Prolonged neonatal jaundice
- Recurrent chest infections
- Malabsorption with diarrhoea or steatorrhoea
- Failure to thrive

Chest X-ray findings

- Findings all become more marked with increasing severity of disease
- Bronchial wall thickening
- Hyperinflation with flattened diaphragm
- Ring and line shadows, increased interstitial markings

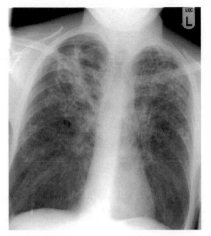

Figure 8.8 Chest X-ray of a child with associated pulmonary changes due to cystic fibrosis (courtesy of Dr Kapila Jain and Dr Simon Padley)

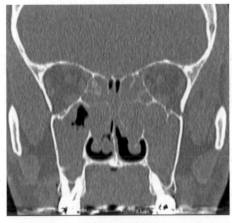

Figure 8.9 Coronal CT scan showing pansinusitis in a child with cystic fibrosis (courtesy of Dr Kapila Jain and Dr Simon Padley)

Investigations

Sweat test	'Gold standard' test for diagnosis
	Sweat is collected in a sweat chamber and the **chloride content** of the sweat is analysed: in cystic fibrosis it is *high* (> 60 mmol/L)
	Two tests are needed to confirm the diagnosis
Immunoreactive trypsin (IRT)	Blood test that can be done in young infants as part of the Guthrie test
	In infants with cystic fibrosis the immunoreactive trypsinogen is elevated
Gene analysis	Commoner CF mutations can be searched for using DNA analysis
	Can be done on the Guthrie test blood, or antenatally in mothers to screen for risk of having a child with CF
	Second pregnancies can be screened with chorionic villous sampling
Stool sample	Children with pancreatic insufficiency have low elastase, absent chymotrypsin and high fat content
Electrolytes	Unwell children may have a **hypokalaemic alkalosis** due to sodium and potassium loss in the sweat

Management

The aims of management are to ensure optimum physical and emotional growth, and to delay the onset of the pulmonary disease. This is achieved by a multidisciplinary team approach and regular review of:

- General growth and development
- Respiratory pathogens
- Frequency and severity of chest infections, and lung function
- Nutrition and gastrointestinal symptoms
- Development of diabetes, liver or joint disease
- Psychosocial problems (school progress etc.)
- Fertility and genetic counselling (later)

Lung disease	Physiotherapy often twice daily, individualized to patient
	Antibiotics:
	■ Long term or pulsed orally as prophylaxis
	■ May be nebulized
	■ Intercurrent infections treated as necessary (oral or IV for 2 weeks)
	Bronchodilators
	Oxygen at home as disease progresses
Gastrointestinal disease	Oral pancreatic enzyme supplements
	Optimum nutrition (high calorie, high protein diet, vitamins, bile acids, salt needed in hot climates and sometimes for babies)
Other treatments	Mucolytics, e.g. DNase or hypertonic saline
	Liver transplant
	Heart–lung transplantation in end-stage disease
	Treatment for complications, e.g. insulin for CFRD
	Gene therapy is still being researched

Clinical scenario

A young girl arrives in the UK from Albania with no medical notes. She is brought to a DGH hospital with a chronic cough which is productive. She is apyrexial; nevertheless a chest X-ray is obtained.

Apparently she takes a number of medicines especially at meal times but her carers are unable to elucidate regarding their specifics.

Her bowel motions are noted to be offensive and she is below the 0.4th centile for weight and height.

1. What test would you organize to establish the diagnosis?
2. If genetic confirmation were needed what gene abnormality would be looked for?
3. Give three staples of medical care which would have fairly immediate impact on her state of health.

ANSWERS

1. Look for evidence of BCG immunization. Mantoux or Heaf test. (Gamma interferon may be an alternative, and early morning naso-gastric aspirates on three separate mornings are sometimes helpful in establishing a diagnosis, but are not pleasant for the child). Sweat test; CF genotype; faecal elastase to assess pancreatic exocrine sufficiency
2. ΔF508, but up to 35 genes are now routinely tested for (if all 35 are negative then for Caucasian children this excludes CF to >98% certainty), and over 300 have been identified coding for abnormalities in the cystic fibrosis transmembrane regulator
3. If TB confirmed: triple or quadruple anti-TB cocktail of antibiotics
   If CF confirmed: exocrine pancreatic supplements; intravenous antibiotic regime appropriate to culture of endobronchial organism identified with its antibiotic sensitivities. Cover staphylococcus, haemophilus and pseudomonas at this age. Thirdly active chest physiotherapy following nebulized bronchodilators

FURTHER READING

Bush A, Davies J. *Paediatric Respiratory Disease: Airways and Infection: An Atlas of Investigation and Management*. Oxford: Clinical Publishing, 2009.

British Thoracic Society Guidelines on asthma management.

Taussig L, Landau L. *Paediatric respiratory medicine*, 2nd edn. London: Mosby, 2008.

Berhman R, Kliegman R, Jenson H, Stanton B. *Nelson Textbook of Pediatrics*, 18th edn. London: Saunders, 2007.

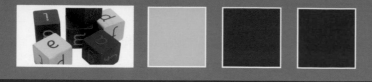

9 Cardiology

- Fetal circulation and birth
- Cardiac evaluation
- Innocent murmurs
- Cardiac failure
- Structural congenital heart disease
- Cardiac surgery
- Rheumatic fever
- Infective endocarditis
- Myocarditis
- Dilated cardiomyopathy
- Arrhythmias
- Further reading

FETAL CIRCULATION AND BIRTH

- *In utero* the fetus obtains oxygenated blood from the placenta via the umbilical vein, which drains via the ductus venosus into the inferior vena cava and from there into the right atrium
- From the right atrium most of the blood passes through the foramen ovale into the left side of the heart, and then to the brain and other organs via the aorta
- Some of the systemic venous return entering into the right atrium will go through the right ventricle into the pulmonary artery
- Blood that enters the pulmonary artery will flow preferentially via the ductus arteriosus into the descending aorta, with a small amount continuing along the pulmonary artery to the lungs
- Blood passes from the aorta via the two umbilical arteries back to the placenta for oxygenation

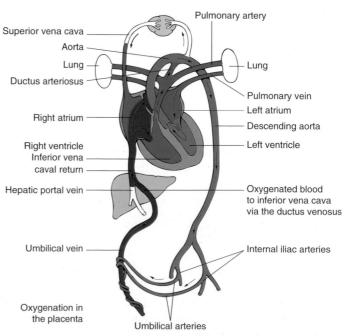

Figure 9.1 Fetal circulation

At *birth* major changes take place after the first breath to establish the postnatal circulation.

- The breath opens up the lungs and reduces the resistance in the pulmonary vascular bed, increasing blood flow through the lungs and return to the left atrium via the pulmonary veins
- This increased blood flow into the left atrium pushes the foramen ovale closed
- The ductus arteriosus also has to close, and this takes place over the first week of life in response to the higher oxygen concentration in the blood

Some forms of congenital heart disease rely on blood flow through a patent ductus arteriosus after birth (**duct-dependent circulations**), and will thus deteriorate rapidly when the ductus closes.

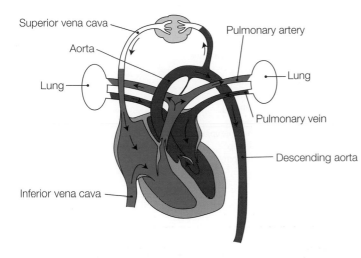

Superior vena cava
Aorta
Lung
Inferior vena cava
Pulmonary artery
Lung
Pulmonary vein
Descending aorta

Figure 9.2 Postnatal circulation. Some forms of congenital heart disease rely on blood flowing through the ductus arteriosus (duct-dependent circulation) and thus will deteriorate rapidly when the ductus arteriosus closes around day 3

CARDIAC EVALUATION

Features to ask about in a cardiac history

Family history	of cardiac disease?
Pregnancy	? Polyhydramnios, ? arrhythmias *in utero*, ? hydrops fetalis, ? abnormal USS ? abnormal karyotype Maternal drug history? Maternal infections?
Neonate	Poor feeding, sweating, tachypnoea, failure to thrive, cyanosis, recurrent chest infections
Infant/older child	Breathlessness, cyanosis, dizziness or fainting, fatigue, recurrent chest infections Chest pains, fluttering (palpitations), sudden collapse, squatting

Features to look for on cardiac examination

- Dysmorphic features, e.g. Down syndrome, Marfan syndrome
- Cyanosis or not (clubbing?)
- Features of heart failure
- Pulse – rate, volume, character, rhythm, femoral pulses
- Auscultation – heart sounds, added sounds, heart murmur?
- Precordial findings – scars, apex beat, thrill, heave, chest symmetry
- Peripheral features – blood pressure, JVP, hepatosplenomegaly
- Respiratory examination

Cardiac scars

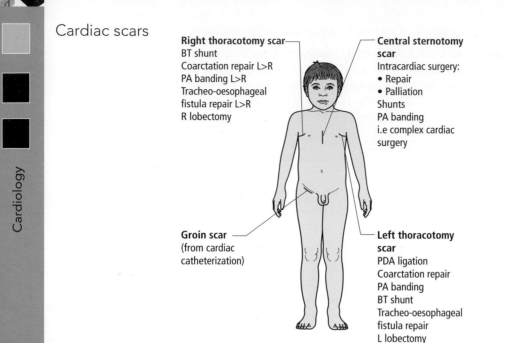

Right thoracotomy scar
BT shunt
Coarctation repair L>R
PA banding L>R
Tracheo-oesophageal
fistula repair L>R
R lobectomy

**Central sternotomy
scar**
Intracardiac surgery:
• Repair
• Palliation
Shunts
PA banding
i.e complex cardiac
surgery

Groin scar
(from cardiac
catheterization)

**Left thoracotomy
scar**
PDA ligation
Coarctation repair
PA banding
BT shunt
Tracheo-oesophageal
fistula repair
L lobectomy

Figure 9.3 Cardiac scars

Vital signs

Children's vital signs alter gradually as they grow.

Table 9.1 **Normal age-related vital signs**

Age (years)	HR	RR	SBP	DBP
< 1 year	120–160	30–60	60–95	35–69
1–3	90–140	24–40	95–105	50–65
3–5	75–110	18–30	95–110	50–65
8–12	75–100	18–30	90–110	57–71
12–16	60–90	12–16	112–130	60–80

SBP, systolic blood pressure; DBP, diastolic blood pressure
Duke J, Rosenberg SG (eds). *Anesthesia Secrets*. St Louis: Mosby. 1996

CARDIAC INVESTIGATIONS

General cardiac investigations are:

- CXR
- ECG (12 lead, rhythm strip, 24-h or 7-day tape, exercise test)
- Echocardiogram
- Oxygen saturation (probe + arterial blood gas)
- Cardiac catheterization and angiography
- Cardiac MRI

These three investigations should be done on any infant in whom cardiac disease is suspected

Chest X-ray silhouette

It is useful to have an idea of how the CXR relates to the heart and lungs.

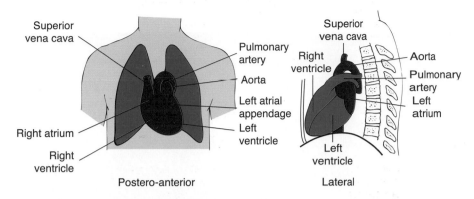

Figure 9.4 Chest X-ray cardiac silhouette

Causes of right-sided aortic arch	**Causes of a big heart**
Tetralogy of Fallot	Heart failure
Truncus arteriosus	Significant left-to-right shunts
Pulmonary atresia with VSD	Dilated cardiomyopathy
Congenital vascular ring	Ebstein anomaly
22q11 deletion	Pericardial effusion

Electrocardiogram (ECG)

The pacemaker of the heart (the **sinus node**) is in the right atrium, and generates an electrical impulse that spreads through the atria causing atrial contraction and reaches the **atrioventricular node** (at the junction between the atria and the right ventricle) where it passes rapidly to both ventricles causing ventricular contraction. The ECG demonstrates this electrical activity in the heart, and may demonstrate conduction defects, arrhythmias, axis deviation or hypertrophy.

Cardiac axis

The cardiac axis is the average direction of spread of the depolarization wave through the ventricles (as seen from the front) and it changes significantly during childhood, from *right and anterior* in infants, to *left and posterior* in adults.

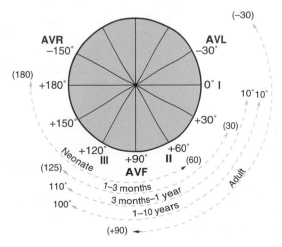

Figure 9.5 Cardiac axis during childhood

Echocardiogram

This is a vital non-invasive tool used in the investigation of cardiac disorders. It is a realtime two-dimensional imaging technique also using Doppler to assess speed and direction of blood flow.

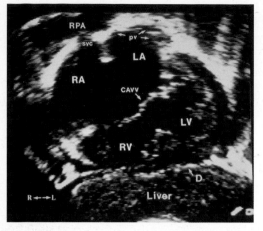

(a)

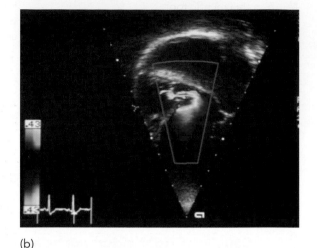

(b)

Figure 9.6 (a) 2D echocardiogram of a child with atrioventricular septal defect (LA, left atrium; RA, right atrium; LV, left ventricle; RV, right ventricle). (b) Colour Doppler image showing right-to-left flow (blue) through a ventricular septal defect during systole in a child with tricuspid atresia (courtesy of Dr Rob Yates)

Cardiac catheterization and angiography

Cardiac catheterization is an invasive procedure employed to measure the pressures and oxygenation within the various cardiac chambers and vessels. Anatomical information is obtained from angiograms (using radio-opaque dye injections at the time of the catheterization).

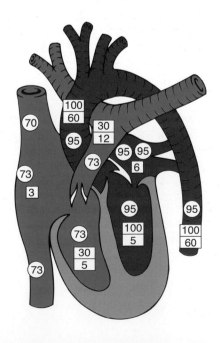

Key

☐ = Blood pressure

◯ = Oxygen saturations

Figure 9.7 Cardiac catheterization data – normal intracardiac pressures

Indications

- Pre-surgical evaluation
- Evaluation of pulmonary vascular resistance
- To monitor progress after surgical intervention
- As a therapeutic tool in interventional cardiac catheterization, e.g. balloon dilatation, embolization and closure of intracardiac defects

Procedure

- Sedation (sometimes)
- Nil by mouth 4 h prior
- X-ray monitoring, ECG connected
- Sterile procedure
- Catheter insertion into peripheral vein (to right side of heart) or peripheral artery (to left side of heart) and pressures measured/samples taken/dye introduced/procedure performed

Complications

- Arrhythmia
- Haemorrhage
- Arterial thrombus
- Embolus
- Device embolization
- Aneurysm formation

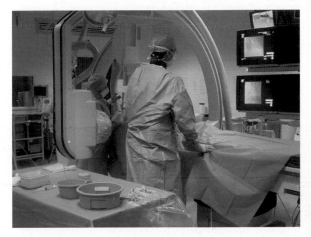

Figure 9.8 Cardiac angiogram being performed

Important cardiac differences between children and adults

Cardiac axis	To the *right and anterior* in a neonate and gradually moves round to the *left and posterior* (as in adults) by teenage years
Vital signs (HR, RR and BP)	*Vary* with age (see Table 9.1)
Heart sounds	*Normal splitting* of the second heart sound (A2 P2) on expiration is audible in children and young adults
	A **third heart sound (S3)** can be normal in children (due to rapid ventricular filling)
Ability to increase **cardiac output**	Children are unable to alter stroke volume very much and rely on **heart rate**

INNOCENT MURMURS

These are heard in around 30% of children. There are two types:

Ejection murmur	Due to turbulent flow in the outflow tracts from the heart
	Buzzing or blowing quality is heard in the 2nd–4th left intercostal space
Venous hum	Due to turbulent flow in the head and neck veins
	Continuous low pitched rumble heard beneath the clavicles
	Disappears on lying down and with compression of the ipsilateral jugular veins

Specific features

- Soft
- Change with altered position, i.e. sitting or lying down

- More pronounced if child tachycardic, e.g. fever, anaemia
- Child asymptomatic
- Normal examination:
  - Normal heart sounds
  - No thrill or radiation
  - Normal pulses
- Normal CXR and ECG

CARDIAC FAILURE

Clinical features

Symptoms	Sweating
	Poor feeding
	Failure to thrive
	Shortness of breath
	Recurrent chest infections
	Abdominal pain (big liver)
	Collapse/shock
	Tachypnoea, intercostal and subcostal recession
Signs	Tachycardia
	Cardiomegaly
	Hepatomegaly
	Gallop rhythm/murmur/muffled heart sounds
	Central cyanosis
	Cool peripheries

! **NB: Lungs often sound clear in neonates and infants, and peripheral oedema is not a feature.**

Management

- Sit child up
- Give oxygen
- Diuretics, e.g. furosemide
- Inotropes (in acute heart failure use IV dopamine or dobutamine, if less severe oral digoxin may be used)
- Vasodilators, e.g. captopril, hydralazine
- Consider intubation and ventilation

STRUCTURAL CONGENITAL HEART DISEASE

Incidence of structural congenital heart disease (CHD) is 8 in 1000 live births.

If CHD is suspected the child should be investigated with:

- CXR
- ECG
- Echocardiogram with Doppler studies
- Cardiac catheterization in some cases for pre-surgical evaluation, etc. (see p. 148–149)

CHD can be divided into *acyanotic* and *cyanotic* conditions.

Causes

CHD may be an isolated phenomenon; however, many syndromes, maternal disorders and drugs taken during pregnancy (teratogens) are associated with specific cardiac defects.

Recurrence risk   If one child affected – 3%
                   If two children affected – 10%
                   If three children affected – 25%

Associations with congenital heart disease

Inherited conditions	Genetics	Cardiac lesion(s)
Down syndrome	Tr21	AVSD, VSD, PDA, ASD
Edwards syndrome	Tr18	VSD, ASD, PDA, coarctation of the aorta
Turner syndrome	XØ	Bicuspid aortic valve, coarctation of the aorta, AS
Marfan syndrome	Fibrillin gene	Dissecting aortic aneurysm, AR, mitral valve prolapse
Noonan syndrome	PTPN11 gene	PS, hypertorphic cardiomyopathy, AVSD, coarctation of the aorta

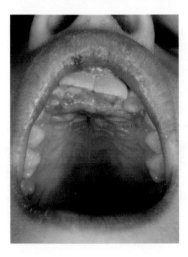

Figure 9.9 High arched palate in Marfan syndrome

Maternal disorders

Diabetes	Increased risk of all types of CHD
SLE, Sjögren	Complete heart block
Rubella	PDA, peripheral pulmonary stenosis

Teratogens

Alcohol	ASD, VSD, TOF, coarctation of aorta
Sodium valproate	Coarctation of aorta, interrupted aortic arch, AS, hypoplastic left heart, ASD, pulmonary atresia with no VSD, VSD

ACYANOTIC CONGENITAL HEART DISEASE

Patent ductus arteriosus

The ductus arteriosus normally closes during the first week of life. This closure is less likely to occur normally in sick premature neonates. Persistence of the arterial duct is also associated with maternal warfarin and phenytoin therapy and congenital rubella syndrome.

Clinical features and signs

Preterm infants	Systolic murmur at left sternal edge (LSE)
	Collapsing pulse (visible brachial or radial artery)
	Heart failure
Older children	Continuous murmur beneath left clavicle
	'Machinery murmur'
	Collapsing *'waterhammer'* pulse
	Heart failure if severe; eventual pulmonary hypertension
ECG	Usually normal
	May show LVH
	Indistinguishable from VSD
CXR	Increased pulmonary vascular markings
	May be normal

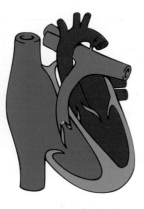

Murmur

S_1 A_2 P_2

(a)

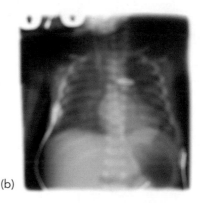

(b)

Figure 9.10 (a) Diagram of patent ductus arteriosus (PDA). (b) Chest X-ray showing clip *in situ* after ligation of PDA

Management

Premature neonate	Fluid restriction
	Indomethacin if < 34 weeks' gestation and within 3 weeks of birth (check renal function, platelets and predisposition to NEC first)
Older child	Transcatheter device occlusion, or
	Surgical ligation

> **!** **NB: A patent ductus arteriosus (PDA) should be closed even if asymptomatic because of the risk of infective endocarditis.**

Ventricular septal defect

This is the most common congenital heart defect (30% of all CHD). The symptoms and signs depend on the size of the hole and any other cardiac defects present. Large ventricular septal defects (VSDs) are less likely to close spontaneously.

Clinical features and signs

- Asymptomatic murmur
- Cardiac failure features
- Recurrent chest infections
- Endocarditis
- Pulmonary hypertension can develop if untreated large defect
- Cyanosis if Eisenmenger syndrome develops (see below). Unusual nowadays; develops around age 15–20 years in large untreated VSDs

Pulmonary hypertension: key findings

- RVH on the ECG
- Loud P2

Eisenmenger reaction

This is when persistently increased pulmonary blood flow causing **pulmonary hypertension** leads to increased pulmonary artery vascular resistance, and eventual **reversal of a left-to-right shunt**. It is becoming rarer as the diagnosis of CHD improves and there is earlier management. **VSD** was one of the commonest causes (Eisenmenger syndrome).

Murmur	Loud *pansystolic* murmur. NB: Smaller holes *may* have shorter, louder murmurs
	Lower LSE
	Parasternal thrill
	+ Mid-diastolic apical flow murmur if large defect (due to increased mitral flow)
Heart sounds	Loud P2 if pulmonary hypertension present
ECG	Normal or LVH
CXR	Cardiomegaly and increased pulmonary vascular markings
	May be normal

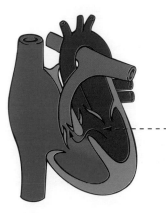

Murmur

S1   A2 P2

Figure 9.11 Ventricular septal defect

Management

Treat cardiac failure if present.

Surgical repair is not always necessary, as many will close spontaneously during the first few years of life. Surgical repair is needed if:

- Severe symptoms with failure to thrive
- Aortic regurgitation develops
- Persistent significant shunting > 10 years of age

Atrial septal defect

There are two types of atrial septal defect (ASD):

Ostium secundum ASD	More common form Defect(s) in the central atrial septum, which may be single or multiple
Ostium primum ASD	Failure of development of the septum primum (which divides the mitral and tricuspid valves) and usually also a cleft in the anterior leaflet of the mitral valve Associated with Down syndrome

	Ostium secundum ASD		**Ostium primum ASD**
Clinical features	Asymptomatic (common) Heart failure (rare until adult life) Atrial arrhythmias (onset 30–40 years)		Many asymptomatic (if small defect) Heart failure recurrent pneumonias (severity depending on A-V valve regurgitation)
Murmur	Ejection systolic Upper LSE ± Mid-diastolic tricuspid flow murmur at lower LSE		As for ostium secundum Also a mitral regurgitation murmur (apical, pansystolic)
Heart sounds	*Wide fixed splitting* 2nd heart sound		As for ostium secundum
ECG	RAD Partial RBBB (in 90%) RVH	*All right sided*	LAD or superior axis Partial RBBB RVH
CXR	Cardiomegaly Large pulmonary artery Increased pulmonary vascular markings		As for ostium secundum but more severe

Ostium secundum atrial septum defect

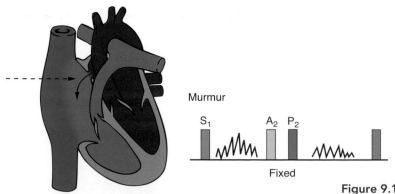

Murmur

Fixed

Figure 9.12 Atrial septal defect

Management

Ostium secundum ASD   Elective surgical or transcatheter device closure is carried out at age 3–5 years (or earlier if necessary) if the child is *symptomatic*

        Small defects will usually close spontaneously

Ostium primum ASD   Surgical repair is always required

Atrioventricular septal defect

This is a severe form of CHD where there is a contiguous atrial and ventricular septal defect, as well as abnormal formation of the atrioventricular valve. It is associated with Down syndrome.

Clinical features

The clinical features are usually severe with early development of heart failure, recurrent pneumonias, failure to thrive, and pulmonary hypertension due to the large left-to-right shunt across both atria and ventricles.

Signs

ECG   LAD or superior axis

               Biventricular hypertrophy

CXR   Cardiomegaly

               Pulmonary plethora

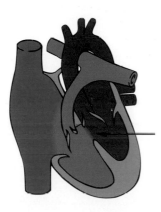

Figure 9.13 Atrioventricular septal defect

Repair is usually needed within the first 6 months of life to prevent pulmonary hypertension becoming irreversible.

Coarctation of the aorta

In coarctation of the aorta the descending aorta is constricted at any point between the transverse arch and the iliac bifurcation, but usually *just distal to the left subclavian artery*.

Associations

- Bicuspid aortic valve (40%)
- Mitral valve anomaly (10%)
- VSD
- Turner syndrome
- Berry aneurysm

Clinical features

These vary as it may present early or late:

Early presentation   Circulatory collapse during first week of life (when the ductus arteriosus closes)

Late presentation	Asymptomatic murmur discovered
	Hypertension in upper limbs only, weak pulses in legs
	Heart failure
	Subarachnoid haemorrhage (subacute bacterial endocarditis or Berry aneurysm)

Signs

- Weak or absent femoral pulses (± left radial pulse)
- Radiofemoral delay *may* be observed in older children
- Four limb BP measurements show higher BP in right arm (+ left arm) than legs
- Murmur – ejection systolic between the shoulder blades

ECG	RVH in neonates (because the right ventricle is systemic in the fetus)
	LVH in older children
CXR	May be normal
	Cardiomegaly + increased pulmonary vascular markings
	Rib notching (due to collaterals developing beneath the ribs) > age 8 years

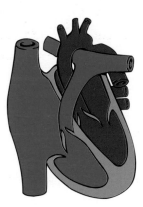

Figure 9.14 Coarctation of the aorta

Management

- In unstable neonates, initial stabilization with prostaglandin E2 (PGE2) is necessary to keep the ductus arteriosus open until the coarctation is repaired
- Then surgical repair with end-to-end repair or left subclavian flap
- Balloon dilatation with or without stenting can be used in older children
- Long term follow-up is necessary as re-coarctation rates are approximately 5%

> **!** **NB: The left subclavian flap procedure leaves the child with a left thoracotomy scar and an absent left radial pulse.**

Pulmonary stenosis

Clinical features

- Usually asymptomatic
- Right heart failure
- Cyanosis in critical neonatal pulmonary stenosis (duct-dependent circulation)
- Arrhythmias (later in life)

Signs

Murmur	Ejection systolic
	Upper left intercostal space
	Right ventricular heave
	No carotid radiation
	No carotid thrill
Heart sounds	Ejection click
	If severe, delayed and soft P2
ECG	RVH
CXR	Post-stenotic dilatation of the pulmonary artery can be seen at any age

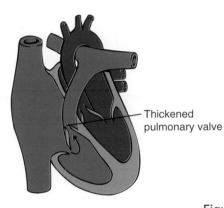

Murmur

S_1 EC A_2 P_2

EC = Ejection click

Figure 9.15 Pulmonary valve stenosis

Management

- If the pressure gradient across the pulmonary valve is > 50 mmHg or there is severe pulmonary valve thickening, then balloon dilatation may be necessary
- Surgical valvotomy is performed if balloon dilatation is unsuccessful

Aortic stenosis

This is usually anatomically a bicuspid valve.

Associations

- Aortic incompetence
- Coarctation of the aorta
- Mitral stenosis

Clinical features

Neonate	Severe heart failure
	Duct–dependent circulation
Older child	Asymptomatic murmur
	Decreased exercise tolerance
	Chest pain, syncope
	Sudden death
	Endocarditis

Signs

Murmur	Ejection systolic
	Aortic area, radiation to the neck
	Carotid thrill

Heart sounds	Paradoxical splitting of second heart sound and soft P2
	Apical ejection click (due to opening of deformed aortic valve)
Pulse	Slow rising plateau pulse
ECG	LVH
CXR	Post-stenotic aortic dilatation

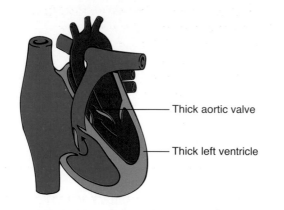

Figure 9.16 Aortic valve stenosis

Management

| Neonate | Valvotomy (balloon or surgical), then valve replacement later on |
| Older child | If symptomatic or resting pressure gradient across aortic valve > 50 mmHg, then valvotomy is required |

CYANOTIC CONGENITAL HEART DISEASE

In cyanotic CHD there is central cyanosis manifest by a blue coloured tongue. The cyanosis occurs because there is:

■ Right-to-left shunting with decreased pulmonary blood flow, e.g. Fallot, TA, PA, Ebstein anomaly, or
■ Abnormal mixing of blood with normal pulmonary blood flow, e.g. TGA, TAPVD, double inlet ventricle, hypoplastic left heart

Many of these disorders need patency of the ductus arteriosus to maintain circulation (they are *duct dependent*), and prostaglandin E2 (PGE2) is used in emergency to maintain the duct open.

Complications

■ Metabolic acidosis
■ Polycythaemia which may lead to thrombosis, embolism, haemorrhage and abscess formation
■ Necrotizing enterocolitis

Tetralogy of Fallot

This is the most common cyanotic CHD. The cyanosis results from left-to-right shunting.

Anatomical features

■ Malaligned VSD
■ RV outflow obstruction (valvular + infundibular stenosis)
■ Overriding aorta
■ RV hypertrophy

Duct-dependent circulations

These are circulations that are dependent on the ductus arteriosus remaining open to maintain pulmonary or systemic blood flow, and therefore deterioration occurs during the first week of life when the duct closes.

Duct-dependent systemic blood flow (cause of collapse in the first week)
Coarctation of the aorta
Critical aortic stenosis
Interrupted aortic arch
Hypoplastic left heart

Duct-dependent pulmonary blood flow (cause of cyanosis in the first week)
Transposition of the great arteries (TGA), and TGA with VSD
Pulmonary atresia with a VSD
Critical pulmonary stenosis
Tetralogy of Fallot (severe)
Tricuspid atresia (TA)
Ebstein anomaly

Prostaglandin E2 (PGE2)

This is a relatively specific ductal smooth muscle relaxant and is used in neonates as an emergency measure (by intravenous infusion) in duct-dependent circulations to keep the ductus arteriosus patent.

Side-effects   Hypotension, fever, apnoea and jitteriness

Associations
- Down syndrome
- DiGeorge syndrome (22q deletion)
- CHARGE syndrome
- VACTERL syndrome

Clinical presentation
- Cyanosis in first few days of life, or
- Murmur detected in first 2–3 months life, or
- **Hypercyanotic spells** (late infancy) where there is *infundibular spasm*:
  - Cyanosis or pallor
  - Occur in the morning and on crying
  - Acidosis
  - Child assumes squatting position (this increases pulmonary blood flow by increasing systemic vascular resistance)
  - Murmur becomes inaudible (due to *no* flow through pulmonary valve)

Signs

Murmur	Ejection systolic
	Upper LSE (due to flow through pulmonary artery)
Heart sounds	Single second heart sound
Cyanosis	
ECG	RAD
	RVH
CXR	Small boot-shaped heart 'coeur en sabot'
	Prominent pulmonary artery bay
	Right-sided aortic arch (30%)
	Pulmonary oligaemia

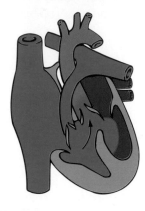

Murmur

Single
A₂

(a)

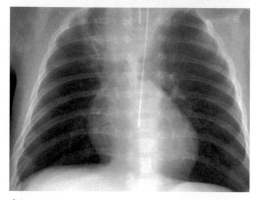

(b)

Figure 9.17 (a) Diagram of tetralogy of Fallot (TOF). (b) Chest X-ray of a 1-month-old child with TOF showing a right-sided aortic arch, elevated cardiac apex and pulmonary bay (courtesy of Dr Simon Padley and Dr Kapila Jain)

Management

- Palliative early surgery in the first few months of life if symptomatic with a modified Blalock–Taussig shunt (Gortex tube between subclavian artery and pulmonary artery)
- Corrective surgery at 4–12 months of age (patch closure of VSD and relief of obstruction of right ventricular outflow tract)

Management of a spell

- Put child in knee–chest position (increases systemic vascular resistance and therefore pulmonary flow, like squatting)
- IV fluids
- Morphine
- Propanolol IV (decreases infundibular spasm)
- May require anaesthesia and ventilation and/or emergency surgery

Tricuspid atresia

- Absence of tricuspid valve
- ASD
- VSD
- Small, non-functional right ventricle

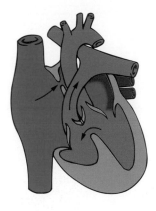

1. *Absence of tricuspid valve*
2. *ASD*
3. *VSD*
4. *Small, non-functional right ventricle*

Figure 9.18 Tricuspid atresia

Clinical features

- Cyanosis usually present at birth and increases with age as pulmonary blood flow decreases
- Systolic murmur at LSE
- Single second heart sound

Signs

ECG Superior axis
Tall P wave in V2
(NB: Severe cyanosis with superior axis can only be TA)
CXR Small heart with pulmonary oligaemia

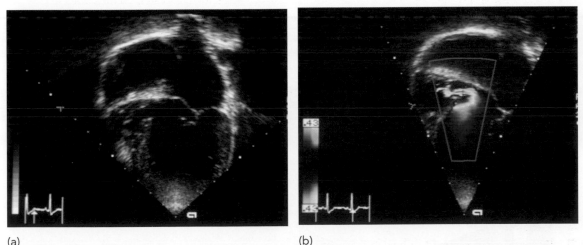

(a)   (b)

Figure 9.19 Echocardiograms. (a) Tricuspid atresia. (b) Tricuspid atresia with flow through a ventricular septal defect (courtesy of Dr Rob Yates)

Management

- Initial palliation with Blalock–Taussig shunt if too little pulmonary blood flow, or pulmonary artery band if too much pulmonary artery blood flow
- Definitive palliation at 2–5 years with the Fontan procedure (SVC and IVC connected to pulmonary artery). There are long term problems, as there is only one effective ventricle and atrial arrhythmias can develop

Hypoplastic left heart

There is underdevelopment of the left side of the heart.

- Small left ventricle
- Small mitral valve
- Aortic valve atresia
- Small ascending aorta

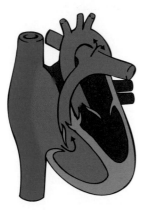

Figure 9.20 Hypoplastic left heart

Neonates present with features of a duct-dependent systemic circulation, i.e. cyanosis, collapse, acidosis and impalpable peripheral pulses, on closure of the ductus arteriosus on day 3.

Management

This condition may be considered inoperable, but a series of surgical procedures to rebuild the aorta and use the right ventricle as a systemic ventricle (the Norwood procedure) can be done.

Transposition of the great arteries

In this condition, the aorta and pulmonary artery arise from the wrong ventricles respectively, creating two parallel circulations. Survival is due to mixing of blood at the:

- Ductus arteriosus
- Foramen ovale
- VSD or ASD if present

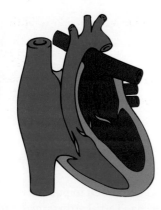

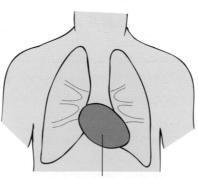

'Egg on side'-shaped heart

Figure 9.21
Transposition of the great arteries

Clinical features
- Cyanosis within hours
- Acidosis
- No murmur (there may be a systolic murmur from increased pulmonary flow)
- Single second heart sound

Signs

ECG   Normal
CXR   'Egg on side' appearance of heart (due to narrow upper mediastinum)
             Increased pulmonary markings

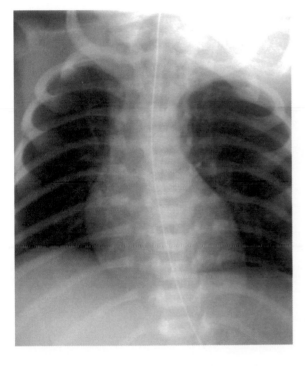

Figure 9.22 Chest X-ray of a 1-month-old child with abnormal mediastinum due to transposition of the great arteries ('egg on side' appearance) (courtesy of Dr Simon Padley and Dr Kapila Jain)

Management
- Emergency neonatal prostaglandin PGE2 infusion
- Atrial balloon septostomy (Rashkind)
- Corrective surgery with anatomical correction (arterial switch procedure) within a few weeks of birth

CARDIAC SURGERY

Cardiac surgery may be *corrective* or *palliative*, i.e. to improve symptoms but not be corrective.

The principles of managing cardiac surgery are:

Pre-operative tests   Blood tests, CXR, ECG, echocardiogram (throat swab, urine specimen)
                       Meet surgeon and sign consent form
Intraoperative care   Heart–lung bypass machine for open heart surgery
Postoperative care   Cardiac intensive care:
- Ventilation (IPPV) or face mask/head box oxygen
- ECMO (extracorporeal membrane oxygenation) may be necessary for a few days

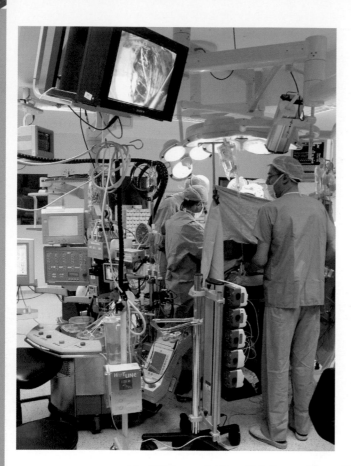

Figure 9.23 Child in theatre having open cardiac surgery

- CVP, arterial line (ABG samples and BP monitoring)
- NG tube, IV lines, urinary catheter
- Pacing wires from heart if previously on bypass

Complications

Immediate	Haemorrhage
	Arrhythmias – temporary pacing with external pacemaker may be necessary
Early	Phrenic nerve damage – treat with diaphragmatic plication
	Infection (wound or chest infection)
	Renal failure (secondary to prolonged bypass, treat with peritoneal dialysis
	Chylothorax (thoracic duct damage) – treat with drainage, low fat diet, TPN or surgical ligation
	Vocal cord paralysis (laryngeal nerve injury) – improves over time
	Brain damage (prolonged hypoxia from unstable postoperative course)

RHEUMATIC FEVER

Rheumatic fever is an inflammatory disease that occurs in response to Group A β-haemolytic streptococcal infection. It is now rare due to antibiotics.

A streptococcal infection, usually a sore throat or scarlet fever, is followed around 2–6 weeks later by a polyarthritis, fever and malaise, and cardiac symptoms (the exact symptoms depending on the organs involved).

Diagnosis is based on the Duckett–Jones criteria, and requires two major or one major plus two minor criteria.

Duckett–Jones criteria

Major criteria		Minor criteria
■ *Carditis* –	endocarditis, i.e. murmur; myocarditis, i.e. heart failure; pericarditis, i.e. pericardial rub, pericardial effusion	■ Fever
		■ Arthralgia
		■ Long PR interval
		■ Raised ESR, CRP
■ *Polyarthritis* –	'flitting' arthritis of medium joints, very tender	■ Leukocytosis
		■ Previous rheumatic fever
■ *Syndenham chorea* –	'St Vitus dance', lasts 3–6 months (involuntary movements)	
■ *Erythema marginatum* –	pale red rings and segments of rings mainly on the trunk (also limbs), in recurrent crops each lasting hours–days	
■ *Subcutaneous nodules* –	hard, painless, pea-like nodules on extensor surfaces	

Investigations

■ To detect evidence of recent streptococcal infection: throat culture, serology, ASOT (positive), blood cultures

■ To investigate the above symptoms and signs: general bloods (FBC, U&E, creatinine), acute phase proteins, ECG, CXR, echocardiogram

Management

■ Bed rest

■ High-dose aspirin

■ Steroids

■ Heart failure treatment

■ Benzathine penicillin intramuscularly or oral penicillin

■ Then **life-long penicillin prophylaxis** (daily oral or monthly intramuscular penicillin)

INFECTIVE ENDOCARDITIS

Infective endocarditis is seen in particular in abnormal heart valves – children with congenital heart disease (especially cyanotic, but not secundum ASD), previously damaged or prosthetic valves. A high velocity flow increases the risk of damage to the endocardium. Endocarditis can be *acute* or *chronic*.

Infecting organisms

■ α-Haemolytic streptococcus (*Streptococcus viridans*) (50% of SBE)

■ *Staphylococcus aureus* (50% of acute endocarditis; central lines and cardiac surgery are risk factors)

■ *Enterococcus faecalis*

■ *Staph. epidermidis* (central lines and cardiac surgery are risk factors)

■ *Candida albicans* (central lines and immunosuppression are risk factors)

■ Aspergillus, brucellosis, histoplasmosis, *Coxiella burnetii* (Q fever) (all rare)

Clinical features

■ Sustained fever, night sweats, malaise

■ Development of *new* cardiac murmur

- Persistence of fever after acute illness (acute endocarditis)
- Splenomegaly and splenic rub
- Small vascular lesions:
  - **Splinter haemorrhages**
  - **Roth spots** (retinal haemorrhages)
  - **Janeway lesions** (red macules on thenar and hypothenar eminences)
  - **Osler's nodes** (hard painful embolic swellings on toes, fingers, soles and palms)
- Major embolic phenomena (cerebral, coronary, pulmonary and peripheral arterial emboli)
- Renal lesions
- Arthritis of major joints
- Clubbing

! NB: Clinical features may be subtle, therefore *always* think of SBE in a child with a known cardiac defect who is unwell.

Investigations

Blood tests	*Serial* blood cultures (at least three sets and more if negative)
	FBC (anaemia almost invariably)
	ESR (↑) and CRP (↑), immunoglobulins
	C3 (low due to immune complex formation)
	Serology (chlamydia, candida, coxiella and brucella) if cultures negative
Urine dipstick	Microscopic haematuria and proteinuria
Echocardiogram	To demonstrate vegetations
CXR and ECG	

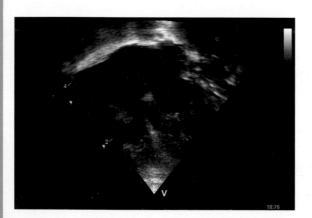

Figure 9.24 Echocardiogram showing vegetation in infective endocarditis (courtesy of Dr Rob Yates)

Management

- 4–6 weeks of antibiotic therapy (initially IV for 2 weeks) with suitable antibiotic
- Antibiotic prophylaxis for future procedures
- Surgery if extensive destructive valve damage, cardiac failure, vegetations or embolism

Antibiotic prophylaxis to prevent infective endocarditis

'At-risk' individuals should receive prophylactic antibiotics for certain procedures to prevent endocarditis. These are children with:

- Heart valve lesions, septal defects, patent ductus arteriosus or prosthetic valves
- Operated congenital heart disease

Different antibiotic regimens are recommended (outlined in the *BNF*) for:

- Dental procedures
- Upper respiratory tract procedures
- Genitourinary procedures
- Obstetric, gynaecological but no longer gastrointestinal procedures

MYOCARDITIS

Myocarditis is inflammation of the heart with necrosis and fibrosis, resulting in serious weakening of the heart muscle, with cardiac and respiratory failure. The most common cause in children is *viral infection*. Most cases of mild inflammation will resolve spontaneously but in a proportion, irreversible devastating damage is done to the heart.

Causes

- Infections:
    – Viral, e.g. coxsackie B, adenovirus
    – Bacterial, e.g. diphtheria, rickettsia
    – Fungal, parasitic
- Toxic, e.g. sepsis, drugs
- Connective tissue disease
- Idiopathic

Clinical features

- Cardiac failure, i.e. tachycardia, weak pulses, respiratory distress
- Arrhythmias
- Sudden death
- May be asymptomatic (in adolescents)

Investigations

Bloods	Cardiac enzymes elevated (CK, LDH, troponin)
	Check viral serology (specific IgM and PCR)
CXR	Gross cardiomegaly, pulmonary plethora
ECG	Arrhythmias
Echocardiogram	Poor ventricular function, large heart, pericardial effusion

Management

This is supportive with management of the cardiac failure and arrhythmias. These children are often seriously unwell, requiring intensive care, and ECMO may be necessary. If there is severe cardiac damage, a cardiac transplant may be needed.

DILATED CARDIOMYOPATHY

Dilated cardiomyopathy (DCM) is the most common type of cardiomyopathy seen in children. It is a disease involving dysfunction of the cardiomyocytes resulting in dilatation and impaired function of the left ± right ventricles. There are many causes and associations; however, most cases remain idiopathic.

Causes/associations

Genetic diseases	Familial, muscular dystrophy, Freidreich ataxia, mitochondrial abnormalities
Infections	Post-viral myocarditis, e.g. coxsackie, echovirus, diphtheria; rheumatic fever, sepsis, HIV, Chagas' disease (trypanosomiasis)
Nutrition	Selenium, carnitine, calcium, or thiamine deficiency, malnutrition Severe chronic anaemia or iron overload, e.g. in thalassaemia
Toxins	Chemotherapy, e.g. doxorubicin, adriamycin, cyclophosphamide

Clinical features

- Heart failure
- Arrhythmias
- Embolism

Investigations

CXR	Cardiomegaly and pulmonary plethora
ECG	LVH, non-specific T wave abnormalities
Echocardiogram	**Large baggy heart** (poorly contracting heart with atrial and ventricular dilatation) Reduced ejection fraction, mitral and tricuspid regurgitation
Other	To look for the cause: metabolic screen, nutritional bloods and genetic screening if indicated

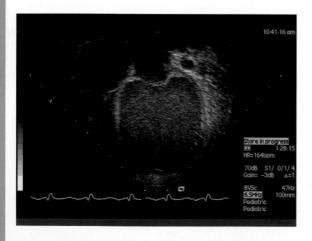

Figure 9.25 Echocardiogram showing grossly dilated left ventricle in dilated cardiomyopathy (courtesy of Dr Rob Yates)

Management

This is supportive (of heart failure and arrhythmias) and anticoagulants (aspirin or warfarin). A cardiac transplant may be needed in severe disease.

ARRHYTHMIAS

SUPRAVENTRICULAR TACHYCARDIA

This is the commonest arrhythmia in children. It is a re-entry tachycardia with premature reactivation of the atria via an accessory pathway.

Supraventricular tachycardia (SVT) rates	
Neonates	> 220 bpm
Older children	> 180 bpm

Causes

Congenital	Accessory pathway, e.g. Wolff–Parkinson–White syndrome
	Structural CHD (unusual)
Stimulants	e.g. caffeine, hot baths, stress

Clinical presentation

In utero	Fetal tachyarrhythmia which can cause hydrops fetalis or intrauterine death
Infant	Poor cardiac output, cardiac failure
Older child	Palpitations, dizziness, shortness of breath, chest pain, collapse

Investigations

■ ECG (particularly of the *tachycardia*; may need 24-h or 7-day recording to ensure a run of tachycardia included)

■ Echocardiogram to exclude structural CHD (although an unusual cause)

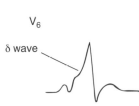

V$_6$

δ wave

- ■ δ-wave
- ■ short PR interval
- ■ wide QRS complex

Figure 9.26 ECG in Wolff–Parkinson–White syndrome (δ-wave, short PR interval, wide QRS complex)

Management

Various techniques and drugs are used to stop an SVT (see below).

■	Vagal stimulation	■ *Diving reflex*:
		Babies – immerse head and face in basin of ice-cold water for 5 s
		Older child – place polythene bag full of ice-cold water on face for 15 s
		or Valsalva manoeuvre
		■ *Unilateral carotid sinus massage* (older children only)
■	Adenosine	Drug treatment of choice in hospital, given by a rapid IV bolus. It temporarily blocks AV conduction so the heart can revert back to normal sinus rhythm
■	Synchronized DC cardioversion	1–2 J/kg, if above fails. Child is sedated or anaesthetized first
■	Other drugs	IV flecanide or amiodarone
		IV or oral digoxin

Maintenance therapy to prevent recurrence may be needed, and this can be achieved with flecanide, propranolol, digoxin or amiodarone.

VENTRICULAR TACHYCARDIA

VT is three or more ventricular beats in a row at a rate of at least 120/min.

Causes

- Metabolic, e.g. calcium, magnesium and potassium imbalances
- Long QT syndrome
- Infantile ventricular tachycardia (VT)
- Post cardiac surgery

Management

- DC cardioversion, IV lignocaine (lidocaine) or IV amiodarone
- Adenosine may be used to slow the rate to allow the diagnosis to be made, but if there is doubt as to whether an arrhythmia is VT or SVT, *always treat it as VT*

Differences between SVT and VT

VT	SVT
Wide complexes	Narrow complexes
Irregular complexes	Usually regular
A–V dissociation	A–V association
Intermittent P waves seen	Regular P waves (if seen)
Fusion and capture beats	
Fusion beat = early beat with abnormal QRS	
Capture beat = early beat with normal QRS	

CONGENITAL COMPLETE HEART BLOCK

Associations

- Maternal SLE or Sjögren syndrome (maternal anti-Rho antibodies cause atrophy and fibrosis of the AV node)
- Structural CHD (15% of cases), e.g. AVSD, corrected TGA

Clinical features

It may be detected *in utero* with fetal bradycardia, hydrops fetalis or intrauterine fetal death, or may present in the neonatal period with bradycardia and heart failure.

Investigations

- 24-h ECG (the heart block may be intermittent)
- CXR and echocardiogram
- Anti-Ro and anti-La antibodies

Treatment

The placement of a pacemaker is necessary if there are *symptoms* or if the daytime *pulse rate* is < 60 bpm in an infant or < 50 bpm in an older child.

NB: **Children are different from adults because of their inability to increase their cardiac output by altering their stroke volume, and their reliance on heart rate.**

Clinical scenario

A 6-week-old girl with trisomy 21 is seen in a children's hospital because of a fever and increasing shortness of breath. She has no respiratory compromise, but a saturation monitor reveals an oxygen saturation of 88% in air. Supplemental oxygen fails to improve the saturation reading.

On examination she has a long systolic murmur which is associated with a thrill, most evident over the left lower sternal border and apex. A left parasternal heave is noted. On dip-sticking her urine she has haematuria.

1. What is the most likely anatomical problem?
2. Why might she have haematuria?
3. What would be your first two most important investigations?
4. What medications would be most appropriate for treatment of these conditions?

ANSWERS

1. AVSD
2. Subacute bacterial endocarditis
3. ECHO, blood culture
4. Appropriate antibiotics following culture of bacteria and sensitivities, diuretics in case of heart failure e.g. furosemide and spironolactone

FURTHER READING

Anderson R, Baker E, Redington A, Rigby M, Penny D, Wernovsky G (eds.). *Paediatric Cardiology*, 3rd edn. London: Churchill Livingstone, 2009.

Archer N, Burch M. *Paediatric Cardiology: An Introduction*. London: Hodder Arnold, 1998.

Berhman R, Kliegman R, Jenson H, Stanton B. *Nelson Textbook of Pediatrics*, 18th edn. London: Saunders, 2007.

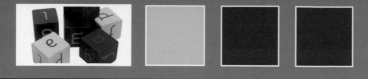

10 Gastroenterology

- Gastro-oesophageal reflux
- Malabsorption
- Gastroenteritis
- Diarrhoea
- Peptic ulcer disease (PUD)
- Inflammatory bowel disease
- Constipation
- Faecal soiling
- Acute pancreatitis
- Gastrointestinal tract bleeding
- Gastrointestinal tract tumours
- Further reading

GASTRO-OESOPHAGEAL REFLUX

This is the passage of gastric contents involuntarily into the oesophagus. It is the result of an incompetent or inappropriately relaxing lower oesophageal sphincter, usually secondary to immaturity.

Associations

- Cerebral palsy
- Hiatus hernia
- Thoracic stomach
- Coeliac disease
- Raised intracranial pressure
- UTIs
- Fictitious or induced illness (formerly called Munchausen syndrome by proxy)
- CHD
- CF

Clinical features

- Vomiting (± altered blood) NB: Possetting is a normal physiological phenomenon
- Crying, food refusal, poor sleeping, irritability
- Usually resolves spontaneously by 12–18 months of age

Complications (in the presence of which GOR is termed gastro-oesophageal reflux *disease* [GORD])

- Faltering growth
- Oesophagitis ± oesophageal stricture
- Apnoea, ALTE, SIDS

- Aspiration, wheezing, hoarseness, recurrent chest infection
- Iron-deficiency anaemia
- Seizure-like events, torticollis

Investigations

These are necessary only if there is failure to resolve with simple measures, or the reflux is complicated (GORD). The investigations are complementary to each other.

Oesophageal pH measurement	% of time pH < 4.0 in 24 h: > 10% = abnormal if < 1 year old > 6% = abnormal if > 1 year old	(NB: only gives information about acid reflux and infants usually reflux in the post-prandial phase when gastric acid is buffered by milk)
Barium swallow and meal	Looking for malrotation, hiatus hernia, oesophageal stricture i.e. anatomical abnormalities only	
Endoscopy	Looking for oesophagitis, stricture, enteropathy or in older children other causes of dyspepsia such as gastritis or peptic ulcer disease	
Other	CXR, urine M, C & S, Hb and iron studies, faecal occult blood. Remember raised intracranial pressure may cause reflux	

Management

Position	Nurse on L side, 30 degrees head up
Thicken feeds	Add thickeners, e.g. Carobel, Nestargel, or use prethickened feeds, e.g. Enfamil AR, SMA Staydown
Change feeds	Consider changing feeds to hydrosylate, e.g. Nutramigen, Pregestamil, Peptijunior, or elemental amino-acid based (Neocate) (see ch. 11)
Drugs	Antacid, e.g. Gaviscon infant Prokinetic, e.g. domperidone H2 blocker, e.g. ranitidine Proton pump inhibitor, eg. omeprazole
Surgery	If medical management fails over a 3-month period, consider an anti-reflux procedure, e.g. Nissan fundoplication, but only if life-threatening reflux as it normally resolves spontaneously by 12–18 months of age in any event

Possetting

This is small volume vomiting during or between feeds. The infant will be thriving and there is no cause for concern. Management is with reassurance.

MALABSORPTION

Malabsorption may be *generalized* or *specific* where individual transport mechanisms or enzymes are defective. Generalized malabsorption presents with faltering growth, growth retardation and often steatorrhoea. Specific malabsorption may present with different features.

Investigations

The list is exhaustive and therefore investigations must be symptom-led. Some investigations to consider are:

Bloods	FBC, iron studies, bicarbonate, U&Es, creatinine, plasma lipids, coeliac screen, CF genotype

Causes of malabsorption	
Generalized	
Gut	Short gut syndrome, blind loop syndrome, chronic infection (giardiasis, immunodeficiency), coeliac disease, food intolerance, (e.g. cow's milk protein, soya), diffuse mucosal lesions, e.g. congenital microvillous atrophy
Pancreas	Cystic fibrosis, chronic pancreatitis, Shwachman–Diamond syndrome
Liver	Cholestasis of any cause, e.g. biliary atresia
Specific	
Protein	Amino acid transport defects, e.g. cysteinuria
Carbohydrate	Disaccharidase deficiencies, e.g. lactase, sucrase–isomaltase, glucose–
Fat	galactose malabsorption
Elements	Abetalipoproteinaemia
Vitamins	Chloride diarrhoea, acrodermatitis enteropathica (zinc)
	Juvenile pernicious anaemia (B12)

Stool	Electrolytes, fats, reducing substances
	Microscopy and culture (cysts, parasites)
	Faecal elastase ($\downarrow$ in pancreatic exocrine insufficiency) and faecal α-1 antitrypsin ($\uparrow$ in protein-losing enteropathy)
	Giardia-specific Ag
Sweat test	Cystic fibrosis
Radiology	AXR, CXR, barium studies
Endoscopy	With duodenal/jejunal biopsies and duodenal juice microscopy (for giardia)
Breath tests	Lactose, sucrose and lactulose breath tests (the latter for bacterial overgrowth)

Management
- Paediatric dietician and a team approach is vital
- Specific approach tailored to condition

FOOD INTOLERANCES

- 'Intolerance': any inability to tolerate a dietary component encompassing 'Allergy': an immunologically mediated food reaction

Dietary protein intolerance

This is most commonly due to **cow's milk protein (CMP) intolerance**. Other protein intolerances occur to soya, wheat, eggs and fish. IgG or T-cell mediated and distinct from Type I IgE-mediated reactions like asthma, eczema or hay fever, although these conditions may overlap in an individual.

Associations
- Atopy
- IgA deficiency and IgG subclass abnormalities

Clinical features

- Diarrhoea (due to associated food-protein induced enterocolitis syndrome [FPIES]), vomiting, faltering growth
- Gastro-oesophageal reflux
- Recurrent mouth ulcers, allergic pancolitis
- History of contact allergy or anaphylaxis (rare) to cow's milk, family history of reaction to foods
- Atopic history (eczema, asthma)

Investigations

Diagnosis may be established by:

- Trial of CMP elimination diet for at least 2 weeks without biopsy, or
- Small intestinal biopsy – patchy, partial villous atrophy, eosinophils in lamina propria
- Other investigations – IgE ↑, eosinophilia

Management

Elimination diet using casein-hydrolysate based formula or amino-acid based formula (see p. 193). Breast feeding mothers need to avoid cow's milk and soya protein. 50% of children recover within 1 year and most of the rest by 2 years.

> **!** **NB: 40% of children with CMP sensitivity also have soya protein sensitivity and need CMP- and soya-free diet, e.g. Nutramigen, Pregestamil, Peptijunior, Aptamil Pepti or elemental amino-acid based milk such as Nescate LCP or Nutramigen AA.**

Post-gastroenteritis intolerance

- Transient condition, occurring after acute gastroenteritis, and resulting in persistent diarrhoea (> 14 days)
- Child has usually developed a temporary intolerance to lactose secondary to CMP sensitization and villous damage
- Diagnosis is made on the history and presence of reducing substances in the stool (positive Clinitest). Test for glucose in the stool (Clinistix) is negative
- Usually resolves on a CMP and lactose-free diet

Lactose intolerance

Lactase, the enzyme necessary for digesting lactose (the sugar in milk), appears late in fetal life and falls after age 3 years. 40% of people from an Oriental background have late-onset (classically age 10–14 years) lactose intolerance.

Primary infant onset lactose intolerance is rare and should not be confused with CMP allergy/intolerance.

Causes

- Transient post-gastroenteritis
- Primary lactase deficiency (very rare)
- Late-onset lactase deficiency (common): 10–14 years

Clinical features

After ingestion of lactose – explosive watery diarrhoea, abdominal distension, flatulence, loud audible bowel sounds.

Investigations

- Stool chromatography positive for lactose, i.e. > 1% present
- Lactose hydrogen breath test

Management

- Lactose-free formula feed for infants
- Milk-free diet with calcium supplements for older children. Powdered or liquid lactose can be purchased over the counter

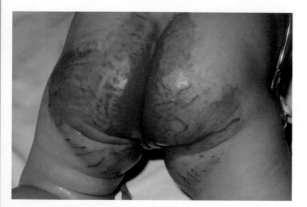

Figure 10.1 Chemical dermatitis secondary to malabsorbed disaccharides

Coeliac disease

A dietary **gliadin** intolerance resulting in small bowel mucosal damage. Gliadin, a fraction of the protein gluten, is found in wheat, barley, oats (marginally) and rye. First presentation may be on introduction of dietary gluten at around 4–6 months of age.

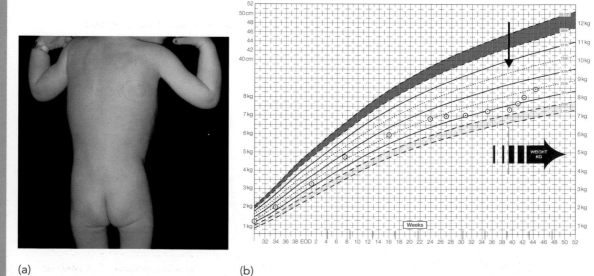

(a)   (b)

Figure 10.2 Coeliac disease. (a) Buttock wasting in a child. (b) Growth chart of an infant. Note the tail-off of growth (faltering growth) after gluten-containing solids were introduced around 6 months of age, and the catch-up growth after a gluten-free diet

Associations

- HLA DQ2, DQ8
- IDDM
- Down syndrome
- Hypothyroidism

Clinical features

- Faltering growth, anorexia, vomiting, diarrhoea
- Irritable, unhappy
- Abdominal pain, rectal prolapse, smelly stools
- Signs of pallor, abdominal distension, clubbing and malabsorption
- More subtle presentation with growth less than expected from parental centiles
- **Dermatitis herpetiformis** – itchy vesicles on extensor surfaces; improves on a gluten-free diet; IgA Abs in normal and perilesional skin, but *not* active lesion. Treatment is with dapsone
- Selective IgA deficiency
- Intestinal lymphoma, bowel carcinoma, osteopaenia in later life

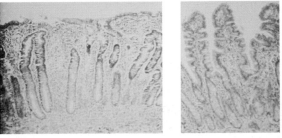

(a)   (b)

Figure 10.3 Small bowel biopsy section showing villous atrophy and crypt hyperplasia in coeliac disease (a) as compared to the normal villi and crypts (b)

Investigations

- IgA anti-endomysial and tissue transglutaminase (+TG) Abs with total IgA level – very sensitive and specific. Antibodies not seen in IgA-deficient individuals +TG IgG also now available. No place for anti-gliadin antibodies
- Jejunal biopsy – 'gold standard'; total or subtotal villous atrophy seen on small bowel biopsy by endoscopy
- Gluten challenge – now only necessary in children diagnosed under 2 years, as they may become normal when > 2 years
- Other findings include anaemia (dimorphic blood film from iron and folate deficiency) and hypoalbuminaemia
- Occasionally water-soluble and fat-soluble vitamin deficiencies, e.g. clotting disturbance secondary to vitamin K malabsorption

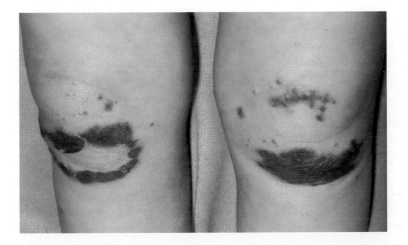

Figure 10.4 Dermatitis herpetiformis in a child with coeliac disease. The vesicles are intensely itchy and almost always burst before they are seen secondary to scratching

Causes of villous atrophy on jejunal biopsy	
Subtotal	**Partial**
Coeliac disease	Cow's milk protein intolerance
Giardia lamblia	Soya intolerance
Tropical sprue	Post-gastroenteritis
(very rare)	Immunodeficiency, e.g. SCID, chemotherapy, AIDS

Management

A lifetime gluten-free diet. This also reduces the risk of complications such as intestinal lymphoma.

SHWACHMAN–DIAMOND SYNDROME

This is an inherited autosomal recessive condition due to a mutation in the *SBDS* gene on chromosome 7q11. Incidence 1 in 50 000 births, male:female = 1:2.

The syndrome involves:

- Pancreatic exocrine insufficiency (with subsequent malabsorption)
- Haematological dysfunction:
  - Neutropaenia, often cyclical, progression to myeloid arrest can occur
  - Neutrophil chemotactic defects
  - Thrombocytopaenia (70%), anaemia (50%)
- Skeletal abnormalities:
  - Metaphyseal dysostosis
  - Short stature and faltering growth

Management is with pancreatic replacement therapy, and steroids or androgens. Average survival time is 35 years. Stem cell transplant and GCSF have been used.

GASTROENTERITIS

Causes

Viral	Rotavirus (winter epidemics, cause 60% of cases in < 2 year olds in winter)
	Norwalk virus, adenovirus (40 and 41), astrovirus
Bacterial	Staphylococcus (exotoxin)
	Watery diarrhoea – enterotoxigenic *E. coli* (ETEC, *traveller's diarrhoea*), *Vibrio cholera*
	Bloody diarrhoea – enteroinvasive *E. coli* (EIEC), enterohaemorrhagic *E. coli* (EHEC), shigella, *Campylobacter jejuni*, *Salmonella enteritidis*, yersinia
Protozoal	Giardia, cryptosporidium, amoebiasis

Clinical features

- Acute-onset vomiting and diarrhoea
- Abdominal pain and distension
- Mild pyrexia
- Invasive bacterial infection – unwell, high fever, blood and mucoid stool

Examination findings

- Assess child for **dehydration**, which is difficult to do accurately. Below 5% dehydration there are no reliable clinical findings. Dehydration is usually hyponatraemic or isotonic

- Other possible findings:
  - Acidosis – tachypnoea
  - Potassium depletion – hypotonia, weakness
  - Hypocalcaemia – neuromuscular irritability
  - Hypoglycaemia – lethargy, coma, convulsions

Hypernatraemic dehydration
- Unusual and potentially serious
- Irritable with doughy skin and relatively good circulation
- Water shifts from *intracellular* to *extracellular*, and therefore the signs of extracellular fluid loss are *reduced*
- Rehydration should be slow (over 48 h) to avoid rapid brain rehydration and subsequent raised intracranial pressure

Dehydration assessment

	Moderate (5–10%)	Severe (> 10%)
Condition	Restless/lethargic	Drowsy
Eyes	Sunken	Very sunken
Fontanelle	Sunken	Very sunken
Tears	Reduced	Absent
Mucous membranes	Dry	Very dry
Tissue elasticity	Reduced	Absent
CRT	2–4 s	> 4 s
Pulse	Tachycardia	Thready, very tachycardic
BP	Normal	Normal or low
Urine output	Reduced	Reduced/absent

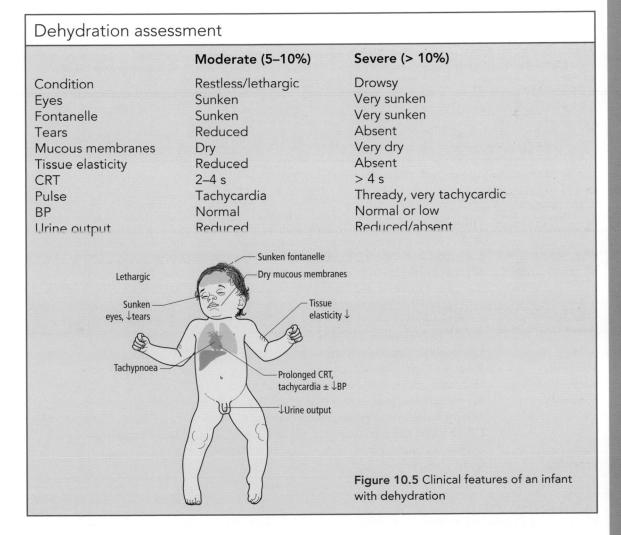

Lethargic

Sunken eyes, ↓tears

Tachypnoea

Sunken fontanelle

Dry mucous membranes

Tissue elasticity ↓

Prolonged CRT, tachycardia ± ↓BP

↓Urine output

Figure 10.5 Clinical features of an infant with dehydration

Investigations

These depend on the clinical state of the child.

Stool	Virology, M, C & S, 'hot stool' for cysts and ova
Bloods	FBC, haematocrit, U&E, creatinine, glucose, capillary blood gas, plasma and urine osmolality, as necessary

Management

Mild (< 5%)   Oral/NG rehydration therapy (ORT) for 24 h or until diarrhoea settles, then milk and light diet. ORT fluid contains glucose and sodium because they are absorbed across even a damaged mucosa by a joint mechanism, and water absorption follows by osmosis

NB: Breast feeding can continue with initial ORT

Moderate/severe (> 5%)   Admit

If the CRT > 3 s or acidotic breathing is apparent, intravenous rehydration is necessary

If in shock, IV volume expansion with 20–30 mL/kg 0.9% saline, then rehydrate over 24 h

---

Rehydration fluids

(1) **Deficit** = % dehydration x weight (kg) + (2) **maintenance fluids** + (3) **continuing losses**

Use 5% dextrose/0.45% saline (or 5% dextrose/0.9% saline) depending on the plasma sodium and calculated total body sodium. If severe acidosis (pH < 7.0) treat with bicarbonate (half the deficit).

For maintenance fluid calculation see p. 480.

Complications

Renal   **Oliguria**, i.e. < 200 mL/m^2/day or < 0.5 mL/kg/h.
- NB: If pre-renal failure – urine osmolality > 500, urine Na < 10 mmol/L, urine urea > 250 mmol/L, urine:plasma osomolality ratio > 1.3
- *Management* – urgent intravenous volume re-expansion. If no recovery of renal function, then give minimal maintenance fluid plus losses only, with no potassium. Dialysis is necessary if the fluid, electrolyte or acid–base status does not correct. Recovery is seen with the polyuric phase of acute tubular necrosis

Renal venous thrombosis (haematuria + renal mass, see ch. 13)

Haemolytic uraemic syndrome (see ch. 13)

Pulmonary oedema   From fluid overload

Convulsions   Several possible causes – hypernatraemia, hypoglycaemia, febrile convulsions, other electrolyte disturbance, cerebral haemorrhage

Check blood glucose, U&E, Mg, Ca and cranial USS, and treat accordingly

Prolonged diarrhoea   > 14 days (see p. 182)

DIARRHOEA

The pathogenesis of most episodes of diarrhoea can be explained by osmotic, secretory or motility disorders, or a combination of these. In **osmotic diarrhoea** the underlying mechanism is a high osmotic load of intraluminal content and in **secretory diarrhoea** the mechanism is active chloride secretion.

Osmotic diarrhoea

Common

Stops when feeding discontinued
Reducing substances in stool
Stool electrolytes ↓ (Na < 50 mEq/L)

Examples:
Lactase deficiency
Drugs, e.g. lactulose
Maldigestion, e.g. Crohn, CF
Transport mechanism disorder,
e.g. glucose–galactose malabsorption

Secretory diarrhoea

Rare

Does not stop when feeding discontinued
Very watery, severe diarrhoea
Stool electrolytes ↑ (Na > 90 mEq/L)

Examples:
Cholera, toxigenic *E. coli*
Congenital chloride diarrhoea
Bile salt/fatty acid malabsorption

Motility disorders

Increased motility	Decreased transit time results in diarrhoea
	Causes include IBS, post-vagotomy and dumping syndrome
Decreased motility	Bacterial overgrowth results in diarrhoea
	Causes include intestinal pseudo-obstruction

Combined mechanisms

- Occurs with *mucosal invasion*, resulting in inflammation, decreased colonic reabsorption and increased motility. This is seen in dysentery from bacterial infection, e.g. salmonella, and amoebic infection
- *Decreased surface area* results in both osmotic and motility disorders, as seen in short bowel syndrome

Causes of diarrhoea

Acute	Gastroenteritis	
	Systemic infection	
	Toxic ingestion	
Chronic	Toddler's diarrhoea	Inflammatory bowel disease
	Post-infectious	Hirschsprung's disease
	Anxiety	Immunodeficiency
	Irritable bowel syndrome	Inborn error of metabolism, e.g. congenital chloride diarrhoea (rare)
	Chronic infection, e.g. giardia, cryptosporidium	Carbohydrate malabsorption, e.g. sucrase–isomaltase deficiency (onset when sucrose introduced into diet with solids)
	Coeliac disease	
	Food intolerance	
	Overflow constipation	Congenital lactase deficiency
	Pancreatic dysfunction	Protein-losing enteropathy, e.g. intestinal lymphangiectasia
		Hyperthyroidism

TODDLER'S DIARRHOEA

A chronic diarrhoea up to 4–5 years of age, with loose stools at a frequency of 3–6/day, and normal growth and nothing abnormal on examination. The cause is not clearly understood and may be due to decreased gut transit time leading to colonic bacterial degradation of partially digested foods and subsequent release of secretagogues.

Management is with reassurance and dietary changes (↑ fat, ↓ fibre, ↓ juice) to increase gut transit time. The condition usually resolves spontaneously by 3 years of age.

CHRONIC DIARRHOEA

Prolonged diarrhoea may be due to any of the above causes, and the child will quickly become malnourished.

Investigations

Stool	M, C & S, reducing substances, fats and electrolytes
	Faecal elastase (pancreatic insufficiency?)
Bloods	FBC (immunodeficiency?), electrolytes, ESR, CRP
	Coeliac screen (anti-endomysial IgA, tissue transglutaminase, and total IgA)
AXR and CXR	Obstruction? Bronchiectasis?
Sweat test	Cystic fibrosis?
Trial off oral feeds	Secretory (diarrhoea will continue) or osmotic diarrhoea (diarrhoea will stop off feeds)
Endoscopy	With small biopsy and duodenal juice culture (enteropathy, infection?)

Management

Nutritional support while the diagnosis is being arrived at. A hypoallergenic modular feed with supplementation, e.g. Neonate, can be tried first. If enteral feeds fail then a period of TPN will be necessary. A trial of metronidazole for 5 days may be considered (as giardia is only detected in stool specimens in 20% of cases).

GIARDIASIS

This is a common infection among children in nurseries and institutions because it spreads rapidly via the faecal–oral route. Caused by the protozoan *Giardia lamblia*.

- Causes diarrhoea and vomiting with abdominal pain
- Illness can be prolonged and result in flattening of the intestinal villi, causing steatorrhoea with malabsorption, weight loss and faltering growth
- Identified by '*hot stool*' microscopy, i.e. sent straight to the lab, but the pick-up rate is only around 20%
- Treatment is with high–dose oral metronidazole for 5–7 days as there is now a 20% resistance rate (empirical treatment may lead to improvement, which is the best diagnostic test)
- Common in HIV and XLA

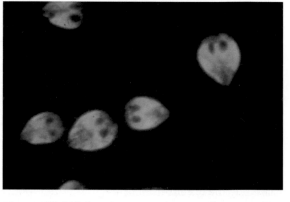

Figure 10.6 Light microscopy immunofluorescence imaging of *Giardia lamblia*

PEPTIC ULCER DISEASE (PUD)

Duodenal ulcers are seen in children, with gastric ulcers being rare. There is an association with *Helicobacter pylori* infection, which can be asymptomatic, or cause chronic gastritis or peptic ulceration, accounting for 90% of duodenal ulcers in children. Intra-familial infection is invoked and occurs early in life. A family history of PUD should be sought. **Zollinger–Ellison syndrome** is multiple ulcers due to a gastrin-secreting tumour, and is rare.

Causes of chronic abdominal pain

Psychiatric	Psychogenic recurrent abdominal pain
Abdominal	Constipation, food intolerance (including lactose intolerance), inflammatory bowel disease, coeliac disease, Meckel's diverticulum, abdominal TB (esp. non-Caucasian or eastern European), peptic ulcer, irritable bowel syndrome
Pancreas/liver	Chronic pancreatitis, cystic fibrosis, cholecystitis, chronic hepatitis
Renal	UTI, pyelonephritis, renal calculi
Metabolic	IDDM, porphyria (rare), lead poisoning (very rare nowadays)
CNS	Migraine
Other	Referred testicular pain, ovarian pain, sickle cell crisis, drug side effects

Clinical features

- Intermittent abdominal pain, worse at night
- Nausea, vomiting
- Iron-deficiency anaemia, gastrointestinal bleeding

Investigations

- Endoscopy with biopsies
- CLO test on biopsy specimen to detect *H. pylori* (*H. pylori* makes urease, which changes the colour of the agar from yellow to pink)

Management

- H2 antagonists or proton pump inhibitor, e.g. omeprazole
- *H. pylori* eradication therapy – omeprazole and a combination of two of amoxycillin, clarythromicin and metronidazole for 1–2 weeks at high dose

INFLAMMATORY BOWEL DISEASE

CROHN DISEASE

Crohn disease is chronic inflammation of the bowel, involving any part from the mouth to the anus, classically the terminal ileum, and the rectum is often spared. The incidence is increasing; male = female.

Differential diagnosis

- Gastrointestinal TB
- Infectious enteropathies, esp. *Yersinia ileitis*
- Small bowel lymphoma

Clinical features

Gastrointestinal	Abdominal pain, diarrhoea, anorexia, aphthous and ulcers
	Abdominal mass, perianal lesions (tags, abscess, fistulae), stricture and fistulae common
	Lip swelling may occur
Systemic	Fever, malaise, oral ulceration, weight loss, anaemia, nutritional deficiencies, growth retardation, amenorrhoea
Extra-abdominal	Pubertal delay (see p. 273)

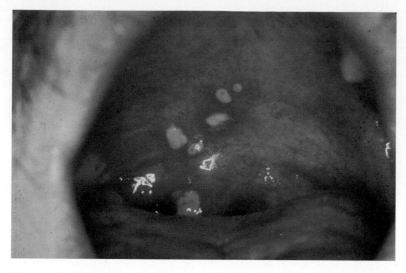

Figure 10.7 Palatal involvement in Crohn disease with multiple oral ulcers

Investigations

Bloods	FBC, iron studies, folate, B12, ESR, CRP, LFTs, serum proteins ($\downarrow$)
	Yersinia and campylobacter serology
Stool microscopy and culture	Enterocolitides (salmonella, shigella, campylobacter, *Entamoeba histolytica*)
Plain AXR	Partial small bowel obstruction
Barium meal and follow-through	*Cobblestone appearance* (linear ulcers), deep fissures, strictures and fistulae common, discontinuous disease with normal *'skip'* lesions
MRT is overtaking barium meal as the small bowel anatomy investigation of choice	
Upper endoscopy and ileocolonoscopy with biopsies and wireless capsule endoscopy	Histology of lesions Non-caseating granulomas, transmural inflammation, patchy involvement

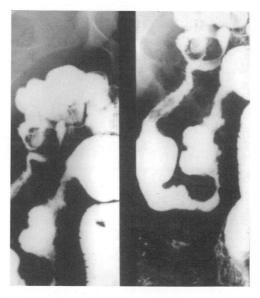

Figure 10.8 Barium meal and follow-through showing a stricture of the terminal ileum in Crohn disease

Management options

Polymeric exclusive diets	Effective as initial therapy instead of steroids. Give exclusive polymeric enteral nutrition, e.g. Modulin IBD, or Alicalm for 6–8 weeks orally or via NG tube, as tolerated
Steroids	High dose for 3–4 weeks, then alternate days and reduce over 4–6 weeks as tolerated
Aminosalicylates	Sulphasalazine, mesalazine, or olsalazine for colon disease
	Delayed release 5-ASA (Asacol) for terminal small bowel disease

Azathioprine	Often now used as part of first line, previously if steroid dependent or not responding
Metronidazole or ciprofloxacin	If fistulae or perianal disease
Methotrexate	Second- or third-line
Tacrolimus/pabecrolimus paste	For perianal disease
TPN	Rarely necessary temporarily
Anti-tumour necrosis factor	(Anti-TNF) monoclonal antibodies, e.g. Infliximab intravenously
Surgery	Reserved for special indications as recurrence risk high
	Resection of disease unresponsive to medical therapy (wide resection margin with right or subtotal hemicolectomy)
	Abscess, perforation, obstruction, bleeding

ULCERATIVE COLITIS

This is a chronic inflammatory disease of the colon with ulceration, classically involving large bowel from the rectum upwards. Small bowel may be involved. Incidence male = female.

Differential diagnosis

- Crohn colitis
- Amoebic colitis
- Bacillary dysentery

Clinical features

Gastrointestinal	Diarrhoea with blood and mucus
General	Anaemia (iron loss from bleeding), growth retardation (malabsorption rare)
Extra-abdominal	See p. 186

Investigations

Blood tests	FBC (Hb ↓, leukocytosis), iron studies, B12, LFTs, ESR, CRP, albumin (↓)
AXR (if abdominal pain)	Decreased haustrations, dilated colon. NB: **Toxic megacolon** = colon width > 2.5 vertebrae
Ileo-colonoscopy with biopsies	Pseudo-polyps, friability with contact bleeding, ulceration
MRI or virtual CT	

Management options

Aminosalicylates	Oral, e.g. sulphasalazine, mesalazine, olsalazine. For mild colitis and prevention of relapses
Enemas	Aminosalicylate or steroid for proctitis
Steroids	Oral or intravenous at 1–2 mg/kg/day (maximum dose 40 mg), to induce remission
Other drugs	Azathioprine, 6-MP, cyclosporin, anti-TNF monoclonal antibodies
TPN	In preparation for surgery
Surgery	Colectomy is performed for fulminant disease unresponsive to medical therapy, or pancolitis – medically uncontrolled with complications and severe symptoms

Extra-abdominal features of Crohn disease and ulcerative colitis

Many extra-abdominal features are associated with inflammatory bowel disease; some are more common in Crohn disease and others in ulcerative colitis.

Crohn (most commonly)
Erythema nodosum
Peripheral arthritis
Aphthous ulcers
Clubbing
Episcleritis
Renal stones (oxalate, uric acid)
Gallstones

Ulcerative colitis (most commonly)
Pyoderma gangrenosum
Ankylosing spondylitis
Sclerosing cholangitis
Autoimmune

Both equally
Uveitis
Conjunctivitis

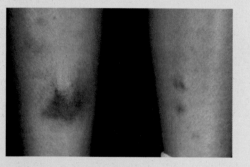

Figure 10.9 Erythema nodosum on the shins in a child with Crohn disease

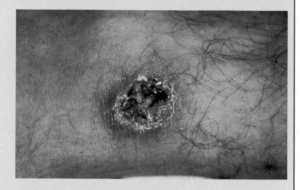

Figure 10.10 Pyoderma gangrenosum

Complications

- Toxic megacolon
- Fulminating colitis
- Colon cancer (long term), therefore regular colonoscopy after > 10 years' active disease.

CONSTIPATION

Constipation is difficulty, delay, or pain in defecation. When prolonged, there may be overflow diarrhoea due to liquid faeces escaping around a hard lump of faeces in the rectum (see Fig 10.11 rectal faecolith). NB: The important differential is Hirschsprung disease.

Causes

Non-organic
Organic   Low residue diet, dehydration, large milk intake
Gut – Hirschsprung disease, stricture, anal fissure
Metabolic – hypothyroidism, cystic fibrosis, hypercalcaemia
Neuromuscular – cerebral palsy, spinal cord lesions, myotonic dystrophy, absent abdominal wall muscles
Drugs – narcotics, antidepressants

Complications

Short term   Constipation quickly resolves with fluids and stool softeners, usually with no sequelae

Long term Constipation leads to:

- Acquired megarectum (decreased sensation of a full rectum)
- Anal fissures
- Overflow incontinence
- Behavioural problems (fear of defecation, embarrassment of overflow)

Investigations

- Abdominal examination – hard faeces
- PR (not always necessary) – faecal mass, soiled anal region, sacral tuft (spina bifida occulta), sphincter tone (↓ in simple constipation, ↑ in Hirschsprung's disease) but not a reliable clinical sign at all
- AXR – loaded with faeces
- Gut transit study

Management

- Positive reinforcement
- Increase fluids and fibre intake
- Oral medications:
  - Softener, e.g. lactulose, liquid paraffin
  - Bulking agent, e.g. Fybogel
  - Non-absorbed laxative irrigative, e.g. Movicol
  - Stimulant, e.g. Senokot, sodium picosulphate
- Enema if necessary for disimpaction, e.g. phosphate enema
- Anal fissure treatment with local topical anaesthetic cream and/or vasodilator (0.2%) glyceryl trinitrate ointment

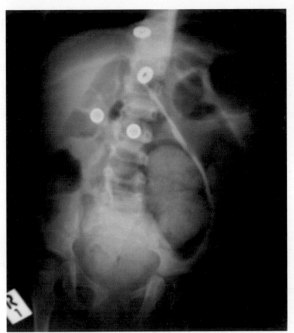

Figure 10.11 Abdominal X-ray showing severe constipation in a 14 month old infant. Note the dilated bowel loops (if small bowel, should be no more than approx. the width of a vertebra) and lots of faeces

HIRSCHSPRUNG DISEASE

Incidence 1 in 5000. Polygenic inheritance, 3–5% recurrence, *RET* oncogene.

This disease is due to the absence of parasympathetic ganglia in Auerbach and Meissner plexi. The unopposed sympathetic activity results in hypertonus of the affected segment of bowel. The disease occurs from the rectum upwards. There are two types:

- Short aganglionic segment – common, male > female
- Long aganglionic segment – rare, male = female, familial

Associations

- Down syndrome
- Lawrence–Moon–Beidel syndrome
- Waardenburg syndrome

Presentation

Neonatal (> 80%)   Acute obstruction, Hirschsprung colitis
Older child   Chronic constipation, history of delayed passage of meconium (> 48 h after birth), faltering growth

Investigations

AXR	Constipation
Barium enema	Narrow aganglionic segment, dilated proximal segment
Anorectal manometry	Failure of internal sphincter pressure to drop with rectal distension
Rectal biopsy	Rectal suction biopsy (mucosa + submucosa) or full thickness biopsy (surgical trans-anal)
Histology of affected bowel	Acetylcholinesterase staining shows *increased* number of hypertrophied nerve bundles that stain positively for acetylcholinesterase

Management

This is surgical, with an immediate definitive repair, or a temporary neonatal colostomy with definitive repair at 3–6 months of age. Definitive repair is with direct resection and anastomosis, or an endorectal pull-through. Ultra-short segment disease can be treated with anal dilatation and partial sphincterotomy.

FAECAL SOILING

Faecal soiling is involuntary soiling. Normal bowel control is achieved by around 2 years (soiling by day: 1–2% 5–12 year olds). Girls are quicker than boys (ratio of boys to girls soiling by day 2:1).

Faecal soiling occurs when there is:

- *Faecal retention with overflow incontinence.* This can happen:
  - After an episode of diarrhoea, then anal fissure causing painful defecation and constipation
  - Due to psychological stress coinciding with toilet training, resulting in refusal to sit on the potty
  - Due to other disease, e.g. Hirschsprung disease, hypothyroidism
  - If the rectum is chronically obstructed with faeces it may enlarge to form a megarectum with decreased sensation of a full rectum
- *Neurological damage* with failure to establish bowel control, e.g. cerebral palsy, learning difficulties
- *Stress* – normal bowel control but soiling in response to stress only

! **NB: Encopresis is the voluntary passage of faeces in an otherwise healthy child beyond the usual age for toilet training. It is due to non-organic causes.**

Management

- Comprehensive history including gastrointestinal and social
- Abdominal (including rectal) and neurological examination
- Plain AXR – faecal retention
- Empty bowel of impacted faeces – microenemas, manual disempaction
- High fibre diet and stool softeners (for soft painless stools)
- For encopresis, psychotherapy (child and family therapy), including a behaviour modification programme (positive reinforcement, defined periods of toilet training, remove fear of the toilet, remove control battle between parents and child)

! **NB: Important to exclude Hirschsprung disease, which is present from birth. If this is suspected, then full investigation is necessary (see p. 187).**

ACUTE PANCREATITIS

This involves inflammation of the pancreas with autodigestion, localized necrosis and haemorrhage. Complications can be severe.

Causes

- Biliary sludging
- Congenital abnormalities
- Blunt abdominal trauma
- Viral infections – mumps, varicella, measles, EBV, coxsackie virus
- Iatrogenic – TPN, steroids, azathioprine

Associations

- Haemolytic uraemic syndrome
- Kawasaki disease
- Diabetic ketoacidosis
- Stem cell transplant
- Brain tumour

The clinical features and management are as for adults.

GASTROINTESTINAL TRACT BLEEDING

Clinical presentations

- Haematemesis – fresh blood or 'coffee grounds' (altered by gastric juices)
- Melaena (altered blood per rectum) – tarry smelly stool
- Fresh rectal bleeding
- Massive bleeding with collapse
- Small bleeds with iron-deficiency anaemia

Causes of gastrointestinal tract bleeding

Infant	Child	Adolescent
Swallowed maternal blood	Colonic polyps (painless)	Bacterial infections
Haemorrhagic disease newborn	Anal fissure	IBD
NEC	Bacterial infections	Anal fissure
Cow's milk protein allergy	Intussusception	Colonic polyps
Anal fissure	Mallory–Weiss tear	Peptic ulcer/gastritis
Intussusception	HUS	Mallory–Weiss tear
Volvulus	HSP	Oesophageal varices
Meckel diverticulum	Oesophageal varices	Telangiectasia
	Meckel diverticulum	
	Oesophagitis	
	Peptic ulcer/gastritis	
	IBD	
	AV-malformation, haemangioma	
	Telangiectasia	
	Sexual abuse	

Investigations and management

- Assess circulation and resuscitate if necessary.
- Bloods – FBC, clotting studies, iron studies
- Faecal occult blood
- Endoscopy – this is the emergency management also. Oesophageal banding for varices. (Sclerotherapy outdated, and insertion of a Sengstaken–Blakemore tube only in extremis)
- Laparotomy and/or mesenteric angiography if necessary

Swallowed maternal blood

This is a common event with small babies. Maternal blood is identified with the APT test. Bloody vomit or stool is mixed with water, centrifuged and the supernatant mixed with 1% sodium hydroxide. If it remains pink = infant blood; if it turns brown = maternal blood.

GASTROINTESTINAL TRACT TUMOURS

JUVENILE COLONIC POLYPS

These occur in 3–4% of the population in the colon only. Symptoms usually occur between 2 and 10 years. Uncommon > 15 years. They are usually benign hamartomas (unless they have an adenomatous element).

Presentation

- Bright red rectal bleeding
- Autolysis
- Prolapse of a polyp
- Anaemia
- Abdominal pain (unusual)

Diagnosis

- Rectal examination
- Colonoscopy with polyp removal
- Barium enema

FAMILIAL POLYPOSIS SYNDROMES
Familial adenomatous polyposis coli

Autosomal dominant, incidence 1 in 8000, pre-malignant condition. The *APC* (adenomatous polyposis coli) gene has been identified on the long arm of chromosome 5: many different mutations may occur within this gene, resulting in familial adenomatous polyposis coli.

Multiple adenomas occur on the distal bowel (100–1000), with onset at age < 10 years. Annual colonoscopy is needed after age 10 years and pan-colectomy after 10 years of disease (usually late teens or early 20s).

Peutz–Jegher syndrome

Autosomal dominant, 50% new mutations. This is a syndrome of:

- Mucosal pigmentation (freckles) of lips and gums
- Stomach and small bowel hamartomas
- Malignant tumours (*not* of the GI tract) develop in 50% of patients

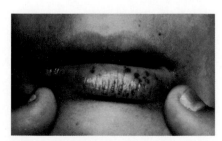

Figure 10.13 Multiple freckles on the lips in Peutz–Jegher syndrome

Clinical scenario

A 4-year-old child presents to the paediatric outpatients with a 2-year history of intermittent diarrhoea, abdominal bloating, lethargy, being generally miserable, and more recently has developed an itchy rash on his elbows.

1. What blood tests would you arrange?
2. If these blood tests were positive for the suspected condition what definitive test would you refer him for?
3. What follow-up, in terms of investigation, would be required?

ANSWERS

1. FBC; total IgA; anti-endomysial IgA; tissue transglutaminase IgA
2. Endoscopic small bowel biopsy
3. Serial serology as above each 6 months for first year and then annually. No need for repeat biopsy if diagnosis is made after age of 2 years. A gluten challenge with pre- and post-challenge endoscopic biopsy may be necessary at 5 years old if diagnosis is made under 2 years of age

FURTHER READING

Kleinman RE, Goulet OJ, Mieli-Vergani G *et al. Walker's Pediatric Gastrointestinal Disease (Fifth Edition).* PMPH USA. 2008.

Walker-Smith JA, Hamilton JR, Walker WA. *Practical Paediatric Gastroenterology (Second Edition).* Philadelphia: B C Decker. 1996.

Wyllie R, Hyams JS. *Pediatric Gastrointestinal Liver Disease (Third Edition).* Philadelphia: Saunders. 2006.

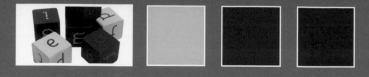

11 Nutrition

- Infant feeding
- Faltering growth
- Specific nutritional deficiencies
- Childhood obesity
- Malnutrition
- Further reading

- Eating disorders, see ch. 24
- Malabsorption and food intolerances, see ch. 10

INFANT FEEDING

- Purely milk feeding for the first 4 months
- Then solid food gradually introduced (**weaning**)

Breast feeding

This, unsurprisingly, is the best option for many reasons (see below), though sometimes mothers have difficulty and prefer to bottle feed.

Initial establishment

- This is critical in the first few days after birth
- It is new to both mother (if first baby) and infant, does not just 'happen' perfectly at once and requires *perseverance*. It is important therefore that the mother is given as much help and encouragement as possible (without being didactic), and that *time* is taken by the midwives and breast-feeding specialists to help establish breast feeding
- Use cup feeds of formula milk if additional feeding is necessary whilst trying to establish breast feeding (the bottle can be easier and therefore the baby may stop trying to breast feed if tried)

Continuation

- Breast feeding continued for the first 4 months has proven benefit to the baby
- Many women commence breast feeding well, but then stop after only a few weeks
- Higher social classes have higher rates of breast feeding
- Help is available from breast-feeding councillors and health visitors in particular

Advantages

- Nutrition optimum, e.g. fatty acids, arachidonic acid and docosohexaenoic acid, needed for infant brain development
- Immunological protection transferred (IgA especially). In the developing world it gives very significant protection against respiratory and gastrointestinal diseases

- Uterine involution (oxytocin release) and maternal weight loss expedited
- Contraceptive (lactation amenorrhoea)
- Convenient and cheap
- Decreases the risk of breast cancer ($\times$ 4.7%/year of breast feeding)
- Reduced incidence of atopy throughout childhood and adolescence
- Helps to establish maternal–infant bonding

There are no real disadvantages of breast feeding:

- It is becoming socially acceptable (and politically correct) to breast feed infants in public places, including restaurants
- Mother need not do all the feeding as expressed breast milk can be given by other carers
- Mother cannot go back to work while fully breast feeding (though some milk may be expressed at work, depending on type of employment)

Twins and higher multiples can be breast fed, although supplemental formula feeds are often necessary.

Reasons for not breast feeding

Maternal	Infant
Maternal drugs, e.g. cytotoxics ⎱ Contraindications Maternal HIV (in the UK) ⎰ Unable to establish feeding Maternal dislike Breast abscess (can use other breast) Maternal acute illness	Acute illness Cleft lip/palate (may manage breast feeding) Metabolic disease, e.g. galactosaemia
NB: Inverted nipples is not a contraindication	

Components of breast milk

- For the first few days, composed of **colostrum** (thick bright yellow–orange) with high protein, phospholipid, cholesterol and immunoglobulin content
- Major differences from formula milk:
  - Casein:whey ratio – high whey in breast milk
  - Fat: higher in breast milk
  - Na, Ca, K ⎫
  - Vitamin K ⎬ Lower in breast milk
  - Iron ⎭
- Cow's milk is vastly different and should not be used as a substitute

Example of types of special infant formula

Milk substitute	Composition
Nutramigen®	Casein hydrolysate (protein hydrolysed to peptides of 15 amino acids or less)
Pregestamil®	Casein hydrolysate
Neocate®	Amino acids

These formulae are used for cow's milk protein (CMP) allergy of varying severity. Soya-based milks are not recommended as there is cross-reactivity with CMP intolerance of approximately 40%.

Weaning

This is the introduction of solid food and is done gradually from around 4–6 months. Different puréed foods are introduced, e.g. mashed banana, one a week initially. Babies generally like sweet things (as breast milk is very sweet), but it is important to introduce a wide variety of flavours early.

Normal cow's milk should *not* be introduced before 1 year of age.

FALTERING GROWTH

This is failure to gain adequate weight or achieve adequate growth during infancy at a normal rate for age. At least two growth measurements are needed 3–6 months apart, which show the child falling across centiles.

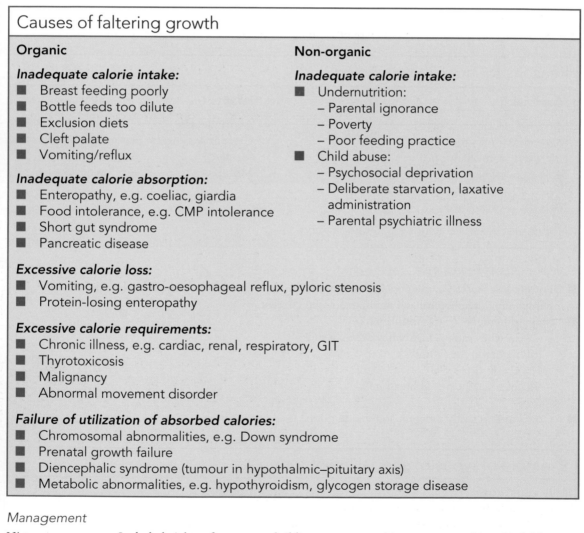

Causes of faltering growth

Organic	Non-organic
Inadequate calorie intake:	***Inadequate calorie intake:***
■ Breast feeding poorly	■ Undernutrition:
■ Bottle feeds too dilute	– Parental ignorance
■ Exclusion diets	– Poverty
■ Cleft palate	– Poor feeding practice
■ Vomiting/reflux	■ Child abuse:
Inadequate calorie absorption:	– Psychosocial deprivation
■ Enteropathy, e.g. coeliac, giardia	– Deliberate starvation, laxative administration
■ Food intolerance, e.g. CMP intolerance	– Parental psychiatric illness
■ Short gut syndrome	
■ Pancreatic disease	

Excessive calorie loss:
- Vomiting, e.g. gastro-oesophageal reflux, pyloric stenosis
- Protein-losing enteropathy

Excessive calorie requirements:
- Chronic illness, e.g. cardiac, renal, respiratory, GIT
- Thyrotoxicosis
- Malignancy
- Abnormal movement disorder

Failure of utilization of absorbed calories:
- Chromosomal abnormalities, e.g. Down syndrome
- Prenatal growth failure
- Diencephalic syndrome (tumour in hypothalmic–pituitary axis)
- Metabolic abnormalities, e.g. hypothyroidism, glycogen storage disease

Management

History	Include heights of parents and siblings, pregnancy history, e.g. smoking, birth history, e.g. gestation and birthweight, dietary assessment and social report
Examination	Weight, height ± head circumference, general examination and developmental assessment
Investigations	Sequence and extent of these is dictated by the clinical history and examination

SPECIFIC NUTRITIONAL DEFICIENCIES

> **!** **NB: Specific vitamin and mineral deficiencies occur rarely by themselves, and are usually part of an overall poor nutrition and many are seen together.**

IRON-DEFICIENCY ANAEMIA

Iron-deficiency anaemia is very common among infants due to insufficient dietary iron. Infants have high iron requirements because they grow rapidly and have small stores.

Causes

Inadequate intake	Most common cause of anaemia in infants
	Infants most at risk:

- Premature infants (lower iron stores and more to grow). Oral iron supplements are recommended for these infants until the age of 2 years (see p. 58)
- Inadequate solid food after 6 months of age (solid foods rich in iron provide more iron than milk), i.e. given too much milk. Seen especially in the developing world in predominantly breast-fed infants after 9–12 months of age
- Formula-fed infants (iron poorly absorbed)
- Those fed cow's milk under 1 year (iron from cow's milk is very poorly absorbed)

Malabsorption	Coeliac disease
Excess loss (bleeding)	Gastrointestinal loss, e.g. Meckel's diverticulum, menstrual loss

Factors which increase iron intake and absorption

- Encourage breast feeding during first 6 months (iron absorbed better than from formula milk)
- If fed formula milk, use those fortified with iron
- Baby cereals contain extra iron
- Standard cow's milk not recommended below 1 year of age
- Fresh fruit and vegetables (vitamin C) enhance iron absorption by changing ferrous (predominant in vegetables) to the better absorbed ferric iron (predominant in meat)
- Food rich in iron (red meat, oily fish, dark green vegetables, beans and pulses, dried fruit and nuts)
- Avoid high-fibre foods and tannins (tea) as they decrease iron absorption

Clinical findings

- Usually asymptomatic – discovered on incidental blood test
- General features of anaemia (see p. 310)
- Nails – brittle, ridged, spoon shaped (koilonychia)
- Mouth – angular stomatitis, painful smooth glossitis
- Gastrointestinal tract – pica (toddlers with iron deficiency), atrophic gastritis, if severe – oesophageal web (Plummer–Vinson syndrome)
- Subtle neurological impairment in toddlers (low motor and cognitive scores and increased behavioural problems)

Specific investigation findings

RBC indices and film	Hypochromic, microcytic, anisocytosis, target cells, pencil cells, moderately raised platelets
Serum iron	↓
Serum ferritin	↓
Total iron-binding capacity (TIBC)	↑
Bone marrow	No iron stores in macrophages, no siderotic granules in erythroblasts

Management

- Investigate and treat underlying cause:
  - Take full dietary and absorption history, do baseline investigations
  - Coeliac screen if necessary
  - Search for blood loss if necessary (endoscopy, colonoscopy, Meckel's scan, haematuria and menorrhagia)
- Give oral iron supplements (elixir or tablets). Dietary management if necessary
- Parenteral iron is rarely needed. It can be given IM or IV. Anaphylactic reactions can occur

RICKETS

Rickets is a failure in mineralization of growing bone. It is most commonly secondary to nutritional causes. In fully developed bone this is called **osteomalacia**.

Daily vitamin D requirement is 400 IU.

Causes

Vitamin D intake inadequate	Nutritional:
	▪ Prematurity (see p. 59 [osteopaenia of prematurity])
	▪ Breast-fed infants more at risk
	▪ Poorly fed infants (malnutrition)
	Malabsorption – coeliac disease, steatorrhoea, cystic fibrosis
	▪ Inadequate sunlight exposure (especially in dark-skinned)
Metabolism of vitamin D	Renal disease. NB: PO_4 ↑
	Liver disease
	Anticonvulsants, e.g. phenytoin (metabolizes vitamin D)
Phosphate excretion increased	Familial hypophosphataemic rickets
	Vitamin D-dependent rickets – type I or type II (receptor defect)
	Fanconi syndrome

Clinical features

- Head – large anterior fontanelle with delayed closure (> 2 years), craniotabes (ping-pong ball skull), frontal bossing
- Chest – enlargement of costochondral junctions (**Rachitic or rib rosary**), Harrison sulcus, pigeon chest
- Thickened wrists and ankles
- Bow legs, knock knees
- Dwarfism, pot belly, muscular weakness, kyphosis, small pelvis, coxa vara
- Late dentition with enamel defects
- Greenstick fractures

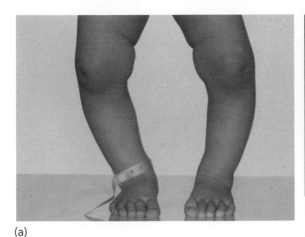

(a)

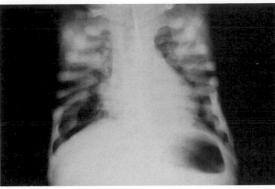

(b)

Figure 11.1 Rickets. (a) Bow legs in a child.
(b) Chest X-ray showing rickety rosary

Table 11.1 Biochemical abnormalities seen in rickets

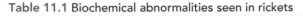

	Ca	PO$_4$	PTH	AP	25(OH)D$_3$	1,25(OH)$_2$D$_3$
Nutritional	N, ↓	↑ or ↓	↑, N	↑	↓	↓
Hypophosphataemic	N, ↓	↓	N	↑	N	↓

AP, alkaline phosphatase; PTH, parathyroid hormone

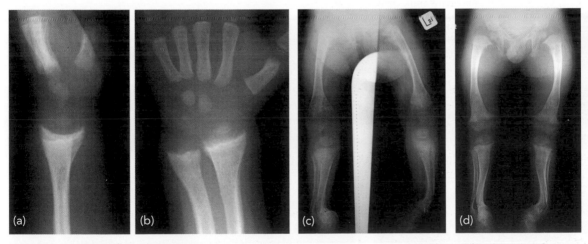

(a)   (b)   (c)   (d)

Figure 11.2 Rickets X-rays. (a+b) 9-month-old infant. Note irregular mineralization and fraying of the provisional zones of calcification at the distal ends of the radius and ulnar. The distal radius is cupped. (c) Advanced rickets in a 2 ½-year-old child. Diffusely osteoporotic shafts with florid fraying, cupping and splaying of the distal end of the femur and proximal ends of the tibia and fibula. Note bowing of the distal shafts of the tibia and fibula. (d) Healing after 6 months of treatment. Note recalcification of the metaphyses at the end of the long bones (courtesy of Dr Kapila Jain and Dr Simon Padley)

Investigations

Biochemical investigations	See Table 11.1
X-ray of left wrist	Widened epiphyseal plate
(or left knee if < 2 years)	Cupping and fraying of the metaphysis
	Increased joint space
	Line of calcification seen when healing
	Cysts, subperiosteal erosions, fractures, Looser's zones, osteopaenia if severe

Treatment

This is with vitamin D in the necessary form:

Nutritional rickets	Calciferol (D$_3$)
Renal disease	Alphacalcidol (1α OHD$_3$) or calcitriol (1,25(OH)$_2$D$_3$)

ACRODERMATITIS ENTEROPATHICA

This is a disorder due to zinc deficiency of various causes:

- *Inherited form* – autosomal recessive; rare condition due to defective intestinal absorption of zinc
- *Acquired transient neonatal form* due to nutritional zinc deficiency from:
  - Breast-fed infants in mothers with low zinc levels
  - Premature infants with prolonged TPN
  - Infants with malabsorption (including cystic fibrosis)

Clinical features

- Inherited form develops when weaned from breast feeding (as breast milk contains a zinc ligand-binding protein and therefore helps zinc absorption) or earlier if bottle fed
- Persistent well-demarcated rash:
  - Nappy rash
  - Around eyes and nose
  - Involves the flexures
- Failure to thrive, listlessness
- Photophobia, diarrhoea, alopecia, nail dystrophy
- *Diagnosis* – plasma zinc levels low (< 50 μg/ml), alkaline phosphatase also low (zinc dependent enzyme)
- Rapid response to zinc supplementation

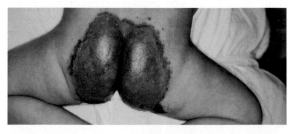

Figure 11.3 Well-demarcated erythematous nappy rash in acrodermatitis

CHILDHOOD OBESITY

Childhood obesity is increasing in incidence in the UK. It is defined as a body mass index (BMI) > 85th percentile; a BMI > 35 is morbid obesity. The International Obesity Task Force (IOTF) has developed specific BMI centile charts

- In infants may be secondary to maternal anxiety with inappropriate overfeeding to comfort the baby and/or postnatal depression
- Bottle-fed infants are more likely to become obese
- In children, commonly due to a combination of inadequate exercise and poor quality nutrition. Treatment can be difficult as underlying familial eating and exercise habits need to be altered
- Other causes – Cushing syndrome, Prader–Willi syndrome

- *Associated problems:*
  - Advanced bone age, increased height (early), early puberty
  - Psychological effects (poor self-image, depression)
  - Sleep apnoea (severe obesity)
  - Obesity throughout life increased
  - Long term effects – hypertension, diabetes, cardiovascular disease

MALNUTRITION

Malnutrition is categorized into the short term response of **wasting** (weight for height ratios) and the long term response of **stunting** (height for age and sex ratios) using standard scores. Weight for age ratios make no distinction between the short and long term effects. Traditionally it has been classified into marasmus, kwashiorkor and marasmic kwashiorkor.

Marasmus

This is a mixed deficiency of both protein and calories, resulting in non-oedematous malnutrition. Decreased weight for age and sex ratios (< 60% of the mean).

- Hungry, listless, emaciated child
- Loose, wrinkled skin, 'old man' appearance, decreased skin turgor
- Muscle atrophy and little subcutaneous fat
- Thin sparse hair, hair colour changes unusual
- Hypothermia, bradycardia, hypotension (basal metabolic rate ↓)

Kwashiorkor

This results in oedema which is due to unknown causes, although it has historically been attributed to a disproportionately low protein intake compared with calorie intake. There is a near-normal weight for age ratio (weight for age and sex ratio < 80%) and oedema.

- Lethargic, miserable, no appetite
- Oedema: hypoalbuminaemic, overall 'fatness' appearance, moon face
- Hepatomegaly (fatty infiltration)
- Cardiomegaly
- Thin, red hair and darkened skin
- Skin lesions (flaking paint rash, ulcers, fissures, pellagra-type rash)
- Infections, secondary immunodeficiency

Marasmic kwashiorkor (mixed type)

A combined type exists where there are features of both marasmus and kwashiorkor, with a weight for age and sex ratio of < 60% with oedema.

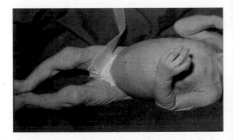

Figure 11.4 Child with severe malnutrition shows a lack of subcutaneous fat stores and muscle wasting

Management

1. Initial rehydration with oral rehydration salt solution or IV fluids if in shock
2. Dilute milk for 5 days, increasing volume gradually to 150 mL/kg/day. Look for and treat hypoglycaemia, hypothermia, electrolyte imbalance, micronutrient deficiencies and infection
3. High-energy feeds as strength builds up. NB: If feeds are too strong too early, hepatomegaly and a slower recovery result

Clinical scenario

A 4-month-old boy is referred for faltering growth (failure to thrive). He is bottle fed; his mother is 16 years of age and confused about how to mix his feeds, he is vomiting frequently, and he has eczema. His nappies are full of mucous diarrhoea 10 times a day. He is pale and has poor muscle bulk with poor subcutaneous fat stores.

1. What three causes of his poor growth can you point to?
2. How would you improve his nutrition?

ANSWERS

1. Poor intake due to vomiting. Poor calorie intake because the feeds may be too dilute. Poor absorption of nutrition due to allergy-related small bowel damage (enteropathy)
2. Education and support of mother in the community either with other family members or with health visitor input. High-energy milk feed with weaning on to solid food high in calories. Perhaps a low-allergy feed would be beneficial

FURTHER READING

Duggan C, Walker JB, Watkins WA. *Nutrition in Pediatrics (Third Edition)*. Philadelphia: B C Decker. 2008.

Kleinman RE, Goulet OJ, Mieli-Vergani G *et al. Walker's Pediatric Gastrointestinal Disease (Fifth Edition)*. PMPH USA. 2008.

Wyllie R, Hyams JS. *Pediatric Gastrointestinal Liver Disease (Third Edition)*. Philadelphia: Saunders. 2006.

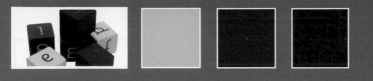

12 Liver

FUNCTIONS OF THE LIVER

Protein	Metabolism – principal site of synthesis of all circulating proteins
	Degradation – amino groups and ammonia are converted to urea
Carbohydrate	Preterm infants have inefficient regulation of this metabolism
Lipid metabolism	Young infants have reduced capacity for hepatic ketogenesis
Bile	Bile acids – synthesis from cholesterol
	Bilirubin metabolism (see Fig. 12.6)
	Bile secretion – neonates have inefficient ileal reabsorption and hepatic clearance of bile acids from portal blood, and therefore raised serum levels of bile acids
Hormone and drug metabolism	Newborn infants have decreased capacity to metabolize certain drugs
Immunological function	

INVESTIGATIVE LIVER BLOOD TESTS

Laboratory tests examine the *functions* of the liver and include markers of liver cell *damage*. As the liver has a very large functional reserve, functional test results change late in disease.

Albumin	Synthetic function marker
Prothrombin time (PT)	Very sensitive synthetic function marker
Bilirubin	Raised bilirubin level may be **conjugated** = 'direct' reading or **unconjugated** = 'indirect' reading
Aminotransferases (transaminases)	**Aspartate aminotransferase (AST)** – mitochondrial enzyme (also in heart, muscle, kidney, brain) **Alanine aminotransferase (ALT)**: cytosol enzyme. More specific to liver than AST (Also in bone, intestine and placenta)
Alkaline phosphatase γ-Glutamyl transpeptidase (λGT)	Microsomal enzyme; increases in cholestasis and induced by some drugs, e.g. phenytoin
Serum proteins	**Albumin, globulins** and **immunoglobulins**
α-Fetoprotein	Normally produced by the *fetal liver*, seen in teratomas, hepatocellular carcinoma, hepatitis and chronic liver disease, and in pregnancy with fetal neural tube defect
Immunological tests	**Anti-mitochondrial antibody (AMA)** in primary biliary cirrhosis and autoimmune hepatitis **Antinuclear (ANA), anti-smooth muscle (ASM)** and **liver/ kidney microsomal (LKM)** antibodies seen in autoimmune hepatitis
Other biochemical alterations	Hypoglycaemia, electrolyte imbalance, hyperammonaemia

CLINICAL MANIFESTATIONS OF LIVER DISEASE

Liver disease may be *acute* or *chronic*.

ACUTE LIVER DISEASE

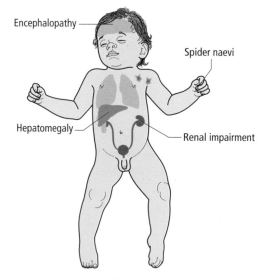

- Asymptomatic
- General malaise (fever, anorexia)
- Hypoglycaemia
- Hepatomegaly
- Jaundice
- Pruritis
- Spider naevi and liver palms (rare)
- Encephalopathy, bleeding disorders and renal impairment may occur

Figure 12.1 Clinical manifestations of acute liver disease

CHRONIC LIVER DISEASE

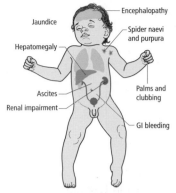

Figure 12.2 Clinical manifestations of chronic liver disease

- Asymptomatic
- Anorexia
- **Liver size** – increased (hepatomegaly), decreased or no change
- Jaundice
- Pruritis – seen in cholestasis due to conjugated hyperbilirubinaemia
- **Other** skin changes – palmar erythema, spider naevi (telangiectasia in the distribution of the superior vena cava, < 5 may still be normal), xanthomata, purpura, clubbing
- **Portal hypertension** – an increase in portal venous pressure to > 10–12 mmHg. Caput medusae, varices, splenomegaly
- **Ascites** – due to hydrostatic pressure from sinusoidal blockade and hypoalbuminaemia
- **Encephalopathy** – portosystemic encephalopathy, a chronic syndrome involving neuropsychiatric disturbance, drowsiness, foetor hepaticus and liver flap. Due to metabolic abnormalities
- **Endocrine abnormalities** – testicular atrophy, gynaecomastia, parotid enlargement
- **Renal abnormalities** – secondary impairment of renal function. Hepato-renal syndrome (renal failure of no other demonstrable cause in a patient with cirrhosis)
- **Gastrointestinal bleeding** – due to coagulation dysfunction and portal hypertension

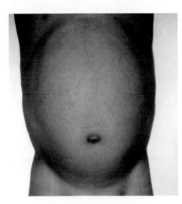

Figure 12.3 Ascitic abdomen

FULMINANT HEPATIC FAILURE

This is an acute clinical syndrome resulting from massive impairment or necrosis of hepatocytes in a patient without pre-existing chronic liver disease. The prognosis is poor with a mortality without transplant of around 70%.

Causes

- Hypoxic liver damage
- Viral hepatitis, combined B and D especially
- Drugs, e.g. paracetamol, sodium valproate
- Metabolic disorders, e.g. Wilson disease, galactosaemia, neonatal haemochromatosis

Clinical features

- Progressive jaundice, foetor hepaticus, fever, vomiting, abdominal pain
- Rapid decrease in liver size with no clinical improvement (ominous sign)
- Defective coagulation
- Hypoglycaemia
- Sepsis
- Fluid overload

- Occult gastrointestinal or intracranial bleeding
- Pancreatitis
- Hepatic encephalopathy with cerebral oedema (lethargy, sleep rhythm disturbance, confusion, progressing to coma)

> **Poor prognostic features**
> - Onset of liver failure < 7 days
> - < 10 years
> - Shrinking liver size
> - Renal failure
> - Paracetamol overdose
> - Hypersensitivity reactions of unknown aetiology

Investigations

- PT ↑
- Transaminases (raised initially, then may decrease with no clinical improvement, indicating little or no functioning liver remaining)
- Ammonia ↑
- Glucose ↓
- Hyperbilirubinaemia (conjugated and unconjugated)
- Metabolic acidosis, K^+ ↓, Na^+ ↓
- EEG (monitor of cerebral activity, occult seizures may be present)

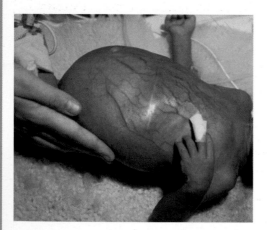

Figure 12.4 Infant with terminal liver failure. Note the abdominal distension secondary to ascites, caput medusae of portal hypertension and poor general nutritional state

Management

The aims of management include close monitoring to prevent complications, maintenance of blood glucose > 4 mmol/L, support of the cardiovascular, renal and respiratory systems, and close monitoring of CNS function. Liver transplant should be considered early if recovery is considered unlikely.

Cerebral complications	Avoid sedation as this masks encephalopathy
	Monitor for ↑ ICP and maintain normal ICP with mannitol, hyperventilation, thiopentone and haemofiltration as necessary
Renal complications	Nephrotoxic drugs and arterial hypotension should be avoided
	Established renal failure is treated with haemofiltration

Sepsis	Daily culturing for infection, and empirical use of broad-spectrum antibiotics with antifungals. Aciclovir if herpetic origin
Bleeding	Vitamin K IV given daily. Avoid invasive procedures if possible
Respiratory complications	ARDS equivalent may occur
Cardiovascular complications	Inotropic support as required
Gastrointestinal complications	Prophylaxis for stress ulceration with IV ranitidine or omeprazole

CIRRHOSIS

This is a histological diagnosis identified by *fibrosis and nodule formation* with *abnormal liver architecture*, and results from necrosis of liver cells. It may be macronodular (nodules up to 5 cm), micronodular (nodules < 3 mm) or mixed. Progressive scarring in cirrhosis leads to restricted blood flow with further impairment of liver function and portal hypertension.

Causes

- Acute viral hepatitis
- Metabolic liver disease, e.g. Wilson disease, tyrosinaemia
- Veno-occlusive disease (especially post-BMT)
- Autoimmune chronic active hepatitis, primary biliary cirrhosis
- Idiopathic

The prognosis is variable and the 5-year survival rate is around 50%, depending on the aetiology.

Causes of hepatomegaly	
Inflammation	Hepatitis – viral, bacterial, toxic
	Autoimmune – chronic hepatitis, SLE, sarcoidosis, sclerosing cholangitis
Tumour	Primary neoplasm – hepatoblastoma, hepatocellular carcinoma
	Secondary deposits – leukaemia, lymphoma, neuroblastoma, histiocytosis
Post-hepatic portal hypertension	Hepatic vein obstruction
	Cardiac failure, pericardial tamponade (constrictive pericarditis, e.g. TB)
Biliary obstruction	Extrahepatic obstruction
Haematological	Sickle cell disease, thalassaemia, spherocytosis
Metabolic disease	Fatty liver – cystic fibrosis, Reye syndrome, TPN, IDDM
	Lipid storage disease
	Glycogen storage disease
	Other – Wilson disease, haemochromatosis, α-1 antitrypsin disease
Cysts	Polycystic kidney disease, hydatid infection
Apparent	Chest hyperexpansion due to lung disease, Reidel's lobe

JAUNDICE (ICTERUS)

Serum bilirubin > 35 μmol/L is clinically detectable.

Jaundice is traditionally classified as pre-hepatic, hepatocellular, and obstructive (cholestatic), but this is inaccurate as cholestasis occurs in hepatocellular as well as obstructive jaundice. It may help to consider jaundice as:

- Haemolytic (pre-hepatic)
- Congenital hyperbilirubinaemias (hepatocellular)
- Cholestatic:
  - Intrahepatic (hepatocellular and/or obstructive)
  - Extrahepatic (obstructive)

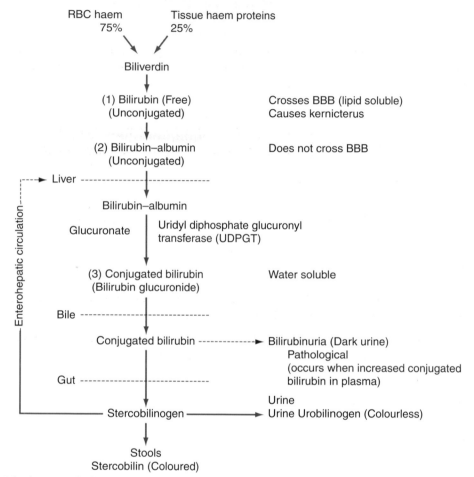

Figure 12.5 Bilirubin metabolism

HAEMOLYTIC JAUNDICE

- Unconjugated bilirubin ↑ (not water soluble, therefore not in urine) = **acholuric jaundice**, i.e. *no bilirubinuria*). Therefore urine and stools *normal* colour
- Urine urobilinogen ↑
- Transaminases, alkaline phosphatase and albumin all normal
- Haemolytic features:
  - Plasma haptoglobins ↓
  - Lactate dehydrogenase (LDH) ↑
  - Reticulocytes ↑
  - Bone marrow erythroid hyperplasia
  - Spherocytes, red cell fragments, sickle cells may be present

- In **intravascular haemolysis**:
  - Haemosiderinuria, haemoglobinuria
  - Methaemalbumin
  - FDPs ↑, haptoglobins ↓

CHOLESTATIC JAUNDICE

- Conjugated bilirubin ↑ (with some unconjugated hyperbilirubinaemia)
- Pale stools
- Dark urine (bilirubinuria)

Altered synthetic function and transaminases may sometimes accompany the picture (see Table 12.1), and vary in intrahepatic, e.g. due to parenchymal disease (hepatocellular) and bile canalicular excretion problem, and extrahepatic disease (large duct obstruction).

Table 12.1 Biochemical features of cholestatic jaundice

	Intrahepatic	Extrahepatic
AST, ALT	↑ ↑	(↑)
Alkaline phosphatase	(↑)	↑ ↑
PT	↑	↑
Albumin	↓	↓
λGT	↑	↑

NEONATAL JAUNDICE

Over 60% of neonates become jaundiced. The cause may be the **unconjugated hyperbilirubinaemia** (more common) (see p. 66) or **conjugated hyperbilirubinaemia** (see below).

Management depends on the bilirubin level and rate of increase, the gestational and chronological age, the clinical condition of the infant and the cause (and type) of jaundice.

Neonatal conjugated hyperbilirubinaemia

Causes

Extrahepatic   Extrahepatic bile duct obstruction:
- Biliary atresia
- Choledochal cyst

Intrahepatic   Intrahepatic bile duct obstruction:
- Intrahepatic biliary hypoplasia, e.g. Alagille syndrome
- Progressive familial intrahepatic cholestasis
- Hepatocyte injury:
  - Infections – hepatitis, e.g. HSV, CMV, enteroviruses, hepatitis B and C; systemic, e.g. listeria, toxoplasmosis, UTI
  - Metabolic disease – galactosaemia, α-1 antitrypsin deficiency, cystic fibrosis
  - Other – idiopathic neonatal hepatitis, hypothyroidism, TPN therapy, chromosomal abnormality, hypoxic–ischaemic damage

> **!** **NB: 'Neonatal hepatitis syndrome' refers to intrahepatic inflammation and cholestasis of many causes (idiopathic, infectious hepatitis, or intrahepatic bile duct paucity).**

Examination and investigations

Examination	Liver and spleen size
	Cystic mass below the liver (choledochal cyst)
	Skin lesions, purpura, choroidoretinitis (? congenital infection)
	Cataracts (galactosaemia)
	Cutaneous haemangioma (hepatic haemangioma)
	Dysmorphic features (trisomy 13, 18 or 21, Alagille syndrome)
Biochemistry	Fractionated bilirubin (conjugated > 20% of total is pathological)
	LFTs
	Blood glucose, U&E, creatinine
	Galactose-1-phosphate uridyl transferase for galactosaemia
	α-1 antitrypsin phenotype
	Metabolic screen (urine and serum amino acids, urine reducing substances)
	Sweat test if feasible, immunoreactive trypsinogen (IRT), CF genotype
	Thyroid function tests
Haematology	FBC, prothrombin time, blood group
Infection screen	Including hepatitis and congenital infection screen
Imaging	USS liver and gallbladder
	Isotope TOBIDA scan
	Direct cholangiography at operation
Liver biopsy	Biliary tract and hepatocellular differentiation (NB: Correct prothrombin time prior to biopsy if abnormal)

Biliary atresia

Incidence 1 in 15 000–20 000 live births.

A condition of *progressive* obliteration of part or all of the extrahepatic biliary ducts (an obliterative cholangiopathy). This leads to chronic liver failure and death. It should be suspected if there is prolonged jaundice beyond 14 days.

Clinical manifestations

- Normal at birth
- Jaundice persisting from day 2
- Pale stools and dark urine
- Hepatosplenomegaly with progressive liver disease

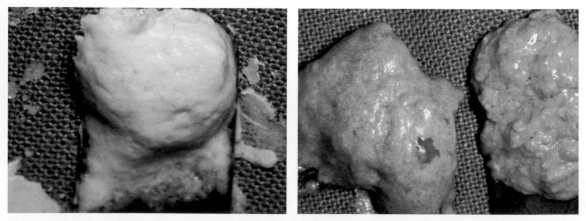

Figure 12.6 Pale and greasy stool of steatorrhoea (left) compared to a normal breast-fed infant stool (right)

Investigations

LFTs	Often normal enzymes, with conjugated hyperbilirubinaemia
USS	May be normal, gallbladder may be absent on fasting USS when it should be present
Fasting TOBIDA radioisotope scan	Isotope uptake into liver unimpaired, excretion into the intestine absent
Liver biopsy	Perilobular oedema and fibrosis, proliferation of bile ductules, bile plugs, basic hepatic architecture intact
Laparotomy with operative cholangiography	

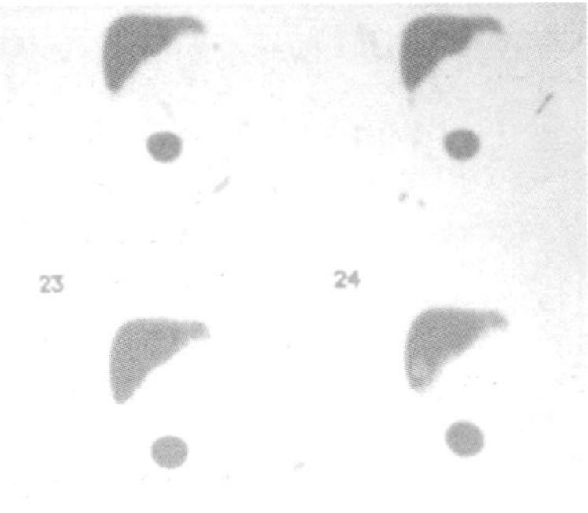

Figure 12.7 TBIDA scan showing no isotope excretion into the bowel in an infant with congenital biliary atresia

> **!** **NB: It can be difficult to differentiate *biliary atresia* (bile duct proliferation present on liver biopsy) from *neonatal hepatitis* (intrahepatic disease with giant cells present on liver biopsy).**

Management

■ Kasai procedure (hepatoportoenterostomy):
  – 80% success rate
  – Later complications – cholangitis, fat malabsorption, cirrhosis, portal hypertension
  – NB: Surgery must be performed < 60 days of life to increase chances of success
■ Liver transplantation usually necessary at a later date

Alagille syndrome (arteriohepatic dysplasia)

Autosomal dominant (gene mapping now possible). Incidence 1 in 100 000 births.

A syndrome of:
■ Bile tree paucity
■ Cardiac defects
■ Tuberous xanthoma
■ Dysmorphism

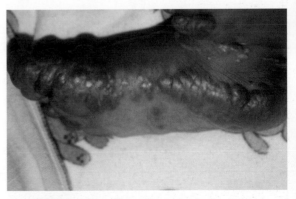

Figure 12.8 Tuberous xanthomas on the feet in Alagille syndrome

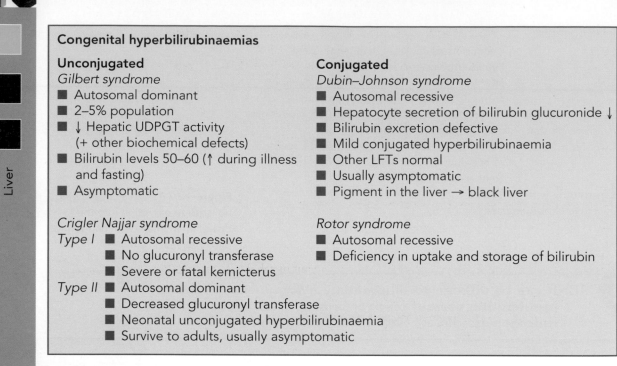

Congenital hyperbilirubinaemias

Unconjugated

Gilbert syndrome
- Autosomal dominant
- 2–5% population
- ↓ Hepatic UDPGT activity
  (+ other biochemical defects)
- Bilirubin levels 50–60 (↑ during illness and fasting)
- Asymptomatic

Crigler Najjar syndrome

Type I
- Autosomal recessive
- No glucuronyl transferase
- Severe or fatal kernicterus

Type II
- Autosomal dominant
- Decreased glucuronyl transferase
- Neonatal unconjugated hyperbilirubinaemia
- Survive to adults, usually asymptomatic

Conjugated

Dubin–Johnson syndrome
- Autosomal recessive
- Hepatocyte secretion of bilirubin glucuronide ↓
- Bilirubin excretion defective
- Mild conjugated hyperbilirubinaemia
- Other LFTs normal
- Usually asymptomatic
- Pigment in the liver → black liver

Rotor syndrome
- Autosomal recessive
- Deficiency in uptake and storage of bilirubin

METABOLIC DISORDERS

WILSON DISEASE (HEPATOLENTICULAR DEGENERATION)

Autosomal recessive. Gene mapped to chromosome 13q14–21. Incidence 1 in 100 000 births.

The underlying problem is a defect in the hepatocytes which prevents entry of copper into the caeruloplasmin compartment. Copper therefore accumulates in the liver and then escapes to the circulation and other organs such as the brain, kidneys and eyes.

Copper metabolism
Ingested copper is absorbed in the stomach and small intestine, and transported bound to albumin to the liver. In the liver it is incorporated into caeruloplasmin for transport to the rest of the body. It is excreted into the biliary system or incorporated into copper storage proteins.

Clinical manifestations

Liver	Manifest > 5 years
	Subacute or chronic hepatitis, hepatomegaly ± splenomegaly, fulminant hepatic failure, cirrhosis, portal hypertension, manifestations of chronic liver disease
Brain	Manifest > 10 years
	Copper deposition in the basal ganglia
	Intention tremor, dysarthria, choreoathetosis, dystonia, behavioural change – bizarre or psychotic, school performance deterioration (occasionally these are the only manifestations)

Kidney	Proximal renal tubular acidosis (Fanconi syndrome), renal failure
Blood	Haemolysis, may be initial presentation, severe
Cornea	Kayser–Fleischer ring is *pathognomonic* (golden brown ring at periphery of cornea due to deposition in Descemet membrane)

Investigations

Urine	24 h copper excretion ↑
	24 h copper excretion after penicillamine given ↑ ↑
Serum caeruloplasmin	↓
Liver biopsy	Characteristic histology and periportal copper deposition present
Serum copper	Raised early in disease, may be normal

Management

Symptoms and signs improve with therapy; pre-symptomatic disease is treated in relatives.

Copper chelation agents	Penicillamine orally (NB: This is an antimetabolite to vitamin B6; therefore, this is also given)
Copper intake	Reduce to < 1 mg/kg/day
	Foods high in copper – liver, nuts, chocolate, shellfish
Liver transplant	If fulminant liver disease

Screening

All family members are screened for pre-symptomatic disease:
- Caeruloplasmin (↓)
- Urine copper (↑)
- Liver biopsy if diagnosis suspected

Antenatal diagnosis is possible.

HAEMOCHROMATOSIS

Autosomal dominant disease of excess iron deposition and absorption. The underlying defect is unknown.

The *clinical manifestations* include:

Liver	Fibrosis, cirrhosis and primary hepatocellular carcinoma
Pancreas	IDDM
Heart	Cardiomyopathy, arrhythmias
Endocrine glands	Pituitary failure, growth failure, hypothyroidism, hypoparathyroidism, testicular atrophy
Skin	Slate-grey discolouration
Joints	Chondrocalcinosis

Clinically significant symptoms are rare before the third decade.

Neonatal haemochromatosis

This is an acquired condition secondary to severe prenatal liver disease. Liver dysfunction is severe, with liver transplantation usually required. An aggressive chelation and antioxidant regimen can, rarely, avoid the need for liver transplantation.

Transfusion-induced haemochromatosis

This occurs with multiple chronic transfusions (as seen in thalassaemia major, see ch. 18), and results in a similar pathology due to the excess iron deposition. Therefore chelation therapy must be given.

ALPHA-1 ANTITRYPSIN DEFICIENCY

Autosomal dominant. Gene located on chromosome 14q31–32.3. Incidence 1 in 2000–5000 live births. Common in Northern Europeans (1 in 10 carries a deficiency gene).

This disease is the result of a deficiency of α-1 antitrypsin in varying degrees of severity. α-1 antitrypsin is a protease inhibitor (Pi) made by hepatocytes; it is a glycoprotein and accounts for > 80% of the circulating α-1 globulin.

The disease results in:
- Liver disease – childhood onset
- Lung disease – onset at 20–40 years

Proteases are inherited as a series of codominant alleles (over 20 phenotypes exist). The genetic variants are characterized by their electrophoretic mobilities as medium (M), slow (S) and very slow (Z). Example genotypes are:

PiMM	Normal phenotype
PiSS	α-1 AT 60% activity
PiZZ	α-1 AT 15% activity. 1 in 3400 births. Most clinical disease. 20% have neonatal cholestasis
Pi null null	Not associated with liver disease. 0% α-1 AT activity

Clinical manifestations

Liver	Very variable
	Neonatal cholestasis, transient jaundice in first few months of life, hepatomegaly, ± splenomegaly, childhood cirrhosis
Respiratory	Emphysema (as adult)
Skin	Persistent cutaneous vasculitis, cold-contact urticaria, acquired angio-oedema

Investigations
- Serum α-1 antitrypsin (↓)
- Liver biopsy (globules of α-1 antitrypsin in the periportal cells)
- Pi phenotype
- Parental genotype

Antenatal diagnosis is possible.

Management
- Liver transplant if severe liver disease
- For lung disease, danazol (increases α-1 antitrypsin) and enzyme replacement therapy available
- Genetic counselling required for future pregnancies

REYE SYNDROME

A syndrome of acute encephalopathy and fatty degeneration of the liver. Incidence has markedly declined over recent years due to decreased aspirin use in children and greater recognition of the differential diagnoses.

Usual age of onset 4–12 years; mortality 40%.

Associations
- Aspirin therapy
- Viral infections (influenza B, varicella)
- Mitochondrial cytopathy

Clinical manifestations

- Prodromal URTI or chicken pox
- 4–7 days later:
  - Vomiting +++
  - Encephalopathy
  - Moderate hepatomegaly, no jaundice, not icteric
  - ± Hypoglycaemia

Differential diagnoses

- CNS infections
- Drug ingestion
- Haemorrhagic shock with encephalopathy
- Metabolic disease, e.g. fatty acid oxidation defects, organic acidurias, urea cycle defects

Investigations

Bloods	Ammonia ↑ (>125 µg/dL)
	AST, ALT, LDH, CK (↑)
	Glucose (↓, in small children especially)
	Clotting deranged (PT ↑)
Liver biopsy	Fatty infiltration, specific mitochondrial morphology on EM

> **!** **Avoid lumbar puncture in Reye syndrome as ICP is raised.**

Management

This is supportive, with correction of hypoglycaemia and coagulation defects, and intensive care as necessary. It is important to:

- Control raised ICP
- Make sure the diagnosis is correct

HEPATITIS

VIRAL HEPATITIS

This may be caused by the hepatitis viruses, CMV, EBV, HSV, varicella, HIV, rubella, adenovirus, enteroviruses and arboviruses.

Hepatitis A (HAV)

This is an RNA picornavirus and is the commonest cause of viral hepatitis.

Transmission	Faecal–oral (especially water, seafood, poor sanitation)

Clinical features

Incubation (2 weeks)	Infective until just after jaundice appears
Prodrome (2 weeks)	Malaise, nausea, vomiting, diarrhoea, headaches
Jaundice (2–4 weeks)	Cholestatic jaundice, mild hepatosplenomegaly, symptoms improving
Rare complications	Fulminant hepatic failure, vasculitis, arthritis, myocarditis, renal failure

Investigations

Prodrome   Serum bilirubin (N)
                    Urine bilirubin and urobilinogen (↑)
                    AST (↑ ↑)
                    FBC (WCC ↓ with relative lymphocytosis, aplastic anaemia)
                    Coombs +ve haemolytic anaemia)
                    ESR ↑
                    Stool EM +ve for HAV
Jaundice   Bilirubin (↑)
                    AST (↑) for up to 6 months
                    Alkaline phosphatase (↑)
                    Anti–HAV IgM

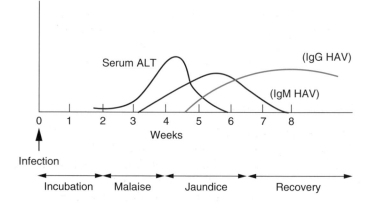

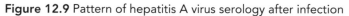

Figure 12.9 Pattern of hepatitis A virus serology after infection

Management
Supportive only. No carrier state.

Prevention
Passive immunization   Standard immunoglobulin, 3 months' protection
Active immunization   Vaccine available

Hepatitis B (HBV)

DNA hepadnavirus.

Transmission   Intravenous, close contact, vertical transmission

Clinical features
These are as for hepatitis A, but are more prolonged and severe.

Investigations
As for hepatitis A.

Specific markers for hepatitis B	
Antigen	**Antibody**
HBsAg	Anti-HBsAg
HbcAg	Anti-HBcAg
	IgM anti-HBcAg
HBeAg	Anti-HBeAg

Disease course

Most make a full recovery

Fulminant hepatitis (1%)	Anti-HbcAg diagnostic in this situation
Chronic infection (10%)	HBsAg (normal carrier state)
	HbeAg (very infectious)
	70–90% asymptomatic → hepatocellular carcinoma
	10–30% chronic hepatitis → cirrhosis → hepatocellular carcinoma
	Common among infants infected < 1 year

Carriers may be treated with pegylated interferon-α which may seroconvert them.

Infants of hepatitis B carrier mothers

These are at risk of contracting hepatitis B.

If mother is: HBsAg +ve Anti-HBeAb +ve	}	Vaccine within 12 h of birth, IM Repeat doses of vaccine at 1 and 6 months
If mother is: HBsAg +ve HBeAg +ve	}	Vaccine within 12 h of birth Hepatitis B immune globulin (HBIG) < 1 h Repeat doses of vaccine at 1 and 6 months

---

Hepatitis C (HCV)

RNA virus with six subtypes. Types I, II and III are common in Europe; Type IV is common in the Far East.

Transmission	Vertical (uncommon)
	Intravenous, close contact

This causes a mild flu-like illness. Rare complications are aplastic anaemia, arthritis, agranulocytosis and neurological problems. Chronic liver disease occurs in 50% →, cirrhosis (50%) →, hepatocellular carcinoma (15%).

Diagnosis is with anti-HCV antibody detection (negative until 1–3 months after clinical onset). Pegylated interferon-α and ribavirin can be given to chronic carriers, the earlier in childhood the better. There is no prophylaxis for maternal transmission.

Hepatitis D (HDV)

Hepatitis D virus (Delta virus) is an incomplete RNA particle enclosed in the HBsAg. Two patterns of infection are seen: *superinfection* in a person already infected with HBV, and *coinfection* with HBV.

Transmission	Close contact, vertical

Diagnosis is by detecting IgM antibody to HDV. Chronic infection is very serious as 70% develop cirrhosis. Interferon-α therapy causes remission only.

Hepatitis E (HEV)

RNA virus.

Transmission   Enteral route

Clinical illness is similar to hepatitis A, although often more severe.

Diagnosis is by HEV RNA detection in serum or stools. No carrier state exists and there is no effective prophylaxis.

CHRONIC HEPATITIS

This is the presence of hepatic inflammation (manifest by elevated transaminases) for > 6 months. There are two subdivisions of chronic hepatitis, distinguished histologically:

Chronic persistent hepatitis   Benign, self-limiting usually
Chronic active hepatitis   Progressive disease with eventual cirrhosis

The clinical manifestations are variable:

- Asymptomatic
- Chronic liver disease
- Hepatic failure

Causes

- Persistent viral infection
- Autoimmune
- Drugs, e.g. isoniazid, nitrofurantoin, sulphonamides, dantrolene
- Metabolic, e.g. cystic fibrosis, Wilson disease, haemochromatosis, α–1 antitrypsin disease

PORTAL HYPERTENSION

This occurs when the portal pressure is elevated > 10–12 mmHg (normal = 7 mmHg). Increased portal venous pressure results in collaterals (varices) developing (porto-systemic shunting) and a hyperdynamic circulation. These together can cause varices to rupture and result in GI bleeds.

Causes

It is caused by obstruction to the portal flow anywhere along the portal system.

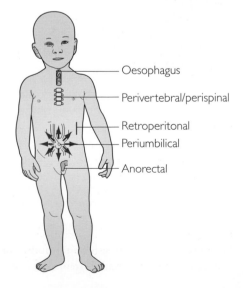

Oesophagus

Perivertebral/perispinal

Retroperitonal
Periumbilical

Anorectal

Figure 12.10 Important sites of collateral vessels (varices) in portal hypertension

Prehepatic	Hepatic	Post-hepatic
Small liver, big spleen	Liver small/large/normal Big spleen	Big liver, big spleen
Portal/splenic vein thrombosis: ■ Neonatal sepsis ■ Dehydration ■ Hypercoagulable state *Increased portal flow:* ■ A-V fistula	*Hepatocellular:* ■ Congenital hepatic fibrosis ■ Viral hepatitis ■ Cirrhosis (any cause, e.g. cystic fibrosis) ■ Hepatotoxicity, e.g. TPN, methotrexate *Biliary tract disease:* ■ Sclerosing cholangitis ■ Choledochal cyst ■ Biliary atresia ■ Intrahepatic bile duct paucity	*Hepatic vein occlusion (Budd–Chiari syndrome):* ■ Congenital venous web ■ Polycythaemia ■ Leukaemia ■ Coagulopathy ■ Sickle cell disease ■ Oral contraceptive pill ■ GVHD *Veno-occlusive disease* (seen with BMT) *Right heart failure* *Constrictive pericarditis*

Clinical features

- Bleeding oesophageal varices
- Cutaneous collaterals (periumbilical, inferior abdominal wall)
- Splenomegaly (depending on site of the obstruction)
- Liver size may be normal, enlarged or small, and there may be signs of underlying liver disease
- Haemorrhagic encephalopathy secondary to massive GI bleed

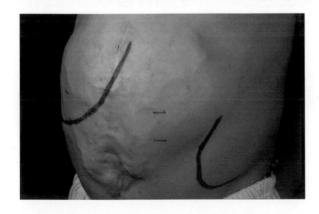

Figure 12.11 Child with hepatosplenomegaly and portal hypertension. Note the caput medusae

Investigations

USS	Outlining portal vein pathology, direction of flow of the portal system, presence of oesophageal varices
CT/MRI scan	Findings as for USS
Arteriography	Can be done from the coeliac axis, superior mesenteric artery or splenic vein
Endoscopy	Outlining oesophageal and gastric varices

Management

Emergency	Resuscitation (clear fluids and blood) Treatment of coagulopathy (FFP, vitamin K, platelets) Nasogastric tube

H2 antagonist or proton pump inhibitor IV
Other drugs if necessary (octeotride, GTN)
Endoscopy – elastic band ligation of varices
Occasionally, in extremis, insertion of a Sengstaken tube (gastric balloon only) may be required

Elective   Endoscopic obliteration (as above)
Porto-systemic shunts, e.g. TIPSS (transjugular intrahepatic porto-systemic shunt)
(Shunts have complication of encephalopathy)
Liver transplantation (for intrahepatic disease or hepatic vein obstruction)

GALLSTONES (CHOLECYSTITIS AND CHOLELITHIASIS)

Gallstones are relatively rare in children. They are of the pigment type in 70% of cases in children and cholesterol stones in 20%.

Associations

- Chronic haemolysis (sickle cell disease, spherocytosis) – pigment stones
- Crohn disease
- Ileal resection
- Cystic fibrosis
- TPN therapy
- Obesity
- Sick premature infants

LIVER TRANSPLANTATION

- Orthotopic liver transplant is available for chronic liver disease or acute/subacute liver failure
- Transplant should be considered before irreversible nutritional deficit, and growth and developmental delay
- Biliary atresia and metabolic liver disease are common indications in children
- Combined small bowel and liver transplantation is now an effective treatment for short-gut or intestinal failure. However, isolated small bowel transplant is recommended unless end-stage liver dysfunction accompanies bowel disease

Indications and contraindications of urgent liver transplantation

Indications	Contraindications
Deteriorating liver synthetic function	Irreversible cerebral damage
INR > 4	Multisystem disease not correctable by transplant,
↓ing transaminases reflecting ↓ing hepatic mass	e.g. peroxisomal disorders
Blood glucose and albumin ↓ing if unsupported	
Emergent and worsening hepatic encephalopathy	

Chronic indications also include:
- Poor quality of life
- Severe pruritus
- Persistent encephalopathy
- Recurrent hepatic complications
- Persistent hyperbilirubinaemia > 120 μmol/L

Complications

Early   Renal impairment, hypertension, GI haemorrhage, graft dysfunction, acute rejection
Late   Infection (especially bacterial, CMV and PCP), organ rejection, lymphoproliferative
       disease

Prognosis

80–90% 5-year survival rate for elective transplantation.

Clinical scenario

An 8-week-old infant is seen by his GP for the first time, as he is part of a travelling family. He was born at home and has had no problems to date except an umbilical infection which was treated effectively by local antiseptic lotion application.

It becomes clear that he has never passed a normally coloured stool and all of them have been pale, whilst his urine has been increasingly dark. He is clinically jaundiced and has a hepatomegaly of 3 cm below the right costal margin.

1. What is the most likely diagnosis?
2. What are the three most important investigations?
3. What is the definitive therapeutic step and how quickly should this be arranged?

ANSWERS

1. Biliary atresia
2. Fasting ultrasound looking for a gallbladder; liver isotope excretion scan; liver biopsy
3. Kasai porto-enterostomy – as quickly as possible, as it becomes rapidly less successful after about 60 days of life

---

FURTHER READING

Kelly D. *Diseases of the Liver and Biliary System in Children (Third Edition)*. Blackwell Publishing Limited. 2008.

Kleinman RE, Goulet OJ, Mieli-Vergani G *et al*. *Walker's Pediatric Gastrointestinal Disease (Fifth Edition)*. PMPH USA. 2008

Wyllie R, Hyams JS. *Pediatric Gastrointestinal Liver Disease (Third Edition)*. Philadelphia: Saunders. 2006.

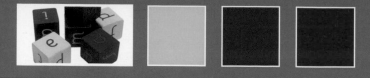

13 Renal Medicine

- Functions of the kidney
- Renal investigations in children
- Congenital structural malformations
- Urinary tract infection
- Nephrotic syndrome
- Glomerulonephritis
- Haemolytic–uraemic syndrome
- Renal calculi
- Renal venous thrombosis
- Hypertension
- Renal failure
- Further reading

Specific additional renal problems arise in children as a consequence of both congenital maldevelopment and functional immaturity of the kidneys and urinary tract.

FUNCTIONS OF THE KIDNEY

- Excretion of waste products
- Regulation of body fluid volume and composition (salt, water and pH balance)
- Endocrine and metabolic (renin, prostaglandins, erythropoietin, vitamin D metabolism)

RENAL INVESTIGATIONS IN CHILDREN

Many renal investigations are common to both children and adults but some differences arise because of collection techniques and difficulty in assessing immature renal/urinary tract function.

URINE TESTS

Urinalysis (dipstick)	Sticks can be used to test for: glucose, protein, ketones, pH, urobilinogen, nitrates and nitrites, leukocyte esterase
Microscopy	White cells, red cells and bacteria (Gram stain) – seen in infection
	Casts and red cells – seen in glomerular inflammation/nephritis
Culture	Bacteria, white cells – seen in infection

Urine sample collection is problematical in children since they cannot void to order, and contamination of samples can both complicate diagnosis and delay treatment.

Methods to collect urine from children		
Specimen	**Indication**	**Potential problems**
Clean catch	Infants	Difficult to time
		Three samples ideally
		needed prior to treatment
Suprapubic aspirate	May use in infants < 1 year	*'Gold standard'* sample
	Standard in sick infants	Invasive technique
Catheter sample	If catheter *in situ*	Contamination possible
	In sick older child	
Mid-stream urine (MSU)	Children > 3 years old	Contamination possible
	(or younger with patience)	

BLOOD TESTS

Creatinine

Creatinine is a *poor* indicator of renal function in children since it is influenced not only by renal function but also by muscle mass; hence, because of their low muscle mass, creatinine levels do not rise in children until significant renal damage has occurred.

! **NB: Immediately after birth neonatal creatinine is a reflection of the maternal creatinine.**

Urea and electrolytes, and bicarbonate

Again, urea is dependent on protein catabolism.

Glomerular filtration

Glomerular filtration (GFR) is the total volume of plasma per minute filtered through the glomerulus:

$$\text{GFR} = \frac{\text{Urine flow} \times [\text{urine}]}{[\text{plasma}]} \qquad [\ \ ] = \text{concentration of substance}$$

GFR is low *in utero* and immediately after birth, but rises to adult levels by 18 months–2 years of age.

An accurate GFR can be obtained using Cr EDTA or inulin (the gold standard, for research purposes only). Alternatively, a rough guide to GFR can be derived using various formulae that include height and/or weight:

$$\text{Approximation of GFR} = \frac{\text{Height (cm)} \times \text{K}}{\text{Plasma creatinine (}\mu\text{mol/L)}}$$

(K = 40–50 in childhood)

RADIOLOGICAL INVESTIGATIONS
Ultrasound scan

The standard imaging procedure generates information on renal size and growth, structure and dilatation (which may be a marker of obstruction). *No* information is obtained on *renal function*.

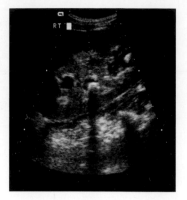

Figure 13.1 Renal ultrasound scan showing echogenic renal calculi in the kidney

Micturating cystourethrography (MCUG)

Contrast medium is instilled into the bladder via a urethral catheter and the urinary tract is visualized while the infant is voiding. This is a sensitive technique to detect and grade reflux, and outline urethral obstruction on voiding with the catheter removed, but is a relatively invasive procedure due to the necessity to place a catheter.

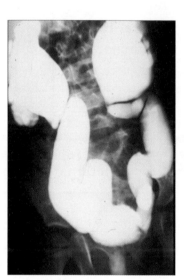

Figure 13.2 Micturating cystourethrography showing severe bilateral vesicoureteric reflux with ureteric dilatation

Static nuclear medicine scan (DMSA)

Static renal scanning with technetium–labelled 2,3–dimercaptosuccinic acid (DMSA). DMSA is taken up by proximal tubules and the functional cortical mass is outlined. Normal results range from > 45% for one kidney to < 55% for the other kidney. DMSA is used to detect renal scarring and pyelonephritis (though it cannot differentiate acute from chronic).

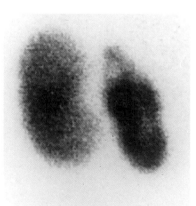

Figure 13.3 Tc-DMSA scan (right posterior oblique projection) showing a defect in the upper pole of the right kidney

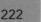

Dynamic nuclear medicine scanning (DPTA and MAG3)

Radioisotope scanning with technetium-labelled diethylenetriaminepentaacetic acid (DTPA) or mercapto-acetylglycine (MAG3). DPTA and MAG3 are freely filtered through the glomerulus. In a normal scan the isotope is quickly excreted, but with pathology the excretion is delayed. Furosemide is then given to differentiate an obstructed system (where delay continues) from an unobstructed system. Used to detect renal blood flow, function and drainage disorders, and reflux in an older child who can control micturition on demand.

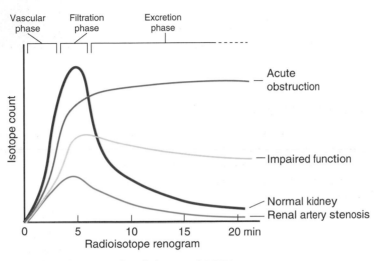

Figure 13.4 Normal and abnormal DPTA scans

Intravenous urography

Intravenous urography (IVU) is used to check detailed anatomy, i.e. renal pelvis, calyces, ureters, stones and obstruction. Contrast is given IV and is excreted via (and hence outlines) the urinary tract. It is rarely needed nowadays.

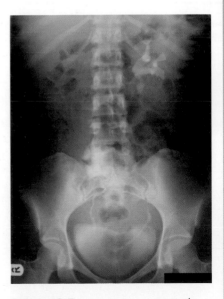

Figure 13.5 Intravenous urography. Contrast visible in normal left renal pelvis, but right kidney is law and malrotated with some obstruction (a pelvic kidney)

CONGENITAL STRUCTURAL MALFORMATIONS

DYSPLASTIC KIDNEYS AND RENAL AGENESIS

Renal dysplasia is a histological term – the kidney contains undifferentiated cells and metaplastic structures such as smooth muscle and cartilage. This is usually due to an early developmental problem leading to aberrant interaction between epithelial cells in the ureteric bud and the surrounding mesenchyme cells. Later, lower urinary tract obstruction can also cause dysplasia (but this is usually less severe since the initial development is normal).

Dysplastic kidneys

Clinical features

- May be large and multicystic, normal size or small
- Initially large kidneys may become small and then disappear *in utero* (= false appearance of renal agenesis)
- May be unilateral or bilateral
- Associated with other renal abnormalities, often with obstruction, i.e. atretic ureters or lower urinary tract abnormalities
- Associated with extrarenal abnormalities
- If urine flow is reduced bilaterally or completely blocked it causes the **Potter sequence**:
  – Oligohydramnios
  – Potter facies (squashed face, low-set ears, flat nose)
  – Pulmonary hypoplasia
  – Limb abnormalities

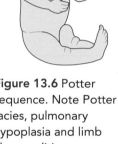

Figure 13.6 Potter sequence. Note Potter facies, pulmonary hypoplasia and limb abnormalities

Diagnosis

- USS (antenatal or postnatal) – bright hyperechogenic kidneys (large and multicystic kidney disease [MCKD], normal size or small), oligo- or anhydramnios
- Abdominal mass in newborn
- Later finding (incidental scanning, family scanning, hypertension or renal failure)

Comparison of unilateral and bilateral dysplasia		
	Unilateral dysplasia	**Bilateral dysplasia**
Incidence	1 in 3000–5000 births	1 in 10 000 births
Diagnosis	May be incidental finding Prenatal detection variable (depends on severity)	Normally diagnosed *in utero* because decreased liquor volume
Other kidney	Abnormal 30–50% (structural or VUR)	N/A
Other renal anomalies	May be present	May be present
Extrarenal anomalies	Less common	More common < 35%
Chromosomal defects	Rare	About 10%
Prognosis	Good if *normal other kidney*: slight risk of CRF, tumour in dysplastic kidney, hypertension Generally involute without problems *If abnormal other kidney*: increased risk of BP ↑, CRF, UTI	*Poor* if ↓ liquor, small kidneys (often die in neonatal period from pulmonary hypoplasia and renal failure) *In less severe disease*: chronic renal failure in long term, recurrent UTIs, hypertension

POLYCYSTIC KIDNEYS

Polycystic kidney disease is caused by defects in terminal maturation of the renal system, with an initially normal nephron and collecting duct, and later cystic dilatation of these and loss of adjacent normal structures. Polycystic kidney disease may be recessive (ARPKD) or dominant (ADPKD); the latter presents in early adulthood.

Autosomal recessive polycystic kidney disease

Gene – fibrocystin on 6p. Incidence 1 in 40 000 births.

Presentation

In utero	Large hyperechogenic kidneys on USS ± oligohydramnios
At birth	Massive kidneys (abdominal mass)

Clinical features

Renal	Bilateral symmetrical renal enlargement with numerous microscopic corticomedullary cysts
	Gradually develop BP ↑ and slow decline in renal function
Liver	Bile duct proliferation, portal fibrosis

Prognosis

Death in the neonatal period (10%) or, if the child survives beyond this, reasonable prognosis with slow decline (50% in renal failure by end of childhood – note these updated figures are much better than quoted in older textbooks).

DUPLEX KIDNEY

Incidence 1 in 100 (very common). Two ureteric buds develop on one side.

ECTOPIC KIDNEY

The kidney fails to ascend from the pelvis, e.g. pelvic kidney. There is usually normal function as long as the other kidney is normal. Increased risk of UTI.

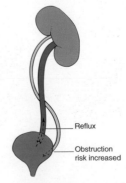

Figure 13.7
Ureteric duplication

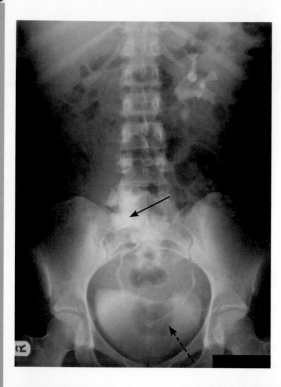

Figure 13.8 Pelvic kidney shown by intravenous urography (arrow). The ectopic right kidney is low and malrotated with obstruction at the pelviureteric junction. Left kidney is in the normal position. Note a ureterocoele at the left vesicoureteric junction (dotted arrow)

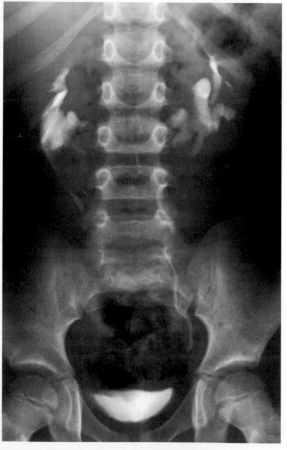

Figure 13.9 Horseshoe kidney in a 6-year-old boy. The IVU study shows typical reversal of the normal renal axis and malrotation of the lower half of both kidneys where the calyces point, instead of laterally

HORSESHOE KIDNEY

Incidence 1 in 500. This is aberrant fusion of the two kidneys at the lower poles, and may also be dysplastic.

There is an increased incidence of UTI, stones and PUJ obstruction.

HYDRONEPHROSIS

Hydronephrosis is dilatation of the renal pelvis. It is relatively common.

Associations
- Reflux
- Obstruction
- Renal dysplasia/hypoplasia

Bilateral significant hydronephrosis (> 15 mm) detected antenatally must be investigated urgently since it may indicate lower urinary tact obstruction, such as posterior urethral valves in boys which often need rapid corrective surgery. There is argument over the size of dilatation that needs full investigation, but > 15 mm definitely does.

VESICOURETERIC REFLUX

Vesicoureteric reflux (VUR) is retrograde flow of urine from the bladder into the ureters ± renal pelvis, due to incompetence at the vesicoureteric junction or abnormality of the whole ureter.

- Very common (1 in 50–100)
- Associated with hydronephrosis and renal scarring
- Familial – multifactorial, several loci found but no specific genes yet
- Usually resolves spontaneously (10–15% improvement in reflux is seen per year)
- Graded in severity – Grades I and II have spontaneous resolution in 80%, Grades II and IV have spontaneous resolution in 15%
- 20% of adult end-stage renal failure is a result of 'reflux' nephropathy

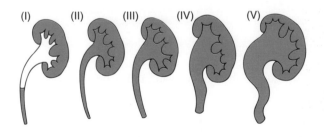

Figure 13.10 Grades of vesicoureteric reflux, divided by degree of reflux and types with normal calibre or dilated ureters

Traditional teaching is that reflux can result in renal scarring (**reflux nephropathy**) because:

- Renal pelvis is exposed to high pressures (during urination)
- Reflux facilitates the passage of bacteria into the renal pelvis

But many of the kidneys are already abnormal at birth because of combined maldevelopment of the lower urinary tract (ureters and bladder) and kidneys, i.e. urinary tract 'field defect'.

Management of reflux and renal scarring
NB: Most centres have specific local protocols, hence this is only a guide.

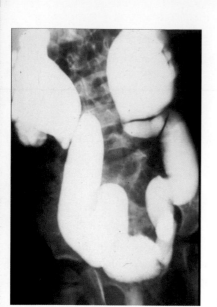

Figure 13.11 Severe bilateral vesicoureteric reflux with gross ureteric dilatation seen on MCUG

- Long term antibiotic therapy, e.g. trimethoprim 2 mg/kg/day. Controversial when to stop, i.e. when reflux resolved, no UTIs for a year, or after the age of 5 when new scarring is very rare
- Routine MSU and when symptomatic
- Consider circumcision in boys if recurrent UTIs and *tight foreskin*
- Cystoscopic injection of reinforcing material around ureteric orifices in the bladder or surgical reimplantation of ureters (old fashioned) if medical management fails (rarely necessary)
- If there is bilateral scarring, perform regular renal growth and function tests

Reinvestigate regularly in early childhood looking at:

- Renal growth (USS)
- If the condition has resolved (MAG3)
- Any new scars (DMSA)
- BP check 6–12 monthly for life

BLADDER EXSTROPHY

Incidence 1 in 40 000 births (rare but severe defect).

Bladder exstrophy is due to failure of growth of the lower abdominal wall, and a breakdown of the urogenital membrane.

Classical features

- Bladder protrudes from the abdominal wall and its mucosa is exposed
- Pubic rami and rectus muscles separated
- Umbilicus displaced downwards
- Epispadias (with undescended testes in boys, clitoral duplication in girls)
- Anteriorly displaced anus and rectal prolapse

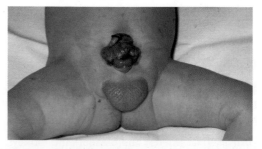

Figure 13.12 Bladder exstrophy in an infant showing the bladder protruding through the abdominal wall

This condition results in urinary incontinence, broad-based gait, increased incidence of bladder cancer, infertility and sexual dysfunction. Management involves complex surgery in a specialist centre.

PRUNE BELLY SYNDROME

Prune belly syndrome is characterized by:

- Deficient abdominal muscles with wrinkly prune-like abdomen
- Undescended testes
- Urinary tract abnormalities (dilated ureters, large bladder, dysplastic kidneys)

It is thought to result from severe urethral obstruction early in fetal life, and oligohydramnios and pulmonary hypoplasia are common.

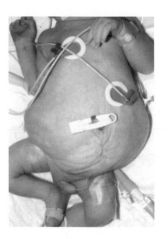

Figure 13.13 Prune belly syndrome. Note the lack of tonicity of the abdominal wall and wrinkled prune-like skin

CONGENITAL URINARY TRACT OBSTRUCTION

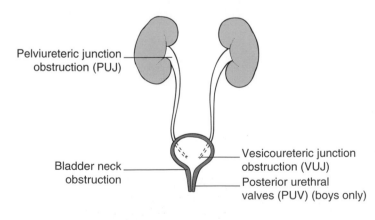

Pelviureteric junction obstruction (PUJ)

Bladder neck obstruction

Vesicoureteric junction obstruction (VUJ)

Posterior urethral valves (PUV) (boys only)

Figure 13.14 Urinary tract obstruction sites

Obstruction results in:

- Dilatation of the urinary tract proximal to the obstruction
- ± Hydronephrosis and hydroureter
- ± Dysplastic or malformed kidneys, often with peripheral cortical cysts

Intrauterine detection of dilatation on antenatal USS is possible, and many cases are detected on routine antenatal scans. It is important to assess infants in whom congenital hydronephrosis has been detected in order to check for *obstruction* and possible *renal damage* and then treat the cause. These infants are commenced on prophylactic antibiotics from birth, which may later be discontinued if all investigations are normal.

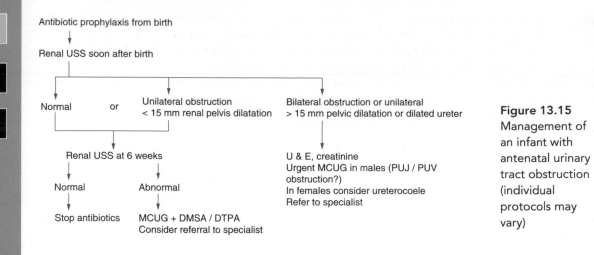

Figure 13.15 Management of an infant with antenatal urinary tract obstruction (individual protocols may vary)

Posterior urethral valve obstruction

- Seen in male infants only
- Outflow obstruction in the posterior urethra causes aberrant bladder development with small capacity and thick wall
- Bilateral hydronephrosis
- There may be associated ureteric and kidney abnormalities
- If severe, oligohydramnios and the Potter sequence can occur
- Important to recognize early as prompt surgical treatment can delay/prevent renal failure (although irreversible renal damage may have already occurred prior to birth)

URINARY TRACT INFECTION

A urinary tract infection (UTI) can present as **acute cystitis**, **acute pyelonephritis** or **septicaemia**, or be picked up as asymptomatic bacteriuria.

Causes

Predisposing factors Urinary tract abnormality (in 50%)
                           Female (occurs in 3% of girls, 1% of boys)
                           Immunosuppression
Common bacteria   *Escherichia coli*
                           Proteus (boys particularly)
                           Pseudomonas aeruginosa (common in structural renal abnormalities)

Clinical features

Asymptomatic bacteriuria
Infant   Sepsis (pyrexia of unknown origin)
                           Failure to thrive, gastro-oesophageal reflux
Older child   Dysuria, frequency, nocturia, abdominal pain, incontinence of urine,
                           haematuria, smelly urine
                           Systemic infection (fever, unwell)

> **NB:** UTI associated with *reflux* in a *growing* kidney can result in renal scarring with later hypertension and renal failure (see reflux nephropathy, p. 224).

Diagnosis

- Urine sample (see p. 220)
- In unexplained fever, and sick infants and children – urine sample, U&Es, creatinine, ESR, CRP, blood cultures
- Urgent USS if there is a known structural malformation and concern of obstruction, or severe localized flank pain (looking for an obstructed kidney)

Features in a urine sample suggestive of a UTI

- Proteinuria, haematuria, nitrite, leukocyte esterase (*dipstick*) ⎫
- Pyuria (almost always) (*microscopy*)   ⎬ *Suggestive*
- Organisms seen on microscopy (*microscopy*)   ⎭
- Single species growth, i.e. > 10^5/mL (culture) = *Diagnostic*

Management

- Antibiotic therapy – IV if unwell or infant, oral if well child
- Optimize hydration
- Commence prophylactic antibiotics until *further investigations* complete
- Drainage procedures are required if infected obstructed kidney

---

Future prevention of UTIs

- High fluid intake
- Girls to wipe themselves after micturition from front to back
- Empty bladder completely and regularly
- Avoid constipation

Further investigations in proven UTI

Further investigation is necessary once a UTI has been diagnosed in a child, in order to check for any renal damage, anatomical or functional abnormality.

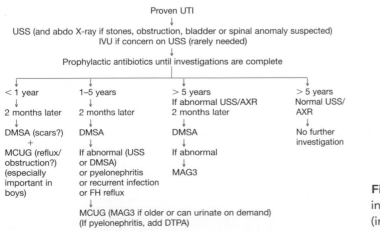

Figure 13.16 Further investigation in proven urinary tract infection (individual protocols may vary)

NEPHROTIC SYNDROME

Nephrotic syndrome is characterized by *heavy proteinuria* and the consequences of hypoalbuminaemia. It occurs in 1 in 50 000 children, is twice as common in boys, and the typical age of presentation is 1–6 years.

Diagnostic triad

- Proteinuria > 40 mg/h/m^2
- Hypoalbuminaemia < 25 mg/L
- Oedema

NB: Hyperlipidaemia (raised LDL and triglycerides) also occurs in most cases, but is not part of the diagnostic triad.

There are three main types of nephrotic syndrome in childhood:

Minimal change disease (85–90%)	No changes seen under normal microscope but podocyte foot process fusion on electron microscopy
Focal segmental glomerular sclerosis (10–15%)	Focal because not all glomeruli affected (usually deeper ones) and segmental because only segments of each glomeruli are affected
Membranous nephropathy (1–5%)	Associated with hepatitis B and malignancy such as lymphomas (more often seen in adults)

Congenital nephrotic syndrome presenting *in utero* or within the first month of life is rare. Several mutations have been found, most notably in the nephrin gene (Finnish congenital nephrotic syndrome).

Other types of nephrotic syndrome fall into an overlap pattern with nephritis, where there is marked inflammation in the glomerulus – hence there will be additional features secondary to the inflammation, such as red and white cells ± casts in the urine. Unlike uncomplicated nephrotic syndrome, it is rare for the plasma albumin to fall below 20 g/dL in these conditions. Causes include:

- Poststreptococcal glomerulonephritis (GN)
- Henoch–Schönlein purpura (HSP), anaphylactoid, drugs
- Heavy metals, malaria, systemic lupus erythematosus (SLE)

Clinical features

- **Classical presentation** is with **dependent oedema**, i.e. oedema collects at the lowest part, particularly of the face and eyes in the morning, since children often sleep face down; frequently misdiagnosed as allergies in the early stages
- As hypoproteinaemia worsens, the **oedema** becomes widespread and does not improve during the day; sites include the ankles and lower legs, scrotum and **sacrum**. Ascites can develop and shortness of breath with pleural effusions
- **Non-specific symptoms** – progressive lethargy and anorexia, occasionally diarrhoea
- **Infections**, particularly encapsulated organisms such as pneumococcus more likely. Peritonitis also possible (primary or pneumococcal)
- **Frothy urine** (rare)
- **Intravascular hypovolaemia** (secondary to hypoalbuminaemia) may present with abdominal pain, circulatory collapse/shock or venous thrombosis

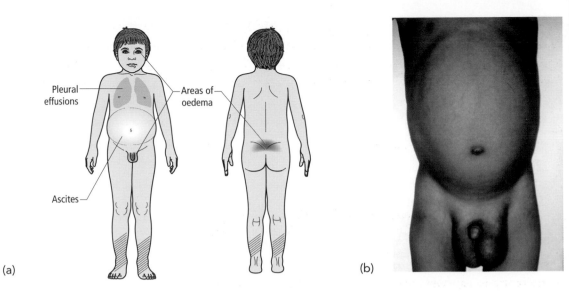

Figure 13.17 Nephrotic child. (a) Clinical features. (b) Note abdominal ascites and bilateral hydrocoeles

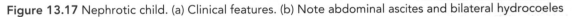

❗ NB: These children do not appear dehydrated because they are so oedematous, but they can have profound intravascular hypovolaemia because their fluid is in the wrong compartments.

Features of intravascular hypovolaemia

Orthostatic hypotension   Tachycardia
Oliguria   Abdominal pain
Cool peripheries   Rising haematocrit
Prolonged capillary refill time   Urine sodium < 20 mmol/L (severe if < 5)
Significant core–periphery temperature gap

NB: The blood pressure will *not* fall in children until there is *severe* hypovolaemia due to their compensatory mechanisms, therefore these features must be checked regularly

---

Causes of proteinuria

Physiological	**Pathological**
Orthostatic, i.e. proteinuria only when standing upright	Tubular disease – hereditary tubular dysfunction, acquired tubular dysfunction
Exercise induced (transient)	Glomerular disease – glomerulonephritis, nephrotic syndrome
Febrile (transient)	Other – UTI, drugs, tumours, e.g. lymphoma, stones

Initial investigations

Urine	Dipstick for proteinuria – will have +3 or +4 proteinuria
	Albumin:creatinine ratio – > 200 mg/mmol
	Sodium concentration – < 20 mmol/L is an indication of hypovolaemia
	Microscopy – no or minimal cells in uncomplicated nephrotic syndrome (cf red and white cell casts in glomerulonephritis)
Blood	FBC, ESR – ↑ haematocrit or haemoglobin (signs of hypovolaemia), ?signs of infection
	U&E, creatinine – raised urea may indicate hypovolaemia
	Albumin – <25 g/L (by definition)
	Cholesterol, triglyceride – ↑; whether treatment is required in acute stages is controversial
	(Hep B S Ag – if membranous GN and from Middle/Far East or at-risk group)

Other investigations if there is a suggestion of overlap with glomerulonephritis:

Blood	Complement factors – C3 and C4 ↓ (except in minimal change)
	ASOT, anti-DNAse B – positive if streptococcal infection
Throat swab	M, C & S – ? streptococcal sore throat
Renal biopsy	Done if:
	– No response to steroids after 4–6 weeks
	– Atypical features at presentation, e.g. hypertension, high creatinine, infant < 1 year

Management

- Oral corticosteroids – 60 mg/m^2/day (2 mg/kg/day) for 4 weeks (NB: this is longer than older regimens, which reduced when clear of proteinuria for 3–4 days, because there is increasing evidence that a longer initial course reduces chance of relapse and hence overall steroid dosage), then 40 mg/m^2/day alternate days for 4 weeks. If no response to steroids consider renal biopsy
- Oral penicillin prophylaxis
- Monitor intravascular volume (see below)
- Daily weight, electrolytes and albumin and fluid input–output chart
- Diuretics as needed (in hospital only)
- Monitor proteinuria (by urine dipstick at home when recovered to assess for a relapse)

Complications

- Hypovolaemia – see above
- Infection – high risk of infection, classically pneumococcal peritonitis, although Gram-negative sepsis now becoming commoner as the penicillin reduces Gram-positive cases (due to low immunoglobulins)
- Intravascular thrombosis – DVT and renal vein thrombosis (due to hypovolaemia and hypercoagulable state)
- Hypercholesterolaemia
- Acute tubular necrosis (if severe hypovolaemia)

Prognosis

Steroid sensitive disease	One-third no relapses
	One-third occasional relapses
	One-third regular relapses
Steroid resistant disease	Alternative immunosuppressive therapy needed
	High proportion (up to 50%) will progress to chronic renal failure

If the child is well, then yearly follow-up is required, checking particularly for BP and growth.

GLOMERULONEPHRITIS

Glomerulonephritis (GN) is the term for numerous diseases that involve *inflammation of the glomerulus*. It is often immune mediated. There are two main mechanisms for immunological injury:

- Deposition of circulating antigen–antibody complexes (95% of GN)
- Deposition of anti-glomerular basement membrane antibodies (5% of GN)

Important causes

- Poststreptococcal glomerulonephritis
- Henoch–Schönlein purpura (HSP)
- IgA nephropathy
- Alport syndrome

ACUTE NEPHRITIC SYNDROME

GN presents with the acute nephritic syndrome, which has four major characteristics:

- **Haematuria** (weak tea through to coca cola-coloured urine)
- **Proteinuria**
- **Oliguria**
- **Volume** overload leading to hypertension because of increased circulating volume (cf often decreased in nephrotic syndrome) and oedema because of increased extravascular fluid

Other features are red cell casts and white cells in urine.

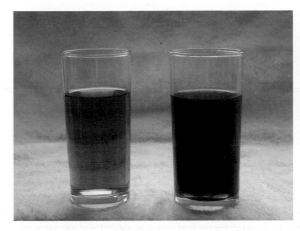

Figure 13.18 Colours of urine in nephritic syndrome range from 'weak tea' to 'coca cola'

General investigations

Urine	Urinalysis (protein, blood, casts)
	M, C & S (haematuria, proteinuria, casts, features of infection)
Blood	FBC, ESR
	U&E, creatinine, LFTs
	Complement levels (C3 and C4)
	Viral titres, ASOT
	HBsAg, ANA
Throat swab	M, C & S (features of infection)

Management

The management is *supportive*:

- Fluid restriction – give **insensible loss** (300–400 mL/m²/day) + **urine output**
- Sodium restriction – difficult in children, hence often use 'no added' salt diet
- Management of hypertension, e.g. diuretics
- Penicillin if positive throat swab or nephrotic range proteinuria
- Renal dialysis if necessary, e.g. if marked hyperkalaemia

POSTSTREPTOCOCCAL GLOMERULONEPHRITIS

This typically presents as the nephritic syndrome 1–2 weeks after group A β-haemolytic streptococcal URTI, or 2–3 weeks after streptococcal skin infection.

Investigations

- As above for nephritis
- Plus specific investigations to look for previous streptococcal infection:
  - Antistreptolysin O titre (ASOT)
  - Anti-DNAse B antibodies
  - Throat swab
- Complement studies show C3 raised and C4 normal

A renal biopsy is only necessary if there are atypical features, i.e. severe hypertension, rising creatinine.

Treatment

Treatment is a 10-day course of penicillin and supportive therapy for the nephritis (as above). Over 95% will spontaneously resolve; however, microscopic haematuria can continue for up to 1 year.

HENOCH–SCHÖNLEIN PURPURA

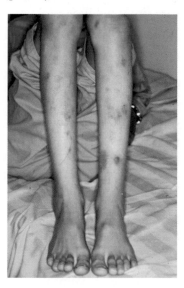

- Vasculitis of small blood vessels
- Usually affects children aged 3–10 years
- Twice as common in boys
- Often a preceding URTI
- Most common in late winter and early summer

Clinical features

There are four classical features:

Rash	Red macular rash becoming petechial over the buttocks and legs, and pressure points, e.g. sock line Often the first sign and can recur over weeks
Joint involvement	Non-destructive arthritis of the large joints (knees, ankles)
Abdominal pain	May have bloody stools due to intussusception or gastrointestinal bleeding from vasculitic lesions and also ileus, protein-losing enteropathy
Haematuria	Secondary to the glomerulonephritis

Figure 13.19 HSP rash on legs is often petechial

Other organs can be affected and there may be oedema.

The renal disease can range between:

- Microscopic haematuria
- Nephritic syndrome
- Nephrotic syndrome

Investigations

- General investigations for nephritis (as per streptoccocal infection), plus
- IgA (elevated in > 50%)
- Clotting and platelet screen (may be deranged)

Treatment

- Treat any suspected infection
- Supportive therapy for the rash, arthralgia, fever and malaise
- Renal disease:
  - Standard treatment of nephritic or nephrotic syndrome
  - Renal biopsy if severe hypertension or rising creatinine

- If severe, intractable abdominal disease, steroids may be effective (whether these mask abdominal pain associated with an intussusception is debatable)

IgA NEPHROPATHY (BERGER NEPHROPATHY)

This is a focal segmental GN with deposits of IgA in the mesangium (and raised serum IgA in around 20%). It is twice as common in boys.

Clinical features

- Microscopic haematuria
- Macroscopic haematuria *during intercurrent infections*, e.g. sore throat

Management

A renal biopsy is required to establish the diagnosis. There is no specific therapy but follow-up for life is necessary as end-stage renal failure (ESRF) develops in up to 25%. (Proteinuria and hypertension are associated with a poor prognosis.)

ALPORT SYNDROME

This is an inherited disease of collagen IV (an integral part of basement membranes, including that in the glomerulus). X-linked dominant and autosomal dominant inheritance reported; spontaneous mutation in 20%. It is more severe in males.

Clinical features

- **Ocular defects** (15%) – cataracts, macular lesions, anterior lenticonus
- **Sensorineural deafness**
- **Hereditary nephritis** – microscopic haematuria, proteinuria, ESRF by age 20–30 years

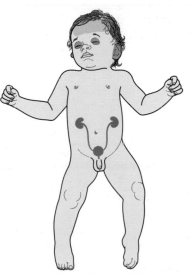

Figure 13.20 Clinical features of Alport syndrome

The disease generally presents as haematuria and a young patient may show none of the above features. Parents and siblings of an affected child should be screened by urine dipstick at least. On electron microscopy of renal biopsy there is a typical '*basket weave*' appearance (due to splitting of the basement membrane).

HAEMATURIA

This may be visible as discoloured urine (**macroscopic**) or invisible but detected on urine dipstick (**microscopic**).

Causes

- Urinary tract infection
- Glomerulonephritis

- Congenital malformations
- Trauma
- Haematological, e.g. coagulopathy, thrombocytopaenia, sickle cell disease, renal vein thrombosis
- Exercise-induced haematuria
- Drugs, e.g. anticoagulants, aspirin, sulphonamides
- Renal stones, urinary stones (rare)
- Renal tumours (rare), urinary tract tumours (rare)

History

- Trauma, drugs, recent illness
- Abdominal pain, dysuria
- Family history of renal disease, haematuria, bleeding disorders, stones

Investigations

Urine	Dipstick, microscopy and culture
Blood	FBC, U&E, creatinine, C3 and C4, ASOT, Hb electrophoresis
Genitourinary tract	USS

HAEMOLYTIC–URAEMIC SYNDROME

Haemolytic–uraemic syndrome (HUS) is a potentially life-threatening disease, and is the commonest cause of acute renal failure in children. It comprises:

- Acute renal failure
- Microangiopathic haemolytic anaemia (red cell fragments and schistocytes on blood film)
- Thrombocytopaenia

Causes

These can be grouped into two types:

Diarrhoea-positive HUS	Verotoxin producing *Escherichia coli* 0157 (10% of infections with this organism result in HUS)
	Other diarrhoea infection, e.g. shigella (shigatoxin), salmonella, campylobacter
Diarrhoea-negative HUS	Familial disease – children with presenting age < 1 have a poor prognosis
	Complement factor H deficiency
	Drug related – cyclosporin

Clinical features of diarrhoea-positive disease

- Usually < 5 years old
- Bloody diarrhoea; may resolve, then 5–10 days later oliguria, pallor, lethargy and petechiae
- Hypertension and hyperkalaemia are major causes of morbidity
- Other organs may be damaged (leading to fits or coma, or pancreatitis)

Investigations

Blood	FBC and film (microangiopathic haemolytic anaemia, thrombocytopaenia)
	Coagulation screen (normal)
	U&E, creatinine, calcium, phosphate (changes in acute renal failure [see p. 238])
Urine	Urinalysis (mild haematuria and proteinuria)
Stool	M, C & S (? infective organism identified)

Management

This is *supportive*:

- Fluid status – assess carefully, may need diuretics

- Hyperkalaemia – treatment as necessary (see p. 242)
- Dialysis – if needed
- Transfusions – blood; rarely platelets since even though count is low their function is good
- NB: Long term follow-up is essential to look for **hypertension** and **chronic renal failure**

> **!** **NB: Haemolytic uraemic syndrome is the commonest cause of acute renal failure in children in the UK.**

RENAL CALCULI

These are unusual in children; overall incidence 1.5 in 1 000 000. The most common types are **calcium oxalate** and **calcium phosphate** stones, which are radio-opaque.

Causes

Calcium stones	Idiopathic hypercalciuria, primary hyperparathyroidism, vitamin D excess, sarcoidosis, immobilization, juvenile rheumatoid arthritis
Uric acid stones	Lymphoma, ileostomies, Crohn disease, Lesch–Nyan syndrome, polycythaemia
Mixed (staghorn)	Infection with urease-splitting bacteria, e.g. proteus

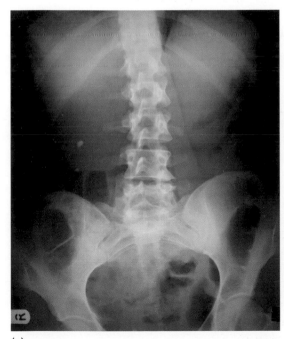
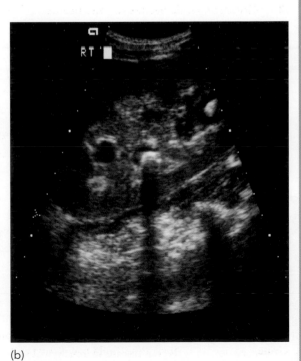

(a) (b)

Figure 13.21 Calculi. (a) Right-sided renal calculi on plain film. Note a calculus in the pelvis which has passed down the right ureter and impacted at the vesicoureteric junction. (b) Ultrasonography in the same patient showing echogenic calculi in the calyces of the right kidney with distal acoustic shadowing. A calculus at the lower end of the right ureter is also clearly identified

Presentation

- Asymptomatic
- UTI
- Haematuria, abdominal pain, renal failure

Management

- Stone removal via lithotripsy or endoscopically
- Maintain a high fluid intake
- Treat the cause if possible

RENAL VENOUS THROMBOSIS

This uncommon problem occurs in sick premature neonates, dehydration, sepsis and congenital cyanotic heart disease, and presents as:

- Gross haematuria and unilateral or bilateral flank masses in neonates
- Micro- or macroscopic haematuria with flank pain in older children
- If it is bilateral, acute renal failure will also be present

Investigations

- USS to check for renal enlargement and extension into the inferior vena cava
- Doppler flow vessel studies, and radionucleotide imaging to assess renal function
- Prothrombotic screen – up to half have an inherited procoagulant defect

Management

- Supportive therapy if unilateral
- If bilateral, fibrinolytic agents or thrombectomy are used

The kidney will become atrophic, and may later need removal if hypertension develops.

HYPERTENSION

Hypertension is the persistent elevation of blood pressure (systolic or diastolic) above the 95th centile. The incidence is around 3% of children.

> **! NB: The correct blood pressure cuff size must be used to record blood pressure. The inflatable bag of the cuff should be > two-thirds the width of the upper arm, and encircle the arm completely.**
>
> **Cuff too small   ↑ BP**
> **Cuff too large   ↓ BP**

Causes

Secondary	Renal disease (parenchymal or renal vascular disease)
	Cardiovascular, e.g. coarctation of the aorta, renal artery stenosis
	Hormonal, e.g. Cushing syndrome, phaeochromocytoma, congenital adrenal hyperplasia
	Drugs, e.g. steroids
Essential	Rare in children (but common in adults)

Clinical features

- Usually asymptomatic
- May have headaches and blurred vision if severe
- Occasional occult presentation as disruptive behaviour, autistic spectrum
- Examine for renal masses/bruits, coarctation of the aorta and eye changes (papilloedema, retinal haemorrhages)

Investigations

These are necessary to identify the underlying cause:

Renal	Urinalysis, M, C & S
	U&E, creatinine, calcium, phosphate, FBC
	Renal USS with Doppler studies, renal function tests, e.g. DMSA
Cardiovascular	Echocardiogram, ECG, fasting lipids
Hormonal	Urine VMA and HVA, oxysteroids and 24-h cortisol
	Plasma renin and aldosterone, cortisol, 21-β-hydroxylase

Management

Emergency	Nifedipine (oral is safer because sublingual can act too rapidly and cause a sudden lowering of BP which can lead to stroke), or IV infusion of sodium nitroprusside or labetolol
Long term	Drug therapy, e.g. vasodilators, diuretics, β-blockers, ACE inhibitors and treatment of the underlying cause

RENAL FAILURE

Renal failure is a failure to maintain adequate fluid and pH balance due to renal insufficiency.

ACUTE RENAL FAILURE

Acute renal failure may be:

- **Prerenal** due to local or general circulatory failure
- **Renal** due to renal parenchymal damage
- **Postrenal** due to outflow obstruction

Causes

Prerenal	Renal	Postrenal
Circulatory failure:	Haemolytic–uraemic syndrome	Bilateral renal obstruction,
■ Hypovolaemic	Glomerulonephritis	e.g. congenital, stones
■ Sepsis	Pyelonephritis	Trauma
■ Cardiac failure	Vasculitis	Neurogenic bladder
Renal artery or vein occlusion	Tumour lysis syndrome	
	Untreated prerenal failure	

Clinical features

- Oliguria (< 1 mL/kg/h or < 300 mL/m^2/day)
- Oedema
- Hypertension
- Vomiting and lethargy

- Electrolyte disturbance and metabolic acidosis
- Urine sodium is a good guide to distinguish prerenal from renal ARF – prerenal < 20 mmol/L; renal > 40 mmol/L. (The normal response is for the kidneys to retain sodium and water if the BP or renal perfusion falls)

Acute tubular necrosis (ATN) is the result of ischaemic tubular damage secondary to hypoperfusion and is the most common pathophysiological finding in established ARF. In ATN there is an initial *oliguric phase* and then *polyuria* during the recovery. The prognosis for full recovery is generally good.

Acute cortical necrosis (ACN) is an irreversible loss of renal function with glomerular damage that heals with scarring. Any cause of severe ATN can lead to ACN.

Management

The management of ARF can be divided into the various problems:

Fluids	Daily weight and electrolytes
	In oliguric phase restrict to insensible loss + ongoing losses
	In polyuric phase be careful to maintain input and electrolytes
Hyperkalaemia	See below
	NB: Medical emergency if ECG changes are present
Hyperphosphataemia	Give a phosphate binder, e.g. calcium carbonate
Hypocalcaemia	Give calcium and 1-α calcidol
Metabolic acidosis	Give bicarbonate, consider dialysis if no response and pH < 7.25
Hypertension	Correct for fluid overload and give antihypertensives
Nutrition	Restrict protein, K, Na and PO_4
Anaemia	Transfuse as necessary (but watch K carefully)
Dialysis	If severe hyperkalaemia, hyponatraemia, metabolic acidosis, fluid overload, symptomatic uraemia or medical management not tolerated, dialysis is necessary. Also allows opportunity to liberalize fluids to improve nutrition

Management of hyperkalaemia

Drug	Onset	Mechanism
10% calcium carbonate (IV)	Immediate	Stabilizes cardiac membrane
Salbutamol (nebulized or IV)	Few min	Shifts potassium into cells
8.4% $NaHCO_3$ (IV)	Few min	Shifts potassium into cells
Furosemide (IV)	Few min	Renal excretion of potassium
Dextrose (IV) (± insulin)	30 min	Shifts potassium into cells
Calcium resonium (rectal or oral)	30 min (rectal)	Potassium excretion via gut
	2 h (oral)	
Dialysis	Rapid (haemodialysis)	Removes potassium
	Slower (peritoneal dialysis)	

CHRONIC RENAL FAILURE

This occurs after a decline in renal function over months or years.

Causes

- Congenital malformations
- Glomerulonephritis

- Inherited nephropathy
- Systemic illness

Clinical features
- Malaise
- Growth failure
- Polyuria, nocturia, oliguria (depending on whether late or acute on chronic), proteinuria
- Uraemia
- Symptoms of anaemia
- Oedema (peripheral and pulmonary)
- Renal bone disease (renal osteodystrophy [renal rickets])

Investigations

Urine	Urinalysis, M, C & S, osmolality
	24-h electrolytes and protein
Blood	U&E and creatinine, phosphate (elevated)
	Ionized calcium ($\downarrow$), bicarbonate ($\downarrow$)
	FBC (anaemia)
	PTH ($\uparrow$)
	GFR (decreased)
Imaging	Left wrist X-ray (bone age and osteodystrophy)
	Renal USS and renal function tests

Management

This can be divided into the specific problems:

Diet	High energy most important, low protein controversial since children need to grow
Osteodystrophy	Manifest as PO_4 $\uparrow$ and Ca $\downarrow$, and secondary hyperparathyroidism
	Aim is to maintain the PTH in the normal range with dietary phosphate restriction, calcium carbonate and vitamin D supplements (1-α calcidol)
Sodium and acidosis	Sodium supplements (unless low urine output)
	Bicarbonate supplements (2 mmol/kg/day)
Anaemia	Subcutaneous erythropoietin therapy
Hormones	Growth hormone given if growth fails to improve with optimal nutritional management
Hypertension	Drug therapy (diuretics, nifedipine, β-blockers)
Dialysis	See below

DIALYSIS

This is necessary in **end-stage renal failure (ESRF)**. There are two methods.

Peritoneal dialysis

The peritoneal membrane is used as a semipermeable membrane. The *dialysate* is run through a tube into the peritoneal cavity and the fluid is changed regularly to repeat the process. It can be done continuously or intermittently:

- **CAPD** (continuous ambulatory peritoneal dialysis) – 2–4 cycles/day done manually
- **CCPD** (continuous cycling peritoneal dialysis) – dialysis only at night with 8–12 cycles done by machine

Peritoneal dialysis is preferred to haemodialysis in children since it is more frequent and can take off more fluid safely; hence fluid restriction is less onerous, which is important to maximize nutrition.

The major complication of peritoneal dialysis is peritonitis.

Haemodialysis

This is technically more difficult. IV access is obtained using an indwelling main venous catheter (most common in children) or by creating an A-V fistula. Blood is directed through a dialysis machine where the semipermeable membrane is located, and the dialysed blood returned to the circulation via the catheter or A-V fistula. It is done around three times per week, for an average of 3–4 h/session.

Haemodialysis is complicated by line infections and sepsis.

RENAL TRANSPLANTATION

This is the preferred option to dialysis as lifestyle is markedly improved. A cadaveric or live-related donor kidney (HLA matched) is transplanted into the iliac fossa (attached to the common iliac vessels), or intra-abdominally in small infants. Long term immunosuppression is necessary. Classical regimens include cyclosporin, prednisolone and azathioprine, but newer agents such as tacrolimus and mycophenolate mofetil are increasingly used.

Complications

- Rejection
- Infection (CMV, varicella)
- Hypertension
- Drug side effects (see below)
- Post-transplant tumours, e.g. post-transplant lymphoproliferative disease (PTLD), may be associated with EBV and tacrolimus

Common side effects of immunosuppressant drugs used in renal transplantation (for more extensive list see *BNF*)

Cyclosporin	Tacrolimus	Azathioprine	MMF
Gum hyperplasia Hypertrichosis Nephrotoxicity (hypertension, hyperkalaemia, HUS)	GI upset (nausea, vomiting and diarrhoea)	Myelosuppression Hepatotoxicity	Nausea and vomiting
Long term increased risk of malignancies, including EBV driven and independent lymphoproliferative disorders, sarcoma (HHV8) (cyclosporin and tacrolimus)			

(a)

(b)

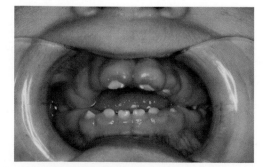

Figure 13.22 Side effects of cyclosporin therapy. (a) Gum hypertrophy. (b) Hypertrichosis

Clinical scenario

A 5-year-old girl has had 3 days of diarrhoea which over the last 12 hours has become bloody. She recovers from this but then 4 days later becomes increasingly drowsy and incoherent and her parents bring her to the Emergency Department. It is found that her blood pressure is 148/98 and this is checked and found to be repeatable. Blood is taken for initial tests and it is noted that significant oozing is occurring from the site of venepuncture.

Tests reveal that her platelets are 45 and Hb is 8.5 with a blood film showing a microangiopathic haemolytic anaemia and thrombocytopaenia.

1. What is the diagnosis?
2. What is the responsible organism?
3. What is the correct treatment strategy?

ANSWERS

1. Haemolytic-uraemic syndrome
2. Enterotoxigenic *E. coli.* Serotype 0157
3. Peritoneal dialysis; strict fluid balance; hypertensive management; platelet transfusion as required; management of incipient disseminated intravenous coagulation; urinary catheterization; assisted ventilation as needed

FURTHER READING

Avner E, Harmon W, Niaudet P, Yoshikawa N (eds.). *Paediatric Nephrology,* 6th edn. Berlin: Springer–Verlag, 2009.

Berhman R, Kliegman R, Jenson H, Stanton B. *Nelson Textbook of Pediatrics*, 18th edn. London: Saunders, 2007.

Rees L, Webb NJA, Brogan PA. *Paediatric Nephrology (Oxford Specialist Handbooks in Paediatrics)*. Oxford: OUP. 2007.

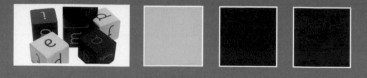

14 Endocrinology

- Pituitary gland
- Adrenal glands
- Thyroid gland
- Parathyroid glands
- Polycystic ovary syndrome
- Glucose metabolism
- Further reading

PITUITARY GLAND

The pituitary gland is divided into:

- Anterior pituitary (developed from the Rathke pouch from an invagination of the oral endoderm)
- Posterior pituitary (which forms a single unit with the hypothalamus and is responsible for the regulation and production of many hormones)

DIABETES INSIPIDUS

Diabetes insipidus (DI) is due to a *deficiency* of vasopressin (ADH) (**cranial diabetes insipidus**) or a *renal insensitivity* (**nephrogenic diabetes insipidus**) to it.

Causes

Cranial	Congenital:
	- Autosomal dominant
	- DIDMOAD (diabetes insipidus, diabetes mellitus, optic atrophy and deafness)
	Newborn:
	- Birth asphyxia, IVH
	- Listeria meningitis
	Infection – TB meningitis
	Tumour – craniopharyngioma
	Infiltration – Langerhans cell histiocytosis
	Ablation – surgery, cranial radiotherapy
Nephrogenic	X-linked recessive
	Renal tubular acidosis
	Hypokalaemia
	Nephrocalcinosis
	Drugs – demeclocycline, glibenclamide, lithium

Clinical features

- **Polyuria, polydipsia and nocturia**

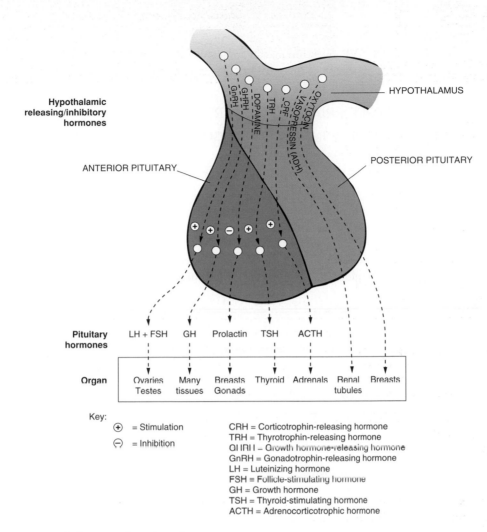

Figure 14.1 Hypothalamic and pituitary hormones

- Anorexia, dehydration, lack of perspiration and large amounts of pale urine
- Rapid weight loss, constant wet nappies and collapse in infants

Diagnosis

Osmolalities	Plasma osmolality − normal or ↑
	Urine osmolality − ↓, i.e. *dilute* (early morning urine osmolality < 280 mOsm/kg after an overnight fast; normal is > 600)
Formal water deprivation test	Deprive patient of water until either a mismatch between urine and plasma osmolality is demonstrated or > 5% weight loss, or urine osmolality is raised
	Then observe failure to concentrate urine
	Then give DDAVP (desmopressin = synthetic vasopressin) and observe urine osmolality rise − a failure of response to DDAVP indicates nephrogenic DI

! NB: Diagnosis of DI is based on demonstration of a *mismatch* between urine and plasma osmolalities.

Management

Cranial diabetes insipidus	DDAVP given intranasally, orally or IM
Nephrogenic diabetes insipidus	Sensitization of the renal tubules with thiazides, carbamazepine or chloramphenicol

SYNDROME OF INAPPROPRIATE ANTIDIURETIC HORMONE SECRETION

Syndrome of inappropriate antidiuretic hormone secretion (SIADH) is characterized by plasma levels of ADH that are *inappropriately high* for the osmolality of the blood.

Causes

CNS	Meningitis, encephalitis, head injury, subdural haematoma, brain tumour, brain abscess, birth asphyxia, hypoxic–ischaemic encephalopathy, IVH, SLE vasculitis
Tumours	Lymphoma, Ewing sarcoma, cancer of the thymus
Infections	Rotavirus, TB, meningitis, encephalitis, brain abscess
Lungs	Pneumonia, cystic fibrosis, IPPV, lung abscess
Drugs	Carbamazepine, chlorpropramide, vincristine, cyclophosphamide, morphine

Clinical features

- Appetite loss, nausea, vomiting, confusion, irritability, fits and coma
- No evidence of dehydration, no oedema, normal blood pressure

> **! NB: Clinical features of SIADH are often vague and non-specific.**

Investigations

Plasma	Electrolytes – Na ↓ (115–120 mmol/L), Cl ↓
	Osmolality ↓ (< 280 mmol/L)
Urine	Electrolytes – Na > 30 mmol/L (i.e. sodium excretion continues inappropriately)
	Osmolality – normal

Treatment

- Fluid restriction
- Daily weight, sodium and osmolality measurements
- Demeclocycline (dimethylchlortetracycline) therapy to desensitize the kidney
- If severe, hypertonic saline with furosemide given under close observation

ADRENAL GLANDS

The adrenal glands produce cortisol, aldosterone and the anabolic and sex hormones.

CUSHING SYNDROME

Cushing syndrome results from a state of increased circulating **glucocorticoids**. It can be secondary to increased ACTH production or a result of autonomous glucocorticoid increase:

Causes

ACTH dependent	Pituitary tumour. NB: This is **Cushing disease**
	Ectopic ACTH production (extremely rare)
ACTH independent	Adrenal adenoma or carcinoma (most often seen in children < 3 years old)
	Exogenous steroids – the *commonest* cause

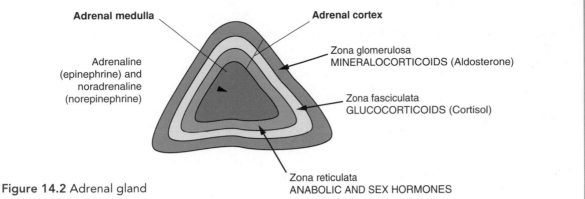

Figure 14.2 Adrenal gland

Adrenal medulla

Adrenal cortex

Adrenaline (epinephrine) and noradrenaline (norepinephrine)

Zona glomerulosa
MINERALOCORTICOIDS (Aldosterone)

Zona fasciculata
GLUCOCORTICOIDS (Cortisol)

Zona reticulata
ANABOLIC AND SEX HORMONES

Clinical features

Growth impairment

Headache, mental disturbance

Hypertension

Proximal muscle weakness

Osteoporosis

Pubertal delay

Impaired glucose tolerance/diabetes (glycosuria)

Moon face (round face, large red cheecks)

Masculinization signs (hirsutism, acne – due to androgen production)

Buffalo hump

Lemon on sticks (truncal obesity)

Striae and bruises

Hyperpigmentation (seen with high ACTH only)

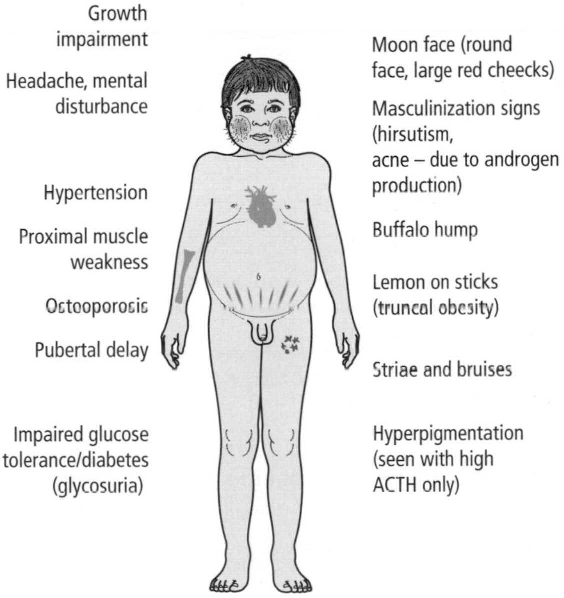

Figure 14.3 Clinical features of Cushing Syndrome

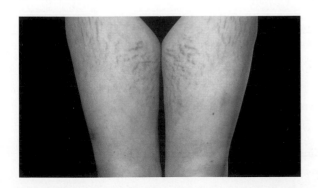

Figure 14.4 Striae distensions on the thighs of a girl with steroid-induced Cushing syndrome

Investigations

Investigations can be divided into those to establish a *diagnosis* and those to establish the *underlying cause*.

Diagnosis	Underlying cause
■ Serum – Na ↑, K ↓, alkalosis	■ ACTH level
■ Cortisol circadian rhythm	< 10 ng/L = ACTH independent
– 0800 and midnight cortisol	20–80 ng/L = normal or high in ACTH dependent
Normal = low at midnight and	> 100ng/L = high in ectopic ACTH
high in the morning	■ Low- and high-dose dexamethasone suppression
Cushing = high midnight levels	tests
■ Urine 24-h free cortisol (↑)	■ CRF test (exaggerated ACTH response = pituitary-
■ Overnight dexamethasone	dependent **Cushing disease**)
suppression test	■ Adrenal CT scan
	■ Pituitary MRI scan

NB: Random cortisol measurement is of no benefit as it fluctuates greatly during the day and is dependent on activity

Treatment

Treatment options include:

- Surgical removal of a pituitary lesion or resection of an adrenal adenoma
- Radiotherapy to the pituitary
- Reduction of exogenous steroids where possible
- Medical therapy with inhibitors of adrenal biosynthesis, e.g. ketoconazole

ADRENOCORTICAL INSUFFICIENCY

This is a deficiency of *all* the adrenal cortical hormones, but the main features are a result of cortisol deficiency.

Causes

Acute   Sudden withdrawal of exogenous steroid
Birth asphyxia
Severe hypotension (causing adrenal infarction)
Sepsis, e.g. Waterhouse–Friderichsen syndrome of adrenal haemorrhage secondary to meningococcal sepsis
Trauma

Chronic   Primary (ACTH ↑):
- Congenital adrenal hyperplasia (CAH)
- Destruction of adrenal cortex (**Addison disease**) due to autoimmune disease or TB
- Leukaemia
- Drugs, e.g. ketoconazole
- Adrenoleukodystrophy (adrenocortical insufficiency and demyelination in the CNS)

Secondary (ACTH ↓):
- Pituitary or hypothalamic disease (tumour, trauma, infection, post–surgical)
- Long term steroid therapy

Clinical features

Acute disease   This presents as an **adrenal crisis**:
- Drowsiness → coma
- Tachycardia, tachypnoea, cyanosis
- Hypotension, peripheral shut-down

Chronic disease   In a baby:
- Apathy, drowsiness
- Failure to thrive
- Vomiting, hypoglycaemia and dehydration leading to eventual circulatory collapse and coma

Older child:
- Weakness, fatigue
- Anorexia, nausea, vomiting, abdominal pain, diarrhoea
- Failure to thrive
- Postural hypotension and salt craving
- Hyperpigmentation of buccal mucosa, scars and skin creases (with primary disease only, secondary to ACTH ↑)

Management

Confirm diagnosis with:
- Serum electrolytes: Na↓, K↑, glucose↓
- Serum hormones: cortisol ↓ (and no diurnal change), ACTH ↑ (in primary disease only)
- Synacthen test (short test and also long if necessary)

Adrenal crisis   IV fluid and salt replacement
IV hydrocortisone
Antibiotics if necessary

Long term therapy   Daily hydrocortisone and fludrocortisone replacement

THYROID GLAND

HYPOTHYROIDISM

Hypothyroidism can be *congenital* (in which there are specific features) or *acquired*. It can be divided into:

- Primary (thyroid gland) – TSH ↑, thyroxine ↓
- Secondary (pituitary)
- Tertiary (hypothalamic) } TSH ↓, thyroxine ↓

Thyroxine controls the metabolic rate and many of the symptoms relate to this with a general '*slowing down*'.

Congenital hypothyroidism

Incidence 1 in 4000.

Causes

- Thyroid dysgenesis (90%) due to:
  - **Thyroid aplasia** (one-third)
  - **Ectopic thyroid** (two-thirds), i.e. lingual, sublingual or subhyoid thyroid
- Dyshormonogenesis (10%) (inborn error of thyroid hormone production)
- Some hypothyroidism is *transient* due to placental transfer of:
  - Antithyroid antibodies (maternal autoimmune thyroid disease)
  - Antithyroid drugs

Clinical features

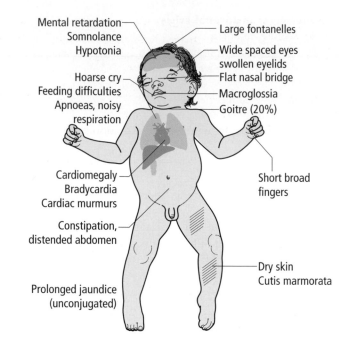

Mental retardation
Somnolance
Hypotonia

Large fontanelles

Wide spaced eyes
swollen eyelids

Hoarse cry
Feeding difficulties
Apnoeas, noisy
respiration

Flat nasal bridge

Macroglossia

Goitre (20%)

Cardiomegaly
Bradycardia
Cardiac murmurs

Short broad
fingers

Constipation,
distended abdomen

Dry skin
Cutis marmorata

Prolonged jaundice
(unconjugated)

Figure 14.5 Clinical features of hypothyroidism

Diagnosis

Usually made with the **Guthrie test** at 5 days of age – a raised TSH (> 100) is found. Confirmation is obtained by checking the serum T4 (low).

Treatment

Thyroxine replacement (oral, 10–15 µg/kg/day).

Acquired hypothyroidism

Causes

Primary	Atrophic autoimmune thyroiditis (microsomal antibodies)
	Hashimoto thyroiditis (microsomal antibodies and goitre)
	Iodine deficiency
	Treatment of hyperthyroidism
	Radiotherapy for lymphoma or leukaemia
Secondary	Pituitary disease
Tertiary	Hypothalamic disease

Clinical features

A gradual onset of:

- Deceleration of growth
- Delayed ossification
- Skin and hair (dry skin and hair, lateral third of eyebrow missing)
- Low energy levels
- Mental slowness at school
- Constipation
- Cold intolerance

HYPERTHYROIDISM

The most common childhood cause of hyperthyroidism is **Graves disease**, where TSH receptor antibodies (TRSAbs) bind to the TSH receptor and cause thyroid hormone production. Transient neonatal disease may be seen secondary to transplacental antibody transfer in maternal Graves disease.

Clinical features

Neurological	Hyperactivity, emotional lability, short attention span and tremor
Gastrointestinal	Increased appetite but no weight gain or loss
Skin	Smooth skin, increased sweating
General	Heat intolerance
Cardiovascular	Tachycardia, palpitations, dyspnoea, hypertension, cardiomegaly, atrial fibrillation (rare)

Investigations

- Free T4 and T3 elevated
- TSH decreased
- TSAbs found in Graves disease

Treatment

Medical	Antithyroid drugs, e.g. carbimazole, propylthiouracil, or radioactive iodine
	Symptomatic control with β-blockers (propranolol)
Surgical	Subtotal thyroidectomy

Graves disease

- Usually a gradual onset of features
- Female > male 5:1
- Features of hyperthyroidism (see above)
- Diffuse toxic goitre
- Thyroid eye signs (exophthalmos, lid retraction, lid lag, impaired convergence, ophthalmoplegia)
- Pretibial myxoedema
- TRSAbs (thyrotropin receptor-stimulating antibodies)

Neonatal hyperthyroidism

- Premature, IUGR
- Goitre, exophthalmos, microcephaly
- Irritable, hyperalert, hyperthermia
- Tachycardia, hypertension, may progress to cardiac decompensation
- Tachypnoea

PARATHYROID GLANDS

The parathyroid glands produce **parathyroid hormone (PTH)**, which is involved in calcium and phosphate homeostasis.

PTH → Plasma calcium ↑
$$\begin{cases} \text{Gut Ca absorption} \uparrow \\ \text{Renal tubular Ca reabsorption} \uparrow \\ 1,25(OH)_2D_3 \uparrow \end{cases}$$

→ Plasma phosphate ↓
$$\begin{cases} \text{Renal phosphate excretion} \downarrow \\ \text{Bone absorption} \uparrow \end{cases}$$

The clinical effects of parathyroid dysfunction are mainly due to **calcium** imbalance.

Goitre

Goitre is an enlargement of the thyroid gland. NB: The child may be euthyroid, i.e. normal, hypothyroid or hyperthyroid

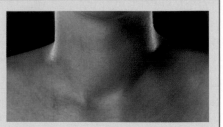

Figure 14.6 Goitre

Causes

Congenital	Older child
Maternal antithyroid drugs	Colloid goitre
Maternal iodine-containing drugs, e.g. amiodarone	Autoimmune, e.g. Hashimoto thyroiditis
Congenital hyperthyroidism	Graves disease
Dyshormonogenesis	Infective thyroiditis
Thyroid teratoma	Iodine deficiency or iodine-containing drugs
	Antithyroid drugs
	Multinodular goitre (seen in McCune–Albright syndrome)
	Thyroid tumour (rare)

Management

■ Assess the goitre – size, consistency, diffuse or nodule/nodular, tenderness. NB: Small infants may have breathing difficulties due to goitre size
■ Check thyroid status
■ Additional investigations – USS thyroid, nuclear thyroid scan, fine needle aspiration

Vitamin D analogues

Vitamin D	= calciferol (D_3)
Alphacalcidol	= 1-α hydroxycholecalciferol
Calcitriol	= 1,25-dihydroxycholecalciferol ($1,25(OH)_2D_3$)

HYPOCALCAEMIA

Causes

PTH ↓ (Ca+ ↓, PO_4↑) Primary parathyroid aplasia or hypoplasia
(**hypoparathyroidism**) DiGeorge syndrome (see p. 103)
Autoimmune
Post-thyroidectomy
PTH ↑ (Ca ↓, PO_4 ↓) Pseudohypoparathyroidism (see below)
Rickets due to:
■ Vitamin D intake and/or calcium intake ↓
■ Vitamin D metabolism ↓ (renal disease, liver disease)
■ Calcium excretion ↓

Clinical features

■ Seizures
■ Cataracts, soft teeth, horizontal lines on fingernails and toenails
■ Muscle cramps, paraesthesia, stiffness

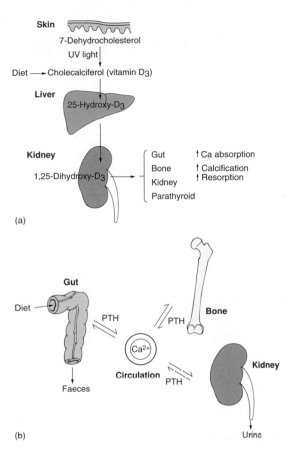

Figure 14.7 Calcium physiology. (a) Vitamin D metabolism and actions. (b) Calcium exchange

- Laryngeal and carpopedal spasm, tetany
- Trousseau's sign (tetanic spasm of hands and wrists with BP cuff above diastolic pressure for 3 min)
- Chvostek's sign (facial muscle twitching on tapping facial nerve)
- Long QT interval, papilloedema

Treatment

Emergency treatment   10% calcium gluconate intravenous
Long term therapy   Oral calcium and vitamin D supplements (calcitriol or alfacalcidol)

Pseudohypoparathyroidism and pseudopseudohypoparathyroidism

Pseudohypoparathyroidism (PHP) is a condition of hypocalcaemia, hyperphosphataemia and elevated PTH levels, usually associated with the physical features listed below. It is due to an end-organ resistance to PTH, which can be secondary to a variety of biochemical defects. Group 1a defects are known to have decreased stimulatory G (Gs) protein activity.

Pseudopseudohypoparathyroidism (PPHP) refers to the *clinical phenotype* with as yet *no demonstrable biochemical defect*, possibly an incomplete expression of PHP.

PHP   Ca ↓, PO_4 ↑, PTH ↑   + phenotype
PPHP   Normal biochemistry   + phenotype

Clinical features

- Short stature, round face, stocky
- Short 4th and 5th metacarpals
- Brachydactyly, bow legs, dimples overlying MCP joints
- Tetany, stridor, convulsions
- Mental retardation, calcification of basal ganglia, cataracts, dental anomalies
- Subcutaneous calcium deposits

Albright's hereditary osteodystrophy is a historical term applying to the clinical phenotype of the skeletal features (short stocky stature, round face, brachydactyly), and calcification and ossification of the skin.

HYPERCALCAEMIA

Causes

PTH $\uparrow$ (Ca$\uparrow$, PO$_4$ $\downarrow$) Primary hyperparathyroidism
Tertiary hyperparathyroidism, i.e. PTH $\uparrow$ after longstanding secondary hyperparathyroidism now treated
Ectopic PTH (some tumours)

PTH $\downarrow$ (Ca$\uparrow$, PO$_4$ $\uparrow$) Vitamin D $\uparrow$ (excess intake, TB, lymphoma, sarcoidosis)
Malignancy (leukaemia, lymphoma, neuroblastoma)
Williams syndrome
Familial hypocalciuric hypercalcaemia

Clinical features

- **Stones** (renal), **bones** (pain), **abdominal moans** (ulcers), **psychiatric groans**
- Anorexia, vomiting, constipation, peptic ulcers, pancreatitis
- Corneal calcification, conjunctival injection
- Polyuria (secondary to nephrogenic diabetes insipidus from nephrocalcinosis)
- Hypertension, arrhythmias, cardiac arrest if levels very high (> 3.75)
- Chondrocalcinosis, subperiosteal bone erosions
- Convulsions

Management

If severe	Intravenous bisphosphonates, e.g. etridronate, pamidronate
	Hydration given with furosemide
If mild	Oral phosphates and/or calcitonin

POLYCYSTIC OVARY SYNDROME

Polycystic ovary syndrome (PCOS) is a common condition of adolescent girls, the essential features of which are:

- Large polycystic ovaries (due to arrested follicular development)
- Increased circulating androgens and a high LH:FSH ratio

Clinical features

The presenting features appear after puberty and vary between individuals:

- Secondary amenorrhoea, irregular menstruation
- Obesity
- Hirsutism

- Mild virilization with acne
- Anovulatory infertility
- Insulin resistance

> **!** **NB: PCOS may present purely with menstrual problems or acne, with no features of the 'classical' overweight hairy girl.**

Investigations

Pelvic ultrasound scan	Large ovaries
	Multiple cysts distributed peripherally within the ovary
	Excessive amount of stroma within the ovary
Main biochemical features	Raised serum androgens
	High LH:FSH ratio

Treatment

There is no cure. The treatment is specific to the *symptoms* present:

Irregular menses/ hirsutism	Ovarian suppression using the oral contraceptive pill or cyproterone (an antiandrogen), or
	Pituitary ACTH suppression with prednisolone
Infertility	Ovarian wedge resection and clomiphene

GLUCOSE METABOLISM

- Blood glucose is generally maintained at a constant level between 3.5 and 8.0 mmol/L
- Glucose is the primary source of energy for the brain. Muscle utilizes glucose for energy and stores it as glycogen. Adipose tissue is also a store for glucose and uses it for triglyceride synthesis. The liver is the principle site for glucose storage as glycogen
- Glucose can be manufactured (**gluconeogenesis**) from glycogen, fat or protein

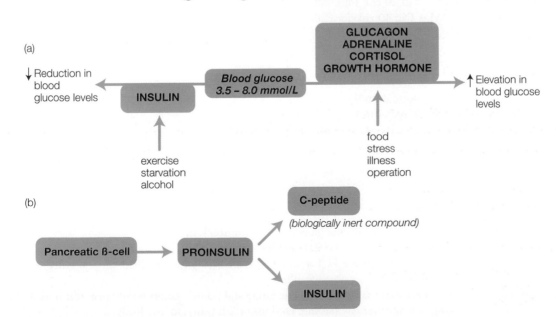

Figure 14.8 Glucose metabolism. (a) Maintenance of blood glucose levels. (b) Insulin production

DIABETES MELLITUS

Diabetes mellitus is a chronic state of hyperglycaemia due to a deficiency of insulin or its actions.

Subtypes of diabetes mellitus

- **Type 1 diabetes mellitus** (previously known as IDDM) insulin deficiency due to an autoimmune process. *The most common form in childhood*
- **Type 2 diabetes mellitus** (previously known as NIDDM) mainly due to failure of insulin action (insulin resistance) and strongly associated with obesity. Although rare in childhood, it is increasing in incidence, particularly in young adolescents
- Other types include those secondary to pancreatic disease (cystic fibrosis) or post pancreatic surgery for **persistent hyperinsulinaemic hypoglycaemia of infancy (PHHI)**
- **Neonatal diabetes mellitus** very rare type that occurs in the newborn period

Type 1 diabetes mellitus

Type 1 diabetes mellitus is characterized by insufficient endogenous insulin and requires exogenous insulin for the maintenance of life. It may develop at any age. Prevalence 1 in 300 and rising.

Insulin levels are finely tuned and fluctuate constantly in order to maintain a stable blood glucose level. In diabetes, the insulin levels are fixed, depending on the latest dose of insulin given, and therefore the blood glucose levels fluctuate, and this leads to both *short* and *long term* consequences. The younger the child is at diagnosis, the longer they have to develop complications.

Causes

- Develops as a result of destruction of the pancreatic β-cells, with consequent insufficient insulin production. It is thought that an environmental insult, e.g. viral illness, results in an antigen cross-reacting and causing autoimmune destruction of the β-cells in genetically susceptible individuals
- There is evidence for genetic, autoimmune and viral factors contributing to diabetes:
  – Father has IDDM – 1 in 20 risk for child
  – Mother has IDDM – 1 in 40 risk for child
  – Sibling has IDDM – 1 in 20 risk for child

Clinical presentations

- Short history (2–4 weeks) of:
  – **Polyuria** (due to osmotic diuresis)
  – **Polydipsia** (due to dehydration)
  – **Weight loss** (fluid depletion, fat and muscle breakdown)
- Ketoacidosis (see below)
- Asymptomatic glycosuria

Diagnosis

Diagnostic confirmation is by:

If symptomatic	Random venous plasma glucose ≥ 11.1 mmol/L or Fasting plasma glucose ≥ 7.0 mmol/L or 2-h plasma glucose ≥ 11.1 mmol/L, 2 h after 75 g glucose load (an oral glucose tolerance test)
If asymptomatic	Venous plasma sample in diabetic range and confirmation with repeat test in diabetic range on another day (fasting, random or 2 h post-glucose load)

Management

Type 1 diabetes requires insulin therapy, but diet is also important. A great deal of support is necessary for the child and the family in managing this chronic disease requiring life-long therapy. A multidisciplinary team is involved incorporating the paediatrician, GP, diabetes nurse, dietician, clinical psychologist, and social worker. Many issues need to be considered, including understanding diabetes, medication, diet, non-compliance, frustration, monitoring, possible complications, hypoglycaemias and emergency advice.

Diet
: This should be high in unrefined carbohydrates, as these have a slow absorption profile (lower glycaemic index, GI) and result in fewer glucose swings
: Refined carbohydrates, e.g. sweets, cause rapid swings in blood glucose levels (high GI)
: Calories are obtained ideally as 55% carbohydrate, 35% fat and 15% protein

Insulin
: Subcutaneous insulin injections are given in the thigh, arm or abdomen
: These are rotated to prevent lipoatrophy or lipohypertrophy
: Different regimens are available to suit different lifestyles:
  - **Twice daily regimen** (used in younger children)
    – **am – before breakfast** give two-thirds daily dose as:
    short acting ⅓, e.g. Actrapid and
    medium acting ⅔, e.g. Monotard
    – **pm – before tea**, give one-third daily dose as:
    short acting ⅓ and
    medium acting ⅔
  - **Multiple dose pen injection regimen** (used in older children). A basal background insulin is given, usually in the evening, and a short acting insulin is given pre meals. This is less rigid and allows more flexibility

Exercise increases the demand for glucose and, as the insulin levels are fixed, a sugar snack taken prior to exercise will provide the energy boost. For prolonged exertion, the insulin dose will need to be reduced.

Insulin utilization rises during illness, though as food intake generally falls, the requirements may not rise.

> **!** **NB: Insulin must be continued during intercurrent illness. Insulin requirements will vary during an illness and close monitoring of blood glucose levels is essential.**

Blood glucose monitoring

- Regular BM stix at home
- Urine glucose unreliable due to variable renal threshold and inability to detect hypoglycaemia
- Glycosylated Hb (HbA1c) or fructosamine give an indication of average blood glucose levels over the previous 6 weeks

The **dawn phenomenon** is the increase in glucose (and insulin requirement) at 4 am due to a growth hormone surge. The **Somogyi phenomenon** is the development of rebound hyperglycaemia after hypoglycaemia at night due to too much insulin given to counteract the 4 am growth hormone surge

Future therapies

New therapies are being developed including stem cell technology, inhaled insulin and other long-acting insulin analogues.

Complications

Hypoglycaemia	Symptoms generally appear when blood glucose < 3 mmol/L
	'Hypos' – sweaty, dizzy, irritable
	Treat with oral glucose drink, glucose tablet or gel (can be placed under tongue if child uncooperative) or glucagon injection
Weight increase	
Behavioural problems	Problems with non–compliance are common in adolescence
	Labelled 'brittle diabetes'
Insulin resistance	Usually due to obesity
Lipoatrophy, lipohypertrophy	Occur at injection sites
Necrobiosis lipoidica diabeticorum	Localized area(s) of waxy atrophic skin on shins
Long term complications	**Renal disease** – microalbuminuria, then proteinuria, then gradual decline in GFR to chronic renal failure

Diabetic eye disease:

- Retinopathy (simple and proliferative)
- Cataracts

Neuropathy, **foot complications** and **cardiovascular disease** later on

Diabetes clinic checks

General health

Growth	Height and weight. Pubertal onset (may be delayed)
Monitoring	Blood sugar monitoring booklet. Look for hypos, high levels and also a 'too perfect' book which may be due to false results being recorded if the child is afraid to admit to problems

HbA1c

Blood pressure

Psychiatric	Any problems adjusting/maintaining compliance
Eye check	Enquire about visual symptoms especially acuity Ophthalmologist	Both done annually if Type 1 DM > 5 years if diagnosed pre-puberty, or > 2 years if diagnosed post-puberty
Urine	Laboratory check for microalbuminuria	

Diabetic ketoacidosis

Diabetic ketoacidosis is a state of *uncontrolled catabolism* associated with insulin deficiency resulting in:

- **Hyperglycaemia**
- **Osmotic diuresis and dehydration**
- **Lipolysis** resulting in free fatty acids that are broken down to ketone bodies which cause a **metabolic acidosis**

Causes

- New presentation of diabetes
- Interruption of insulin therapy
- Intercurrent illness

Clinical features

■ Hyperventilation (Kussmaul respiration, to correct metabolic acidosis)
■ Dehydration
■ Nausea and vomiting, abdominal pain
■ Eventual drowsiness and coma

Management

1. General resuscitation if necessary
2. Take bedside glucose (BM Stix) and urinalysis for ketonuria
3. Take blood for glucose, U&E, FBC, PCV, arterial/venous blood gas, CRP
4. Take blood and urine cultures, CXR (and if clinically indicated a lumbar puncture)
5. Keep the child nil by mouth (due to gastric stasis and vomiting), place nasogastric tube if impaired consciousness and record fluid input–output chart
6. Admit to HDU if necessary
7. Give fluid and insulin therapy under close observation of clinical state and blood parameters

Fluid	Circulating volume expansion with a bolus of 10–20 mL/kg 0.9% saline
	Then rehydrate calculated volume deficit + maintenance fluids over 48 h with 0.45% saline, adding potassium when electrolyte results back (with careful monitoring)
	Change fluid to 0.18% saline 4% dextrose when blood glucose < 12 mmol/L
	Bicarbonate infusion is given in severe acidosis
Insulin	Insulin infusion of soluble insulin 0.01–0.1 U/kg/h to reduce blood glucose at a rate of < 5 mmol/h
	Check blood glucose hourly and U&E 2 hourly initially
	When child is able to eat, transfer to subcutaneous insulin regimen of 0.5–0.7 U/kg/day

NB: Although the serum potassium is initially high, this is only due to potassium leaking out of the cells, and total body potassium is greatly depleted. There is a risk of **hypokalaemia** and **hypophosphataemia** as potassium and phosphate are pushed back into the cells with insulin treatment.

> **!** **NB: Diabetic ketoacidosis must be *corrected gradually* to avoid rapid compartmental fluid shifts that can result in cerebral oedema.**

HYPOGLYCAEMIA

Hypoglycaemia is a blood glucose level < 2.6 mmol/L.

Low glucose levels → Insulin ↓ → Lipolysis
(< 2.6 mmol/L)   Ketogenesis

Causes

Hypoglycaemia can be clinically divided into common transient neonatal hypoglycaemia, and the rarer persistent hypoglycaemia (see below).

Transient neonatal hypoglycaemia ■ Substrate deficiency – prematurity, IUGR
(see p. 69)   ■ Hyperinsulinaemia – infant of diabetic mother
Persistent hypoglycaemia   ■ Hyperinsulinism:
         ■ Persistent hyperinsulinaemic hypoglycaemia of infancy (PHHI, formerly known as neisidioblastosis)

- ■ Insulinoma
- ■ Diabetic child given relatively too much insulin
- ■ Deliberate insulin administration (fictitious and induced illness)
■ Hormone deficiency states – Addison disease, hypopituitarism
■ Metabolic – galactosaemia, fatty acid oxidation defect, organic acidaemia
■ Other:
  - ■ Poisoning (aspirin, alcohol)
  - ■ Liver failure, Reye syndrome

Persistent hyperinsulinaemic hypoglycaemia of infancy (PHHI) is a developmental disorder with hyperplastic, abnormally dispersed β-cells, resulting in inappropriately high levels of plasma insulin.

Clinical features

Neonate	Apnoea, cyanosis
	Lethargy, poor feeding, hypotonia and seizures
Older child	Pallor, anxiety, nausea, tremor, sweatiness, headache
	Dizziness, poor concentration, behavioural change
	Tachycardia
	Diplopia, decreased acuity
	Seizures, reduced conciousness, coma

Management

Check BM Stix, and send blood glucose and U&E. Then, in a child:

If conscious	Give a sugary drink
If reduced consciousness	Insert IV line and give 3–5 mL/kg 10% glucose bolus, and then infusion of 10% glucose at 5 mL/kg/h until blood sugars are stable

For neonate see p. 69

PHHI (hyperinsulinism) is treated with diazoxide and a thiazide diuretic, followed by octeotride. Subtotal pancreatectomy may be necessary if medical management fails.

Clinical scenario

A 9-year-old girl is seen by her GP with nocturnal enuresis and given a bell and pad alarm and the parents are told to use a star chart.

Two weeks later the problem is continuing, and it is noted by her parents that she is drinking a lot of fluid, seems lethargic, has lost some weight, and has developed sweet-smelling breath.

1. What tests would you do to establish a diagnosis?

Prior to any tests being arranged she is admitted to the local paediatric unit by her GP with a drowsy confused state and has, on examination, a capillary refill time of 4 seconds, with vomiting and abdominal pain.

2. What is the most likely diagnosis?
3. Detail the first eight parts of your initial management?

She is stabilized and is around 25 kg and is started on the appropriate treatment.

4. What regime might be ideal for this child?

ANSWERS

1. Urinalysis, blood glucose
2. Insulin-dependent diabetes mellitus
3. ABC and IV normal saline bolus of 20mL/kg
   Insulin infusion at 0.05U/kg/h
   NG tube
   Antibiotics
   Urinary catheter
   Strict fluid balance chart
   Hourly blood sugar and U and Es
   Possibly arterial line
4. Insulin Actrapid pre-meals on background of long-acting insulin twice daily

FURTHER READING

Brook C, Clayton P, Brown R. Brook's *Clinical Pediatric Endocrinology*, 6th edn. Oxford: Blackwell, 2009.

Raine J, Donaldson M, Gregory J, Savage M. *Diabetes and Endocrine Disorders in Childhood*. Oxford: Wiley-Blackwell, 2001.

15 Growth and Puberty

- Growth
- Puberty
- Ambiguous genitalia (sexual differentiation disorders)
- Further reading

GROWTH

- Normal growth is an essential feature of a child's health and well-being
- Slow or fast growth indicates pathology
- Short or tall stature may be due to a pathological cause

Monitoring growth

Height and growth rate vary between individuals.

There are three main phases of growth:

Infantile phase	From birth to 2 years Characterized by rapid, but rapidly decelerating, rate of growth (the average length at birth is 50 cm, 75 cm at 12 months and 87.5 cm at 24 months) Dependent on nutrition
Childhood phase	From 2 years to puberty Characterized by a fairly constant rate of growth (approximately 5–6 cm/year) Dependent on hormonal factors (such as growth hormone)
Pubertal phase	Characterized by an accelerated rate of growth, reaching a peak and then slowing down as growth comes to an end Dependent on growth hormone and sex hormones

Linear growth is complete when the *epiphyses have fused*.

The **expected height** of a child is calculated from his/her **parents' height** (see below). Growth is monitored during childhood to check whether the child falls within the normal range for his/her parents and for the general population, and to check whether he/she is deviating from that range (moving up or down the centiles). There are specific reasons for short and tall stature, and for abnormal growth rate.

Essential growth measurements are **height**, **weight**, (and **head circumference** if < 2 years). Other measurements may be taken for specific reasons, e.g. sitting height and skinfold thicknesses.

Assessing growth

- Need to measure and plot height to assess if height is normal for parents and age-appropriate general population

> ■ Need to look for growth pattern, by re-measuring the child's height over a 6–12-month period to assess:
> – Rate of growth
> – Deviations from a centile

Growth charts

There are charts for height, weight and head circumference ('**growth charts**') at various ages from infancy to adulthood. Similarly, there are charts for the *rate* of change ('**growth velocity charts**'). The newly developed UK growth charts show the normal limits of growth of the population at various ages, from extreme prematurity (23 weeks' gestation) through to 20 years of age. These have been constructed from a much larger sample size (30 000 children of each sex) and from various parts of the UK.

■ Charts outline centiles of children ranging from the 0.4th centile to the 99.6th centile (= ±2.67 standard deviations from the mean)
■ Nine equidistant centile lines 2/3 of a standard deviation apart
■ Children whose height falls within the shaded area (0.4–2nd centile and 98–99.6th centile) need close monitoring
■ Children falling outside the range expected for their parents (target centile range), below 0.4th centile or above 99.6th centile should be formally assessed

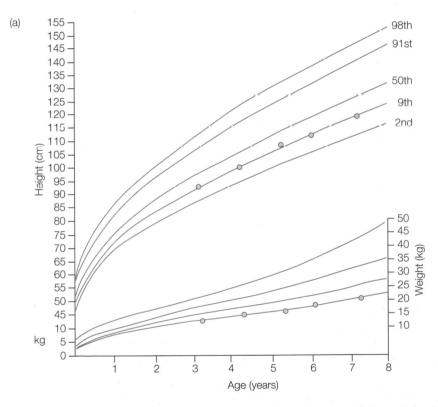

Figure 15.1 Growth charts. (a) Normal growth of a girl between 3½ and 8 years, following the 9th centile. Her mother is on a centile half-way between the 2nd and 9th and her father is on the 25th centile. (b) Growth of a girl with Turner syndrome. Parental heights are on the 75th (mother) and 91st (father) centiles, while the girl is below the 0.4th centile. (c) Growth for girl with hypothyroidism. Note the gradual drifting down the centiles between ages 6 and 9½

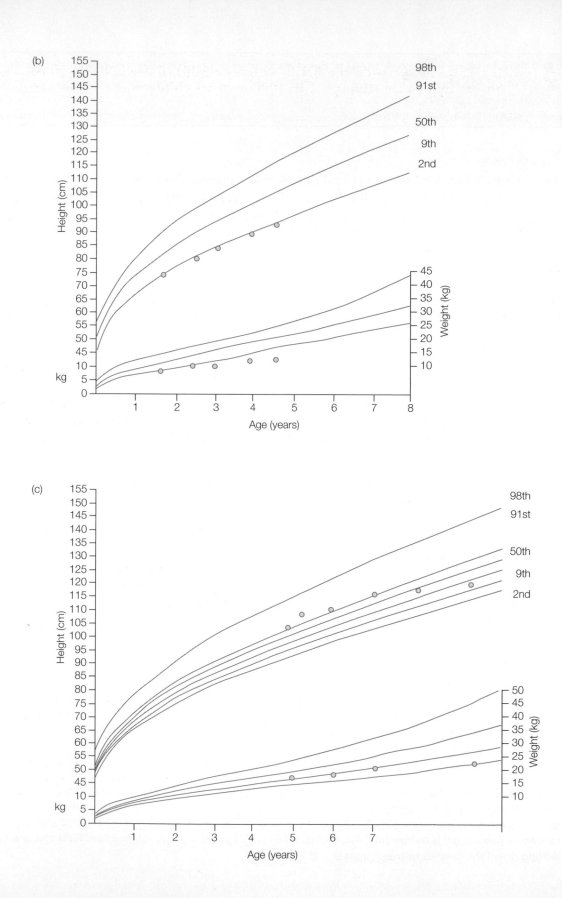

> **NB: If a child lies outside the 0.4th–99.6th centiles, there is likely to be an organic cause (though 4 in 1000 normal children are below the 0.4th centile).**

Predicted adult height

This is an estimate made on the basis of a child's height and assessment of his/her bone maturation (bone age).

The median expected height for any child, the **mid-parental height centile**, and the range of normal height for a child born to a particular set of parents, the **target centile range**, are calculated from parental heights to take into account genetic factors.

Boy's expected height (mid-parental height centile) $= \dfrac{(\text{mother's height} + 12.5\ \text{cm}) + \text{father's height}}{2}$

Girl's expected height (mid-parental height centile) $= \dfrac{(\text{father's height} - 12.5\ \text{cm}) + \text{mother's height}}{2}$

Bone age (skeletal maturity)

- Shows how far the skeleton has matured, i.e. physical development, and can give an idea of potential height, and clues as to the cause of short stature
- Delayed bone age in the absence of pathology = slow maturation = more potential growth remaining
- Bone age is usually assessed by rating a number of epiphyseal centres in the wrist (visualized on an X-ray) from which the rate of ossification is seen. It is then compared to the chronological age

Causes of delayed and advanced bone age	
Delayed	**Advanced**
Familial delayed maturation, i.e. a 'slow grower'	Growth advance
Delayed puberty	Precocious puberty
Severe illness	Excessive androgen production
Hypothyroidism	Hyperthyroidism
Growth hormone deficiency	

Growth velocity

- Sensitive indicator of growth problems and the 'gold standard' for assessing whether growth is progressing normally or otherwise. There is no equivalent sensitive or specific biochemical serum marker of growth
- Age-dependent (see above)
- Two measurements are needed at least 4 months apart, although clinical decisions are often made on the basis of growth data collected over 12 months. The difference between the two height measurements is divided by the time interval between them to give the velocity in cm/year and this is plotted on a growth velocity chart at the mid-point in time
- Growth velocity should vary between the 25th and 75th velocity centiles in order for height to remain normal. If growth velocity is too *slow* (< 25th height velocity centile) or too *fast* (> 75th height velocity centile) investigations should be performed

Catch-up growth

This is a rapid period of growth seen after illness and in babies who had intrauterine growth retardation. Most premature/low birthweight infants will 'catch up' by 2 years of age. They should therefore have their growth charts adjusted for their post-conceptional age until age 2 years.

> **Chronological age** = age since birth date
> **Post-conceptional age** = age since conception

SHORT STATURE

Short stature is height < 2nd centile (approximately 2 standard deviations below the mean).

Causes

Familial	Most common cause – calculate expected height from parental height (see above)
Constitutional delay of growth	'*Slow grower*' – delayed bone age and also a tendency to have delayed puberty and a family history of this pattern of growth Final height is within the norm for child's parents
Psychosocial deprivation	Can result in a small child (who may also be underweight). Child may have a biochemical picture of growth hormone deficiency
Chronic illness	Any chronic illness such as cystic fibrosis, asthma, rickets, malabsorption and also inadequate nutrition
Endocrine (rare)	Growth hormone deficiency:

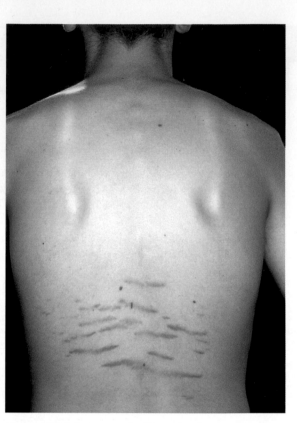

Figure 15.2 Striae on the lower back of a normal boy who has just had the pubertal growth spurt

- Isolated growth hormone synthesis or release defects
- Pituitary deficiency/hypopituitarism/hypothalamic defect
- Post cranial irradiation or chemotherapy
- Laron dwarfism (growth hormone insensitivity)

Hypothyroidism
Pseudohypoparathyroidism and PPHP (see p. 255)
Cushing syndrome (usually iatrogenic)

Chromosomal/gene abnormality	Turner syndrome, Down syndrome, Prader–Willi syndrome
Intrauterine growth retardation	Russell–Silver syndrome
Skeletal dysplasias	Achondroplasia

Investigations

These are determined by the history and clinical findings.

General	Bone age
	TFTs
	FBC, ESR, biochemistry profile, bone profile
	Urinalysis
Specific	Coeliac screen
	Karyotype
	Insulin-like growth factor 1 (IGF-1) and IGF-binding protein-3 (IGFBP-3)★
	Ultrasound of uterus and ovaries
	CT or MRI brain
	Skeletal survey
	Pituitary provocation tests

★IGF-1 levels correlate well with growth hormone status and this together with IGFBP-3 are the initial screening tests for suspected growth hormone deficiency. Random growth hormone levels are unhelpful because growth hormone is secreted in a pulsatile manner and is likely to be low in normal children during daytime.

Treatment

Treatment depends on the underlying pathology. Growth hormone deficiency, Turner syndrome, Prader–Willi syndrome and children who have suffered from IUGR can be treated with daily recombinant growth hormone injections.

TALL STATURE

Tall stature is height > 98th centile.

> **!** **NB: Tall stature is much less common as a clinical problem than short stature, mainly because of its perceived social acceptability.**

Causes

Familial	The most common cause. Tall expected height (from parental heights), the reverse of familial short stature
Hormonal	Precocious puberty
	Congenital adrenal hyperplasia
	NB: In the above two conditions the final height is *short*, although the child is taller than their peers while growing because the growth spurts are reached earlier
	Pituitary gigantism (growth hormone secreting tumour – rare)
	Hyperthyroidism
Syndrome	Klinefelter syndrome (47, XXY)
	Marfan syndrome
	Homocystinuria
	Soto syndrome (*'cerebral gigantism'* – learning difficulties, clumsiness, big hands and feet, large ears, prominent forehead)
	Beckwith–Wiedemann syndrome

Investigations

The investigations are determined by the history and the clinical findings.

General	Bone age
	TFTs
	Karyotype

Specific	Insulin–like growth factor 1 (IGF-1) and IGF-binding protein 3 (IGFBP-3) (see above)
	Ultrasound of uterus and ovaries
	CT or MRI brain
	Homocystine
	17-hydroxyprogesterone/urine steroid profile

Treatment

Treatment depends on the underlying cause. It is possible to treat/limit the final adult height in those with familial tall stature by inducing puberty early (using oestrogen therapy in girls and testosterone therapy in boys) which limits the childhood growth phase and causes premature fusion of the epiphyses.

PUBERTY

Pubertal staging

Pubertal stage is assessed using the sexual maturity rating devised by Tanner in 1962.

Pubertal stages

Puberty onset (timing is variable)

Girls	8–13 years	Breast stage 2	(First sign – breast development)
Boys	9–14 years	Testes volume 4 mL	(First sign – testicular enlargement)

Pubertal growth spurts

Girls	At breast stage 3
Boys	At testicular volume 10–12 mL

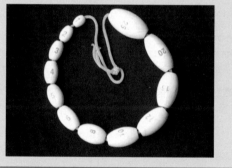

Figure 15.3 An orchidometer

G = Genitals (boys)

 Stage 1 Pre-adolescent

 Stage 2 Scrotum pink and texture change, slight enlargement of the penis

 Stage 3 Longer penis, larger testes

 Stage 4 Penis increases in breadth, dark scrotum

 Stage 5 Adult size

B = Breasts (girls)

Stage 1   Pre-adolescent

Stage 2   Breast bud

Stage 3   Larger, but no nipple contour separation

Stage 4   Areola and papilla form secondary mound. NB: Menarche usually commences at this stage

Stage 5   Mature (papilla projects, areola follows breast contour)

P = Pubic hair   **A = Axillary hair**

Stage 1   Pre-pubertal   Stage 1 No hair

Stage 2   Few fine hairs   Stage 2 Some hair

Stage 3   Darkens, coarsens, starts to curl   Stage 3 Adult hair pattern

Stage 4   Adult type, smaller area

Stage 5   Adult type

Boy's stages G (1–5), P (1–5), A (1–3) + testicular volume (2–25 mL)
Girl's stages B (1–5), P (1–5), A (1–3) + menarche

Definitions

Menarche	Commencement of menstruation. Occurs at breast stage 4. Average age = 12.2 years
Thelarche	Breast development
Adrenarche	Pubic and axillary hair development

PRECOCIOUS PUBERTY

Girls   Secondary sexual characteristics developing < 8 years is abnormal
Menarche < 10 years warrants investigation
Mostly **familial** causes

Boys   Secondary sexual characteristics developing < 9 years is abnormal
Mostly **pathological** cause, e.g. congenital adrenal hyperplasia, intracranial tumours, dysgerminomas

True (gonadotrophin-dependent) precocious puberty is *gonadotrophin-dependent* development of secondary sexual characteristics at a young age in a normal progression accompanied by a growth spurt, leading to full sexual maturity from activation of the hypothalamic–pituitary–gonadal axis (central axis).

False (gonadotrophin-independent) precocious puberty is *gonadotrophin-independent* development and there may be an unusual progression of sexual maturity. Isolated premature thelarche, adrenarche and menarche can occur.

Causes

True (LH ↑, FSH ↑)	Familial
(central axis activated)	Central – congenital, e.g. neurofibromatosis, hydrocephalus
	Acquired – post-sepsis, surgery, radiotherapy
	Brain tumours
False (LH ↓, FSH ↓)	Adrenal – congenital adrenal hyperplasia, adrenal tumour
(excess sex steroids,	Gonadal – ovarian tumour, testicular tumour
not driven centrally)	McCune–Albright syndrome (see below)
	Exogenous sex steroids
	Hypothyroidism

Investigations

Always check:

- Clinical pubertal stage
- Bone age
- Pelvic USS (girls) and orchidometer (boys)
- Features of intracranial mass – visual fields and optic discs

> **! NB: For boys there should be a low threshold for cranial imaging (? tumour), and AFP and hCG measurement (? testicular tumour) due to the high incidence of pathological causes.**

Treatment

Treatment depends on the underlying condition. *True precocious puberty* can be treated with GnRH analogues, and *false precocious puberty* with androgen inhibitors (boys) or oestrogen inhibitors (girls).

McCune–Albright syndrome (polyostotic fibrous dysplasia)

This is a syndrome comprising:

- Precocious puberty
- Polyostotic fibrous dysplasia
- Café–au–lait spots (large ones with very irregular borders and often stopping at the midline)

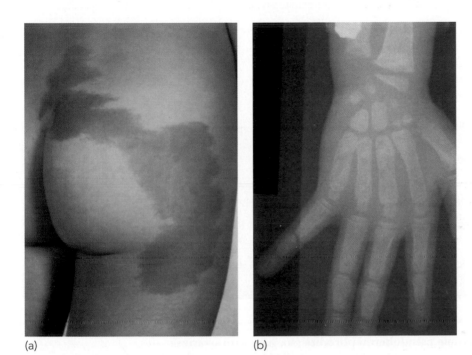

(a)   (b)

Figure 15.4 McCune–Albright syndrome. (a) Large unilateral geographical café-au-lait macule. (b) Hand X-ray showing fibrous dysplasia

It is due to a defect in the *G-protein* controlling cAMP in cells, which results in activation of receptors with a cAMP mechanism and autonomous glandular hyperfunction. Multiple hormonal overactivity may be seen, e.g. ovary, thyroid, adrenal glands and pituitary.

DELAYED PUBERTY

Delayed puberty in *girls* is failure of onset of any signs of pubertal development by 13 years, and in *boys* by 14 years.

> **!** **NB: Mainly boys are affected by delayed puberty, and the cause is usually *constitutional delay* (short child with delayed bone age and family history).**

Causes

Gonadotrophin secretion low	Constitutional – familial or sporadic
	Hypothalamic–pituitary – panhypopituitarism, GnRH deficiency
	Hypothyroidism

Gonadotrophin secretion high	Intracranial tumour, e.g. prolactinoma
	Systemic disease – any severe disease, e.g. renal failure, malnutrition
	Emotional – anorexia nervosa
	Gonadal dysgenesis – Turner syndrome
	Gonadal disease – trauma, torsion or radiotherapy
	Steroid hormone enzyme deficiencies – CAH 3β-deficency (see below)
	Chromosomal – Klinefelter syndrome

Investigations

- Bone age
- Routine haematology/biochemistry/ESR/coeliac screen
- Thyroid function tests
- Gonadotrophin and sex steroid hormone levels
- Karyotype
- Occasionally, LHRH test and hCG test to check testicular responsiveness in terms of testosterone production
- MRI brain and hypothalamic–pituitary area

Treatment

This depends on the underlying condition. For constitutional delay boys can be given low-dose testosterone to induce puberty, and girls ethinyl oestradiol.

AMBIGUOUS GENITALIA (SEXUAL DIFFERENTIATION DISORDERS)

Disorders of sexual differentiation can be due to:

Virilization of a female	**Female pseudohermaphrodite** (46, XX, **with ovaries**):
	■ Congenital adrenal hyperplasia (CAH): 21-hydroxylase deficiency, 11β-hydroxylase deficiency
	■ Maternal virilizing tumours (adrenal, ovarian)
	■ Maternal virilizing drugs
Undervirilization of a male	**Male pseudohermaphrodite** (46, XY, **with testes**):
	■ Defect in testes differentiation: gonadal dysgenesis or agenesis
	■ Defect in testicular hormones: CAH-3β-hydroxysteroid dehydrogenase deficiency
	■ Defect in androgen activity: androgen insensitivity syndrome
	■ 5α-reductase deficiency
True hermaphrodite	(46, XX; 46, XY, mosaic karyotypes, e.g. 46, XX/XY (chimera), XO/XY; **both ovarian and testicular tissue present**)

> **!** **NB: The basic pattern in development is *female*. The presence of testosterone causes the external male sexual characteristics to develop.**

Investigation

- Karyotype
- Pelvic and abdominal USS (to assess internal genitalia and adrenal glands)
- Adrenal steroid profile
- Testosterone and dihydrotestosterone (DHT)

- Other tests such as LHRH test, hCG test, synacthen test
- Occasionally need to perform EUA or laparoscopy to determine external and internal genitourinary structures

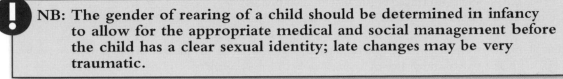

> **NB: The gender of rearing of a child should be determined in infancy to allow for the appropriate medical and social management before the child has a clear sexual identity; late changes may be very traumatic.**

CONGENITAL ADRENAL HYPERPLASIA

Congenital adrenal hyperplasia (CAH) is a group of autosomal recessive conditions resulting from various defects in the enzymes involved in the adrenal steroid synthetic pathways. Incidence 1 in 10 000.

21-Hydroxylase deficiency

This is the most common cause (genetic defect on chromosome 6). The enzyme defect causes the steroid pathway to be deflected from cortisol synthesis down alternative mineralocorticoid and androgenic pathways, with the resultant excess or deficiency of other steroids. Incidence 1 in 10 000.

Clinical features

- Virilization of a female baby (cliteromegaly, etc.)
- Adrenal crisis may occur in first 1–2 weeks of life (NB: They lose salt)
- May present late with precocious puberty, advanced bone age, tall stature in childhood (but eventual short stature as adults), hypertension, hirsutism and skin hyperpigmentation

Investigations

Hormones: ACTH, Testosterone, Androstenedione $\uparrow$ Aldosterone, Cortisol $\downarrow$

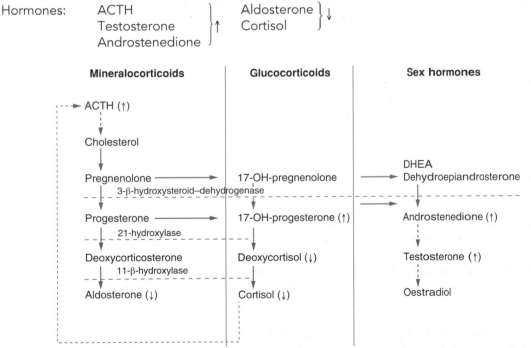

Figure 15.5 Effects of congenital adrenal hyperplasia on steroid biosynthesis

- Plasma 17-OH-progesterone ↑
- Urine pregnanetriol ↑
- Serum electrolytes – Na ↓, K ↑, glucose ↓
- Karyotype
- Pelvic USS (looking for female organs in a masculinized female)
- Urine steroid profile

Antenatal diagnosis is possible, and dexamethasone can be given to the mother in order to decrease fetal ACTH and hence reduce the chance of having a virilized female infant.

> **!** **NB: Boys with CAH are more likely to be diagnosed late because the androgen excess does not cause a clearly abnormal appearance in the newborn period.**

Treatment

- Drugs – hydrocortisone and fludrocortisone replacement
- Surgery if necessary to improve female anatomy
- Monitor growth and skeletal maturity

Clinical scenario

A boy who is 14½ years old is referred for short stature and pubertal delay. His mother is 152 cm and his father is 158 cm. He is 151 cm.

1. What is his expected height and range in respect of his parents' mid-parental height?
2. What do you tell the parents?
3. Would a bone age X-ray be useful?

ANSWERS

1. (Mother's height 152 cm (+12 cm) + Father's height 158 cm)/2 = expected average height attainment on mid-parental height, then +/- 12 cm is the range
2. He is within his expected range and familial short stature may be the only issue – it would be useful to know testicular volume, which if it is less than 5 mL with an orchidometer is reflective of pre-pubertal state and a pubertal growth spurt would still be expected. The age at which his father went through puberty would be helpful in reassuring them
3. A left wrist X-ray for assessment of bone age and hence future potential duration of growth is often a reassuring investigation

FURTHER READING

Kelnar C, Stirling H, Saenger P, Savage M (eds.). *Growth Disorders*, 2nd edn. London: Hodder Arnold, 2007.

Prescovitz O, Walvoord E. *When Puberty is Precocious: Scientific and Clinical Aspects*. New Jersey: Humana Press, 2010.

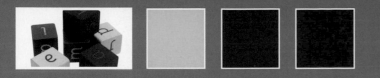

16 Metabolic Disorders

- Basic underlying mechanism
- Classification
- Group 1 disorders: rapid toxic accumulation of a small molecule
- Group 2 disorders: lack of energy
- Group 3 disorders: defects in the synthesis of large molecules resulting in a dysmorphic child
- Group 4 disorders: defects in the metabolism of large complex molecules
- Group 5 disorders: mitochondrial diseases
- Further reading

Inborn errors of metabolism are inherited biochemical disorders, and are generally autosomal recessive and caused by *single gene disorders*. They are individually rare yet collectively not uncommon.

BASIC UNDERLYING MECHANISM

- The molecular anomaly leads to a defect in an **enzyme** (see Fig. 16.1) (or cofactor), or less commonly a **structural protein** such as a transmembrane transporter
- Decreased enzyme activity results in
    - an *accumulation* of the biochemical substrate or a
    - *deficiency* of a product (see Fig. 16.1). This can be particularly harmful if the former is toxic or the latter is essential for cellular function
- The enzyme may require a particular **cofactor** such as a vitamin to function and deficiencies of this cofactor can lead to symptoms similar to those caused by deficiency of the enzyme

Metabolic disorders usually affect children, although increasingly adult phenotypes are being described.

Normal enzyme C function

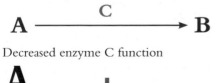

Decreased enzyme C function

Figure 16.1 Mechanism of metabolic disorders. Decreased function of enzyme C leads to an accumulation of A and/or a deficiency of B

Owing to the rarity of the individual conditions, the multitude of possible presentations and the perceived complexity of the investigations required, metabolic disorders are frequently undiagnosed. This is unfortunate as, once suspected, they are generally relatively easy to diagnose and subsequent treatment is often inexpensive yet effective.

CLASSIFICATION

Metabolic disorders can be classified into five main groups.

Small molecule diseases

Group 1 **Rapid toxic accumulation** of a small molecule – organic acidaemias, urea cycle defects, aminoacidopathies

Group 2 **Lack of energy** – glycogen storage diseases, fatty acid oxidation defects

Large molecule diseases

Group 3 **Defect in the synthesis of a large molecule** resulting in **a dysmorphic child** – peroxisomal disorders, congenital disorders of glycosylation

Group 4 **Slow accumulation** of a large complex molecule resulting in **slowly progressive symptoms** – lysosomal storage disorders

Group 5 **Mitochondrial diseases**

GROUP 1 DISORDERS: RAPID TOXIC ACCUMULATION OF A SMALL MOLECULE

- Organic acidaemias
- Urea cycle defects
- Aminoacidopathies

ORGANIC ACIDAEMIAS

Organic acids are produced by the removal of the amino group (nitrogen) from amino acids, and metabolized in the cell to produce energy. *Enzyme defects* in these pathways lead to an accumulation of the *preceding organic acids*. This occurs particularly during periods of increased protein turnover either from *dietary sources* or *intercurrent illness* (endogenous catabolism ↑). A natural catabolism occurs in the *early neonatal period*, making this a particularly vulnerable time.

Examples: Methylmalonic acidaemia, propionic acidaemia

Clinical features

Neonate	Lethargy, poor feeding, vomiting, severe ketoacidosis
Infancy	Intermittent acute attacks of above symptoms during illness or certain diets (episodes are often initially mistaken for sepsis)
Long term	(If untreated) Mental retardation, movement disorders, faltering growth, renal impairment

Investigations

Routine	Blood gas (acidosis)
	Ketones (↑)
	Ammonia (↑)
	Glucose (↓)
Special	Urine organic acids
	Acylcarnitine profile

Management

- Low protein diet
- Vitamin cofactors, e.g. carnitine

- Haemofiltration
- Avoid catabolism (see below)

UREA CYCLE DISORDERS

Similar acute episodes can occur in the urea cycle disorders, a group of conditions caused by enzymological defects in the conversion of *toxic* ammonia and nitrogen waste into *non-toxic* urea (the urea cycle). Deficiencies of all the enzymes in the urea cycle can occur, resulting in urea cycle defects.

Protein feed (amino acids) $\longrightarrow$ Ammonia **Urea cycle** Urea
Toxic *Non-toxic*

Example: Ornithine transcarbamylase deficiency (OTC; X-linked recessive)

Clinical features

Neonate (common)	Severe **hyperammonaemia** and subsequent encephalopathy (lethargy, poor feeding, seizures and coma)
Childhood	Faltering growth, cyclical vomiting and encephalopathy Developmental delay (some types)

Investigations

Routine	**Plasma ammonia** ↑↑ (> 200 µmol/L). This is the key investigation Blood gas – may have respiratory alkalosis
Special	Amino acids Orotic acid

Management

Acute	Urgent haemofiltration to lower the toxic ammonia and related compounds
Long term	Low protein diet and ammonia-lowering medication, e.g. sodium phenylbutyrate, arginine

---

Episodes of metabolic decompensation

Despite treatment, children with organic acidaemias and urea cycle diseases may have frequent episodes of **metabolic decompensation**. These often occur during periods of intercurrent viral infections. Prompt instigation of a high carbohydrate–low protein diet (the emergency regimen) can prevent or at least curtail these, although hospital admission for IV glucose and medications is often required.

AMINOACIDOPATHIES

Investigations

- Amino acid profile (plasma or urine), e.g. PKU – phenylalanine ↑
- Enzyme or molecular test confirmation may be necessary

Management

- Very low protein diet
- Specialized medications
- Supplementary specialized formula (vitamins, minerals, carbohydrates and all essential amino acids except one[s] the patient cannot metabolize to make a complete diet), e.g. for PKU, low-phenylalanine diet for life (*some* phenylalanine must be given as this amino acid is not synthesized in the body). During pregnancy the diet must be strictly adhered to because high phenylalanine levels result in fetal abnormalities, e.g. CHD, and mental retardation

Phenylketonuria

The most common metabolic disorder: incidence 1 in 15 000.

Phenylketonuria (PKU) is caused by a defect in the breakdown of phenylalanine. The enzyme phenylalanine hydroxylase is low or absent and phenylalanine and its alternative pathway metabolites accumulate in the tissues.

$$\text{Phenylalanine} \xrightarrow{\quad \times \quad} \text{Tyrosine}$$

Phenylalanine hydroxylase

Clinical features

NB: These only develop if the condition is untreated:

- Slowly progressive mental retardation
- Spastic cerebral palsy, athetosis, hyperactivity, acquired microcephaly
- Fair hair and skin, blue eyes

Neonatal screening is well established for PKU (Guthrie test – phenylalanine levels ↑) and the classical phenotype is now rarely seen.

Maple syrup urine disease

This is an inability to break down the branched chain amino acids isoleucine, leucine and valine. It usually presents in the neonatal period with encephalopathy.

Tyrosinaemia

This presents with acute or chronic **liver disease** and **renal disease** with renal rickets.

GROUP 2 DISORDERS: LACK OF ENERGY

- Glycogen storage diseases (GSDs)
- Fatty acid oxidation defects

GLYCOGEN STORAGE DISEASES

In order to maintain blood glucose, normal fasted children rely initially on the breakdown of hepatic glycogen and later on the oxidation of fat. Children with GSDs can *make glycogen* but *cannot effectively catabolize it*. **Glycogen** is thus stored in huge quantities in the liver. During periods of starvation, e.g. during an intercurrent viral illness, the children become hypoglycaemic and lethargic. There are several different types involving different enzyme deficiencies.

Clinical features

GSD I and III Hypoglycaemia
Massive hepatomegaly in first few months of life
Long term complications – short stature, hepatoma, osteoporosis and cardiac disease if untreated

GSD VI and IX Milder disease
Hypoglycaemia if significantly stressed, often only have mild–moderate hepatomegaly and have an otherwise excellent prognosis
Long term complications – short stature, hepatoma, osteoporosis and cardiac disease if untreated

Investigations

- *Enzyme activity* (blood or liver) and/or
- Molecular analysis of appropriate *gene*

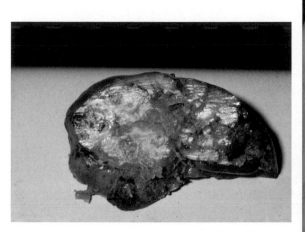

Figure 16.2 Hepatoblastoma in the liver from a patient who died at 3 months of age (courtesy of Dr Callum Wilson)

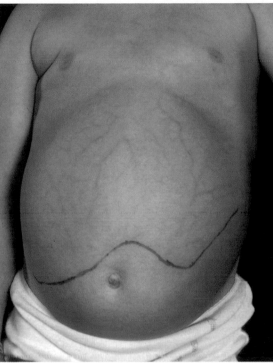

Figure 16.3 Typical massive hepatomegaly in a patient with glycogen storage disease type I (courtesy of Dr Callum Wilson)

Management

Regular high carbohydrate meals during the day, and continuous feeds during the night (or uncooked cornstarch, a slow release form of glucose, every 4–6 h).

Prognosis depends on the degree of metabolic control. It is hoped that with modern management the complications of short stature, hepatoma, osteoporosis and cardiac disease can be mostly avoided.

GALACTOSAEMIA

Incidence 1 in 60 000.

Galactosaemia is an autosomal recessive disorder caused by mutation in a gene on chromosome 9p13. Various mutations are seen and these cause deficiency of the enzyme galactose-1-phosphate uridyl transferase (mnemonic = GAL-I-PUT), resulting in inability to metabolize galactose or lactose (glucose + galactose). Accumulation of galactose-1-phosphate results in damage to the brain, liver and kidney.

Clinical features

Newborn/infant   Vomiting, hypoglycaemia, feeding difficulties
                               Seizures, irritability, developmental delay
                               Jaundice, hepatomegaly, liver failure
                               Cataracts, splenomegaly

Speech and language problems (especially dysarthria) and ovarian failure are almost inevitable, even with therapy.

Investigations

- Enzyme assay in red blood cells
- Urine – non-glucose reducing substances present when milk fed, i.e. Clinitest positive, Clinistix negative (specific for glucose)

Management

Lactose and galactose-free diet.

FATTY ACID OXIDATION DEFECTS

During fasting *fats or fatty acids* are metabolized to *ketones*. These are used as an alternative energy source to glucose and are the main source of energy during starvation. Fatty acid oxidation defects (FAODs) are defects in this pathway and are more variable than the GSDs in their presentation. As children may not be exposed to significant catabolic stress during early life, some cases may not present until mid-childhood or even adulthood.

Examples	Medium-chain acyl-CoA dehydrogenase deficiency (MCAD)
	Very long-chain acyl-CoA dehydrogenase deficiency (VLCAD)
	Long-chain L-3-hydroxyacyl-CoA dehydrogenase deficiency (LCHAD)
	Carnitine palmitoyl transferase 1 deficiency (CPT1)

Clinical features

Typical presentation	Hypoglycaemia and encephalopathy during fasting
Other initial findings	Rhabdomyolysis, cardiomyopathy, arrhythmia (as skeletal and cardiac muscle is particularly reliant on fatty acids for cellular metabolism)
During metabolic stress	Hypoglycaemia with inappropriately low ketones (hypoketotic hypoglycaemia)

Investigations

Diagnosis relies on a strong clinical suspicion and specialized tests:

Measurement of fatty acids	*Urine* organic acids
Fatty acid derivatives	*Blood* acylcarnitine profile (can be done on Guthrie test)

Management

Management is relatively easy, cheap and effective:

- Regular oral feeds
- Regular intake of a carbohydrate solution, either orally or IV, during periods of catabolic stress is essential

> **!** **NB: Many of the small molecule metabolic diseases can now be screened for on the Guthrie test and hopefully this will result in the classical presentations described above becoming much less common.**

GROUP 3 DISORDERS: DEFECTS IN THE SYNTHESIS OF LARGE MOLECULES RESULTING IN A DYSMORPHIC CHILD

- Enzyme defects in the synthesis of large molecules
- Peroxisomal biogenesis disorders
- Congenital disorders of glycosylation (CDG disorders, or carbohydrate deficient glycoprotein disorders)

This is a relatively new yet rapidly expanding group of metabolic disorders. These children tend to be *abnormal at birth* although recognition of this may not be until later. Treatment of all these conditions is generally disappointing.

ENZYME DEFECTS IN THE SYNTHESIS OF LARGE MOLECULES

The defective enzyme in these conditions is involved in the synthesis of large molecules, e.g. cholesterol (e.g. Smith–Lemni–Opitz syndrome) or glycoproteins.

Clinical features

Symptoms	Failure to thrive
	Mental retardation
Signs	Upturned nares
	2–3 toe syndactyly
	Small penis/ambiguous genitalia in males

PEROXISOMAL BIOGENESIS DISORDERS

There is a defect in the transport of enzymes into the peroxisome and thus normal peroxisomal anabolic function is not possible, e.g. Zellweger syndrome. **Peroxisomes** are intracellular organelles and are important in cell membrane formation, synthesis of bile acids and breakdown of very long chain fatty acids (VLCFAs).

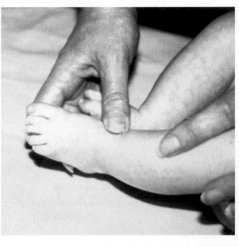

Figure 16.4 Syndactyly of the second and third toes in Smith–Lemni–Optiz syndrome (courtesy of Dr Callum Wilson)

Clinical features

Symptoms	Poor feeding
	Seizures
	Mental retardation
Signs	Hypotonia
	Large fontanelle
	Hepatomegaly
	Corneal clouding, cataracts, retinopathy
	Dysmorphism
	Chondrodysplasia punctata on X-ray (stippled appearance of epiphyses)

CONGENITAL DISORDERS OF GLYCOSYLATION

Before a protein is exported from a cell, carbohydrate moieties are attached by the endoplasmic reticulum and Golgi apparatus in a process known as **glycosylation**. This requires a huge variety of enzymes and defects in any one of these lead to a CDG.

Preliminary diagnosis is made by studying the glycosylation pattern on **transferrin** (a glycoprotein).

Clinical features

Symptoms	Mental retardation
	Abnormal eye movements
Signs	Abnormal fat pads, inverted nipples
	Cerebellar hypoplasia
	Hypotonia, multiorgan dysfunction

GROUP 4 DISORDERS: DEFECTS IN THE METABOLISM OF LARGE COMPLEX MOLECULES

LYSOSOMAL STORAGE DISEASES

Lysosomes are cell organelles important in the recycling of sphingolipids, mucopolysaccharides and oligosaccharides. These large complex molecules are made up of fatty acid chains, carbohydrate moieties and amino groups, and are important as structural components of cells and organelles. They are catabolized in a stepwise fashion by a series of enzyme reactions in the lysosome. A defect in any one of these enzymes leads to a *slow accumulation of the preceding compound* and a corresponding *slowly progressive clinical phenotype*.

Mucopolysaccharidosis type I (Hurler disease)

Symptoms (all progressive)	Cognitive regression
	Skeletal anomalies
Signs	Coarse facial features
	Dysostosis multiplex (skeletal deformity)
	Hepatomegaly
	Cardiomyopathy, valvular lesions
	Corneal clouding
	Skin thickening
Diagnosis	Urine glycosaminoglycans
	White cell enzymes

Tay Sachs disease

Symptoms (all progressive)	Early neurological regression
	Visual impairment
	Seizures
	Decerebration
Signs	Truncal hypotonia
	Hyper-reflexic
	Cherry red spot (retina)
Diagnosis	White cell enzymes
	Hexosaminidase A

Metachromatic leukodystrophy

Symptoms (all progressive)	Ataxia
	Muscle spasms
	Speech, swallowing difficulties
	Neurological regression
Signs	Hypertonia
	Hyper-reflexic
Diagnosis	White cell enzymes
	Arylsulphatase A

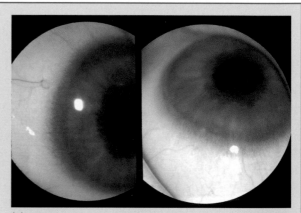

(a)

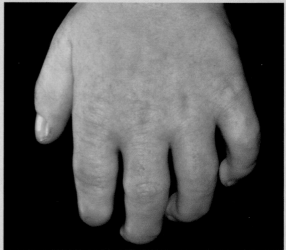

(b)

Figure 16.5 Hurler syndrome. (a) Corneal clouding. (b) Typical 'claw' hand with broad short phalanges (courtesy of Dr Callum Wilson)

The lysosomal storage diseases (LSDs) can show considerable locus and allelic heterogeneity. Different enzyme defects can result in a similar phenotype; alternatively, various lesions in the same gene can result in a severe infantile disease or relatively mild adult onset depending on the degree of residual enzyme activity. There are over 40 known LSDs.

Examples: Hurler disease, Tay Sachs disease, metachromatic leukodystrophy

Clinical features

CNS   **Neurological regression**
Other organs   All organ systems can be affected by the accumulation of these compounds:

- Hepatosplenomegaly
- Cardiomyopathy, valvular lesions
- Bone disease   } All frequently seen
- Infiltrative lung disease
- Renal impairment
- Progressive dysmorphic facial features

Management

- Traditionally treatment has been supportive only
- Organ transplantation (SC or liver) is successful in some conditions
- Recombinant enzyme replacement therapy is becoming increasingly available (expensive yet effective)

GROUP 5 DISORDERS: MITOCHONDRIAL DISEASES

Mitochondrial disease usually refers to defects in the **respiratory chain**. This electron transport chain is responsible for the production of ATP via the transport of electrons from NADH and FADH obtained primarily from the Krebs cycle. Defects in this pathway lead to a failure of ATP production and/or an accumulation of oxidative stress and thus cell death.

Tissues that have high energy demands appear to be particularly vulnerable to mitochondrial cytopathies. The **CNS**, especially the brainstem and basal ganglia, is often affected. The **eye**, **heart**, **liver** and **renal tubules** are also vulnerable, and multiorgan involvement is common.

Inheritance – The respiratory chain involves five enzyme complexes each composed of a number of subunits. These subunits can be encoded by the nuclear DNA in the traditional manner or alternatively by the 16-kb circular DNA present in mitochondria. As mitochondria are inherited from the mother, this leads to the possibility of the unique concept of **inheritance of disease through maternal lines** (see ch. 3). Without a molecular diagnosis genetic counselling can thus be difficult.

Examples   **Congenital lactic acidosis**
                  – floppy neonate, often
                  with cardiomyopathy, liver
                  dysfunction and renal tubular
                  dysfunction. Lactate very
                  high. Death in infancy

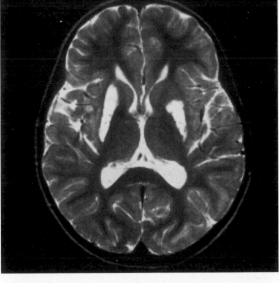

Figure 16.6 MRI of the brain in a patient with Leigh disease, showing typical bilateral lentiform nuclei and right caudate nucleus infarcts (courtesy of Dr Callum Wilson)

Leigh syndrome – initially normal child, progressive basal ganglia and brainstem dysfunction

Investigations

1. **Plasma lactate**   If elevated (and especially an elevated CSF lactate), strongly suggestive of mitochondrial disease (if characteristic signs and symptoms)

2. **Muscle biopsy**   The next investigation in most childhood cases. Should be sent to a recognized laboratory for specific histochemistry and enzymology

3. **Molecular diagnosis**   May then be sought based on the results of the muscle biopsy. Recent rapid advances in mitochondrial genomics and DNA technology suggest that a molecular approach may be more rewarding and could be regarded as the first-line investigation in the near future

Management

Current treatment is generally disappointing. A variety of vitamins, antioxidants and special diets. While there is theoretical, laboratory and anecdotal support for these treatments there is, as yet, little objective evidence of clinical benefit.

Clinical scenario

A 3 month old presents having had a viral infection with lethargy and sweating. The blood sugar level is obtained and noted to be 2 mmol/L glucose. On examination of the abdomen a 5 cm lever edge is palpable below the right costal margin. There is no pyrexia and no skin rash. The parents are second cousins.

1. What is the most likely diagnosis?
2. What are two relevant investigations?
3. What is the usual treatment approach?

ANSWERS

1. Glycogen storage disorder
2. Blood or liver enzyme activity assessment; genetic analysis
3. Correction of hypoglycaemia is a priority. Regular good meals during the day. Corn starch or other long-acting slowly absorbed carbohydrate, especially at night

---

FURTHER READING

Nyhan W, Barshop B, Ozand P. *Atlas of Metabolic Diseases,* 3rd edn. London: Hodder Arnold, 2010.

Saudubray J, van den Berghe G, Walter J (eds.). *Inborn Metabolic Diseases: Diagnosis and Treatment.* Berlin: Springer-Verlag, 2011.

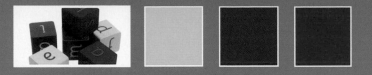

17 Dermatology

- Dermatological history and examination
- Terminology
- Common neonatal skin disorders
- Common skin problems
- Infections
- Cutaneous reactions
- Vascular birthmarks
- Involuting tumours
- Pigmented naevi
- Pyogenic granuloma
- Pigmentary disturbance
- Alopecia
- Rare inherited disorders
- Further reading

DERMATOLOGICAL HISTORY AND EXAMINATION

History of a rash

- Is it congenital? Is there a family history of a similar rash?
- Rash:
  - Onset? How long has it been present? Development: has it changed/spread? Stages?
  - Itchy or painful? Relation to exposure to sunshine?
- Any exacerbating factors?
- Is the child well or unwell? Is there a fever?
- Other symptoms?
- Any contacts? Any travel?
- Any medications (regular or new)? Any other illnesses?
- Any treatments applied and their effect?

Examination

- Examine the *whole child*, i.e. all the skin, do not miss bits
- Remember examination of the skin includes: teeth, nails, hair, mucous membranes and skin (see Fig. 17.1)

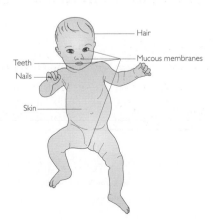

Figure 17.1 Examination of the skin includes hair, teeth, nails and mucus membranes

Describing rashes

- Draw a *diagram*
- Describe individual *lesions* (type [see below], shape, colour, margination and consistency)
- Draw the *arrangement* and *distribution* (linear, annular, localized, diffuse, confluent, symmetrical, mucous membranes involved?)

TERMINOLOGY

Specific terminology is used to describe rashes, and it is worth learning some basic descriptive terms as applying these can often help you to focus more clearly and identify a rash.

Types of lesion

Papule	Nodule	Macule	Plaque	Wheal	Vesicle	Bulla
Elevated lesion < 0.5 cm	Elevated lesion > 0.5 cm	Flat lesion	Elevated area > 2 cm	Transient dermal oedema	Small fluid-filled lesion < 0.5 cm	Larger fluid-filled lesion
Molluscum contagiosum	*Viral wart*	*Vitiligo, freckle*	*Psoriasis*	*Urticaria*	*Herpes simplex (chicken pox)*	*Bullous impetigo*

Further descriptions

Scales	Flakes of stratum corneum, e.g. psoriasis
Excoriation	Damage to skin due to scratching, e.g. any pruritic condition
Lichenification	Thickening due to rubbing, e.g. chronic atopic eczema
Petechiae	Haemorrhagic lesions, e.g. meningococcal rash
Erosion	Loss of epidermis. Heals without scarring, e.g. eczema
Ulcer	Loss of both dermis and epidermis
Scar	Fibrous tissue replacing normal tissue after injury or disease
Pustule	Visible accumulation of pus, e.g. folliculitis
Telangiectasia	Visible small blood vessels, e.g. steroid side effect
Maculopapular	Containing both flat and raised lesions, e.g. measles

COMMON NEONATAL SKIN DISORDERS

ERYTHEMA TOXICUM NEONATORUM (TOXIC ERYTHEMA OF THE NEWBORN)

- 50% of term infants develop this during first few days of life (< 4 days normally)
- Possibly an inflammatory response to sebum

- Blotchy red papules ± pustules (intrafollicular eosinophilic)
- Anywhere on body and face (mostly trunk), except palms and soles
- Infant *well*
- Resolve spontaneously < 3 days
- May recur over first few weeks of life

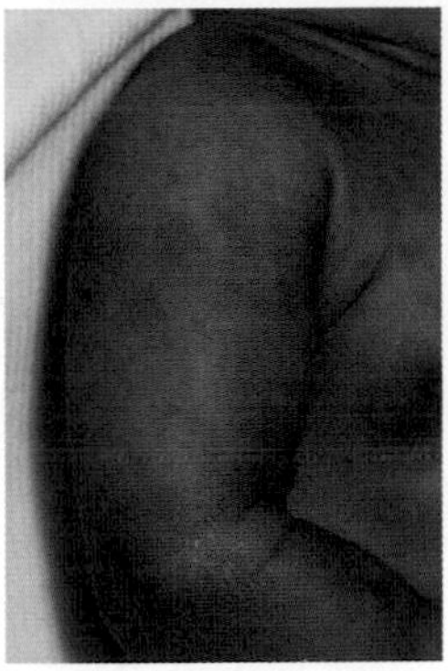

SEBACEOUS GLAND HYPERPLASIA AND MILIA

Sebaceous gland hyperplasia occurs in most neonates and is secondary to maternal androgens.

Pinpoint white papules over the nose, cheeks, upper lip, forehead

Around 40% of infants also have minute 1–2 mm follicular epidermal (keratin filled) cysts (**milia**), which resolve in a few weeks. (At the same sites as sebaceous gland hyperplasia ± scrotum, labia majora and areolae.)

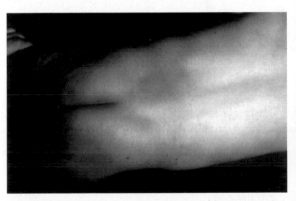

Figure 17.2
Erythema toxicum in a 2-day-old infant

Epstein's pearls (85% neonates) are milia in the mouth (white keratinous cysts) along the alveolar ridge and at the junction of the hard and soft palate.

MONGOLIAN SPOT

This congenital pigmentation is due to melanocytes arrested in the dermis on their way to the basal layer of the epidermis.

- Congenital blue–grey macule(s) of pigmentation on trunk ± limbs
- Common in Orientals (80%) and Afro-Caribbeans
- Slowly fade over first 10 years of life, may be permanent

Figure 17.3 Mongolian blue spots on the back of a black infant

COMMON SKIN PROBLEMS

NAPPY RASH

The main causes of nappy rash are:

Irritant dermatitis	Due to irritant effect of urine and faeces
	Skin creases spared
Candida infection	*No sparing* of skin creases
	Satellite lesions seen
Seborrhoeic dermatitis	Red moist rash with fine yellow scale
	Non-pruritic ± rash elsewhere and cradle cap
Atopic dermatitis	May present as nappy rash due to increased irritability
Psoriasis	Rare. *Intractable* nappy rash. Bright red and well-defined

Treatment is with topical antifungal ± hydrocortisone ointment (and emollients in seborrhoeic and atopic dermatitis). With irritant contact dermatitis, regular nappy changing and a barrier ointment are also necessary.

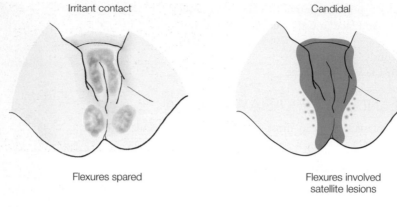

Irritant contact

Flexures spared

(a)

Candidal

Flexures involved
satellite lesions

(b)

Figure 17.4 Types of nappy rash

SEBORRHOEIC DERMATITIS

- Develops in the first few weeks of life, and generally resolves within a few weeks
- Infant is well and *non-itchy*
- Red moist skin and fine yellow scales
- Nappy area, face (cheeks, eyebrows, forehead, behind ears), neck folds, flexures, scalp

They quite often progress to atopic dermatitis.

Treatment
- Daily baths with bath oil
- Wash with emollient, e.g. aqueous cream BP (*no* soap)
- Topical combined antifungal and hydrocortisone

Cradle cap

This resembles (or is thought to be a limited form of) seborrhoeic dermatitis.

- Thick greasy scales and red moist skin on the scalp
- Usually resolves with emollient therapy alone. Use aqueous cream BP as shampoo daily. Occasionally requires 1% hydrocortisone lotion to be applied after washing

ATOPIC DERMATITIS (ATOPIC ECZEMA)

Atopic eczema is an itchy recurrent or chronic skin disease that can begin any age (usually > 6 months) and is often associated with other atopic diseases (for features of atopy, see p. 132). It has an incidence in childhood of around 20% in the UK.

- Itchiness
- Dry skin
- Hyperlinearity of palms and soles
- Dennie–Morgan fold (fold under eyes, not specific to eczema but indicative of atopy)
- Dry irritated swollen eyelids

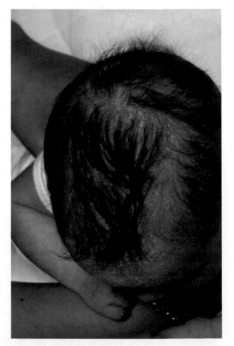

Figure 17.5 Cradle cap in an infant

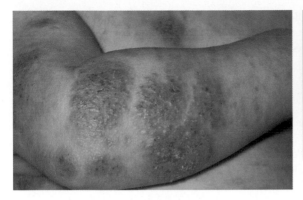

(a)

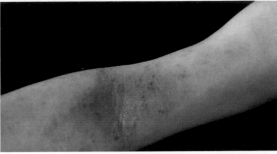

(b)

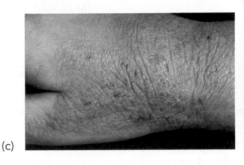

(c)

Figure 17.6 Eczema. (a) Infantile eczema over the elbow – extensor surfaces are involved in infancy. (b) Flexural eczema in an older child – antecubital fossae and popliteal fossae usually affected. (c) Lichenified eczema secondary to scratching

- Lymphadenopathy
- *Acute and subacute eczema* – erythema, weeping and crusting of excoriated areas
- *Chronic eczema* – lichenification (thickening from scratching) and post-inflammatory hyper- and hypopigmentation

The distribution varies with age:

Infants	**Face**, **extensor surfaces** knees and elbows, feet and hands
Older child	Elbow and knee **flexures**, **wrists**, **ankles**, neck ± lichenification

Complications

Secondary bacterial infection	Usually *Staphylococcus aureus* or *Streptococcus pyogenes*
Viral infection	Several viral infections affecting the skin can be more severe and widespread in children with eczema

- **Eczema herpeticum** – herpes simplex virus infection in a child with atopic eczema. Can be widespread; a potentially serious infection.
  Must be treated with antivirals (IV aciclovir if concern) if seen while still extending (< 5 days after onset)
- Molluscum contagiosum
- Viral warts
- Varicella (chicken pox)

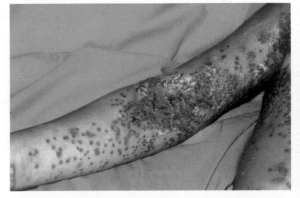

Figure 17.7 Eczema herpeticum on a child's arm

Growth impairment An intrinsic feature of atopic children; more common in severe eczema. It can also be secondary to overzealous dietary restrictions, associated allergic enteropathy with malabsorption, prolonged courses of systemic steroids or, rarely, if too much potent topical steroid is given.

Treatment

First-line therapy

General advice	Detailed advice about eczema, environmental factors and how to use topical treatments
	Keep nails short
	Use only loose cotton clothing
	Stop adults smoking in the house
Reduction of triggers	Avoid **allergens**, e.g. house dust mite reduction (regular hoovering, hard flooring is better than carpets, mattress, duvet and pillow covers), pets (dogs, cats, horses), and **irritants**, e.g. hot and cold conditions, soaps, detergents, wool
Emollients (moisturizers)	In the bath, e.g. emulsifying ointment BP instead of soap
	After baths on skin, e.g. white soft paraffin BP
Topical corticosteroids	Use *minimum strength effective* steroid to minimize side effects
Antihistamines	Regular oral antihistamines reduce eczema severity
Antibiotics	If infected – flucloxacillin (covers *Staph. aureus*) and/or penicillin (*Strep. pyogenes*) or erythromycin are usually the treatments of choice

> **NB: Ointments are generally preferable to creams:**
> **Ointments – greasy, more effective and less liable to irritate than creams**
> **Creams – less greasy, can be drying and additives can cause irritation, but more cosmetically acceptable.**

Topical steroids: groups and side effects

Potency	Example
Mild	Hydrocortisone®
Moderate	Eumovate®
Potent	Betnovate®
Very potent	Dermovate®

Side effects

- Thinning of skin (atrophy)
- Petechiae
- Telangiectasiae
- Striae distensiae
- Growth retardation (if used to excess)

Second-line therapy

Topical immunomodulator Given if topical steroids are insufficient (tacrolimus or pimecrolimus)

Food allergy management	In some children certain foods worsen eczema (onset may also be clearly related to introducing certain foods). A trial avoiding them may be undertaken with the dietician's help to maintain growth and nutrition, e.g. milk, soya, wheat or egg avoidance. (Immediate hypersensitivity reactions to foods [especially contact urticaria] are common. Avoidance in these children is essential as there may be a risk of severe reaction)
Wet wraps and bandages	Wet wraps are double-layer cotton wraps, the inner layer of which is applied wet, under which topical emollients and/or steroids are applied. They are changed 12–24 hourly. They (1) provide physical protection, (2) prolong the effect of emollients and (3) increase the penetration of topical steroids. They also reduce pruritus, probably via cooling. Paste bandages may be used on the limbs with ichthamol impregnated into them which helps reduce lichenification

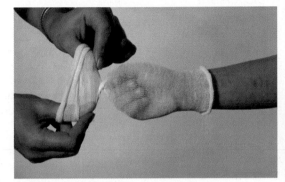

Figure 17.8 Putting wet wraps on the hand

Third-line therapy

Phototherapy	A 6–8 week course of narrow-band ultraviolet-B phototherapy
Chinese herbs	Many parents try Chinese herbs privately (often given as tea). These are not regulated as medicines and there have been problems with renal and liver toxicity
Immunosuppressive drugs	For severe eczema courses of these drugs may be needed, e.g. oral cyclosporin, azathioprine

ACNE

Acne is a common inflammatory disorder of the pilosebaceous unit, most common in teenagers and young adults. It is primarily due to increased sebum production from high androgen levels (oily skin, greasy hair). Androgen levels are high directly after birth which can cause **infantile acne** (due to maternal androgens which rapidly fall), and increase from age 9 years to teenage years. Lipophilic bacteria (especially *Propionibacterium acnes*) colonize the hair follicles. The face, upper back and chest are most commonly affected.

Lesions of acne

- Comedones (plugs of sebaceous material within hair follicle unit)
  (open comedones = blackheads; closed comedones = whiteheads)
- Papules, pustules
- Nodules, cysts
- Scars

Treatment

Topical	Antibacterial and keratolytic, e.g. benzoyl peroxide
	Antibiotic, e.g. erythromycin
	Retinoic acid (can irritate the skin)

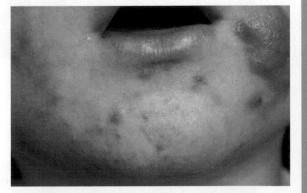

Figure 17.9 Infantile nodulocystic acne

Oral	Antibiotics, e.g. erythromycin. Given for 6–12 months
	Anti-androgens (girls only) – certain oral contraceptive pill formulations
	Retinoid – isotretinoin, given at 1 mg/kg dose usually over 4–6 months. This decreases size of the sebaceous glands, and reduces sebum production and follicular hyperkeratosis. It is very effective, however side effects include dry skin and lips, muscular aches and teratogenicity. Elevated serum lipids and hepatitis (idiosyncratic) may occur (monitor serum lipids and LFTs)

PSORIASIS

Psoriasis is an inflammatory disease where there is increased turnover of the skin with epidermal hyperkeratosis (patches of thickened skin). It affects 2% of the population and around 10% of these will present as children. In children the onset is most commonly 7–8 years. There is often a positive family history.

- Thick white silvery scales
- Face, scalp, elbows, knees and napkin area most common

In children there are two common forms:

Chronic plaque psoriasis	Scaly red plaques mainly on extensor surfaces, usually with scalp involvement
Guttate psoriasis	Lots of small plaques on the trunk. '*Raindrop*' psoriasis. Often precipitated by a streptococcal sore throat (therefore throat swab and antistreptolysin O titre [ASOT] indicated)

Treatment

The mildest effective treatment is used:

Emollients	These may contain keratolytics. In baths as soap, after baths
Topical treatments	Applied once or twice daily:
	Mild or moderate topical steroids
	Steroid and tar mixtures
	Vitamin D3 analogues, e.g. calcipitriol

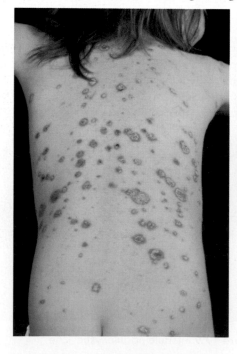

(a)

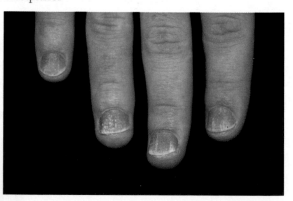

(b)

Figure 17.10 Psoriasis. (a) Guttate psoriasis. Note scattered small plaques with silvery scale. (b) Nail psoriasis (nail pitting)

Phototherapy   Often used for guttate psoriasis, as the plaques are too small for topical therapy to be applied
6–8-week course of narrow-band ultraviolet-B phototherapy is given

INSECT BITES

The most common culprits are cat and dog fleas (tend to form a *row* of bites). Ask about pets.

These may cause:

- No reaction in young infants, or
- Papular urticaria
- Also, commonest cause of blisters in children

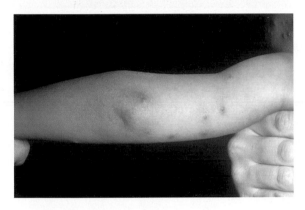

Figure 17.11 Insect bites on an infant

PITYRIASIS ROSEA

- Common rash in children
- Sometimes preceded by mild malaise and fever
- Classically a large pink patch (2–5 cm) called a **'herald patch'** develops first
- Followed by lots of smaller pink patches each with a peripheral collarette of scale. Over the back they form a symmetrical pattern along the rib lines said to resemble the foliage of a Christmas tree
- Cause is unknown but possibly viral and it resolves spontaneously after 6–8 weeks
- Mild topical steroids can be applied to speed up resolution

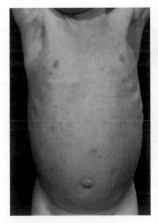

Figure 17.12 Herald patch (central chest) of pityriasis rosea

INFECTIONS

IMPETIGO

A common contagious bacterial epidermal skin infection, due to:

- *Staph. aureus* (NB: Bullous impetigo is usually due to phage group II *Staph. aureus*), or
- Group A β-haemolytic streptococcus (*Strep. pyogenes*), or
- Both

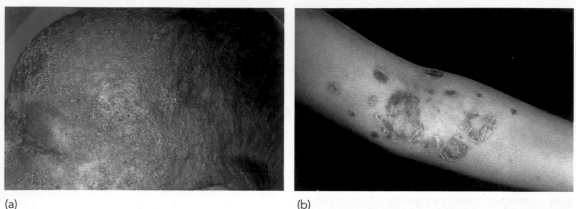

(a)

(b)

Figure 17.13 Impetigo. (a) Yellow crusts over the forehead. (b) Bullous impetigo – bullae have burst

There are two forms:

- **Impetigo contagiosa** – classical annular lesions of honey-coloured crusts + localized lymphadenopathy
- **Bullous impetigo** – fragile vesicles and bullae (localized staphylococcal scalded skin syndrome [SSSS])

Treatment

- Topical antibiotic if mild, or
- Oral antibiotic, e.g. flucloxacillin and penicillin, if more severe

! **NB: Late complication is post-streptococcal glomerulonephritis (see p. 235).**

STAPHYLOCOCCAL SCALDED SKIN SYNDROME

Staphylococcal scalded skin syndrome (SSSS) is a rare skin condition caused by epidermolytic toxin (ET) producing strains of *Staph. aureus,* usually group II phage types 3A, 3C, 55 and 71. It is most common in young infants and, as it is potentially life-threatening due to sepsis and fluid loss, it must be treated rapidly.

- Infant febrile and unwell
- Skin red and extremely tender (intraepidermal blistering), followed by
- Superficial desquamation of the epidermis in sheets

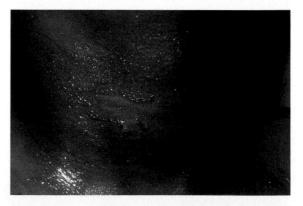

Figure 17.14 Staphylococcal scalded skin syndrome

Treatment

- Take skin swabs of potential site of causative infection, e.g. nose, umbilicus, and blood cultures
- *Frozen section* of denuded skin or skin biopsy can be helpful when there is diagnostic doubt
- Admit the infant with close monitoring of vital signs and fluid balance

- Keep the infant in a warm side-room, place on low pressure mattress
- Regular frequent emollient and non-adherent dressings such as Vaseline gauze
- IV antibiotic therapy to cover *Staph. aureus*, and check cultures as soon as through

MOLLUSCUM CONTAGIOSUM

A common infection with a DNA poxvirus. More widespread infection can occur in children with atopic eczema.

- Pearly umbilicated papules
- Live virus in centre of lesions
- Spread by scratching

The condition will resolve spontaneously in 6–9 months, and treatment is generally contraindicated.

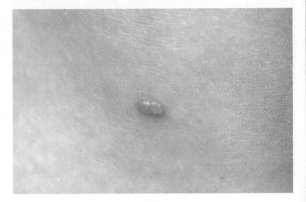

Figure 17.15 Molluscum contagiosum

VIRAL WARTS

These are extremely common in childhood and are spread by contact with people or objects. The various wart viruses (human papillomaviruses [HPV]) are associated with different forms of viral wart:

- **Common warts** (often on fingers)
- **Plantar warts** (*'verrucas'*)(on soles, often painful)
- **Anogenital warts** (if occur and suspect sexual abuse, refer to community paediatrician)

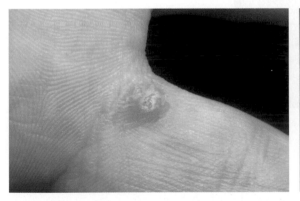

(a)

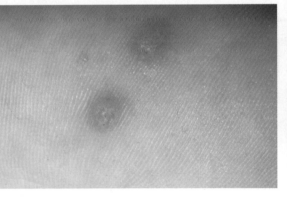

(b)

Figure 17.16 Viral warts. (a) Common. (b) Plantar

Treatment

Warts will eventually disappear spontaneously (from months to years); however, treatment to speed up resolution can be used:

- Wart paints (keratolytics) daily together with paring the warts down
- Cryotherapy (freezing). NB: This is *painful* and therefore usually best avoided

RINGWORM (TINEA)

Ringworm is caused by superficial fungal infection with dermatophytes. The areas most affected in children are:

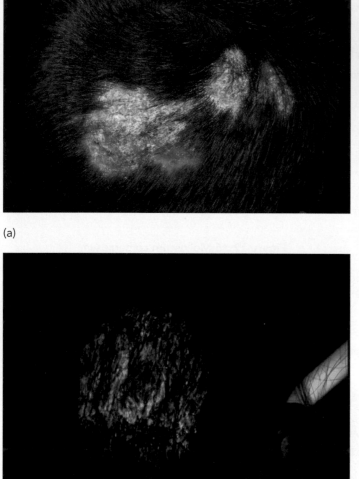

(a)

(b)

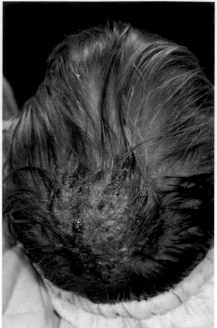

(c)

Figure 17.17 Tinea capitis.
(a) Patchy hair loss with visible scale.
(b) Fluorescent tinea seen under
ultraviolet light. (c) A kerion

Scalp	**Tinea capitis** (very common)
	Patches of alopaecia with scaling, inflammation ± pustules. A common cause is
	Trichophyton tonsurans (this species invades the hair shaft)
Body	**Tinea corporis** (very common)
	Scaly red annular lesions on trunk and/or limbs
	Trichophyton rubrum is a common cause

Management

- ■ Take fungal *skin scrapings* or hair pluckings (in tinea captitis) for microscopy and then fungal culture
- ■ **Tinea corporis** – topical antifungal for 2–4 weeks, e.g. terbinafine cream, unless widespread when oral treatment may be necessary
- ■ **Tinea capitis** – systemic antifungal course is needed, usually for a minimum of 6 weeks

**! NB: Remember to check and treat any siblings, parents or other
contacts who are affected.**

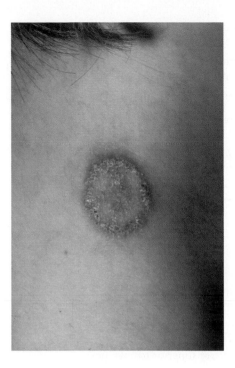

Figure 17.18 Tinea corporis – annular lesion with peripheral scale

SCABIES

Scabies rash is due to infestation with scabies mite (*Sarcoptes scabiei*) and is acquired from close physical contact. The mite makes a burrow under the skin and lays her eggs there. There are usually very few (< 10) mites on the body.

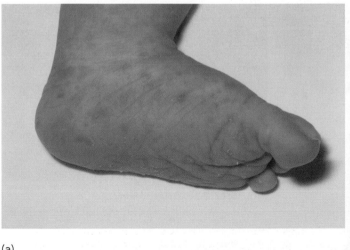

(a)

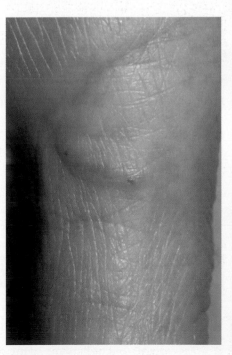

Figure 17.19 Scabies. (a) Prominent rash along the sides of the feet in an infant. (b) Scabies burrow

(b)

- Widespread itchy papular rash (result of *allergic reaction* to the mites, their eggs and excreta)
- Burrows most likely to be found:
  - *Infants*: sides of feet, palms, scalp, often widespread itchy papules and pustules
  - *Older children*: finger and toe webs, wrists, ankles, axillae, scrotum and penis

Management

- Apply KOH solution to one area over a burrow and take scraping, then identify mite or eggs under the microscope
- Topical scabicide, e.g. permethrin cream, after a bath to whole body (and head in infants < 2 years)
- Treat all close contacts
- Bedding and immediate clothes to be hot washed
- Note that the itching usually improves rapidly but may take a few weeks to resolve completely

HEAD LICE (PEDICULOSIS)

Infestation with *Pediculus humanus capitis* (head louse) is usually confined to the scalp, and is *very common*. Resistance to treatment is a problem.

Eggs are firmly stuck to the hair shaft. It causes the scalp to itch. Adult lice are 3 mm in size.

Treatment

- Comb hair with special lice comb to remove eggs and lice
- Chemical applications (malathion, permethrin, carbaryl, lindane) are superior to shampoos

> **!** **NB: Regular head examinations of the whole family are necessary to prevent re-infestations.**

PITYRIASIS VERSICOLOR

A common superficial yeast infection caused by *Pityrosporum ovale* (*Malassezia furfur*) and seen in adolescents.

- Pinkish-brown patches on upper trunk and arms
- Fine scale present
- (Hypopigmented patches if suntanned)

Treatment

Resolves with topical anti-yeast cream, e.g. keta-conazole 2% cream or shampoo.r

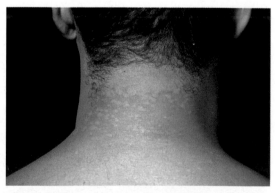

Figure 17.20 Pityriasis versicolor in an adolescent – pale areas on the back of the neck

CUTANEOUS REACTIONS

ERYTHEMA MULTIFORME

Erythema multiforme is a cutaneous reaction with a variable appearance:

- *Target lesions* (red or purpuric centre, then paler ring and surrounding red ring) anywhere on the body (classically extremities initially – hands and feet). Typical target lesions are not always seen

- No treatment is required and the rash resolves spontaneously in 2–3 weeks, but often recurs
- Secondary to *herpes simplex virus infection* (cold sores – most common cause), drugs, e.g. sulphonamides, or post-infection

Stevens–Johnson syndrome

This is a more severe reaction usually caused by various infections, including *Mycoplasma pneumoniae*, or drugs:

- Cutaneous erythema multiforme
- Fever
- Profound mucous membrane involvement, i.e. mouth, conjunctiva and genital area

URTICARIA

Urticaria may be *acute* or *chronic and recurrent* (a cause is only rarely found). Possible causes include infection (often viral), drugs or food, e.g. cow's milk protein.

- Usually an acquired type 1 hypersensitivity reaction, i.e. mediated via IgE, causing itchy red wheals anywhere on the body
- Each wheal usually lasts a few hours before fading and new ones forming

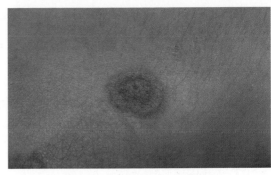

Figure 17.21 Target lesion in erythema multiforme

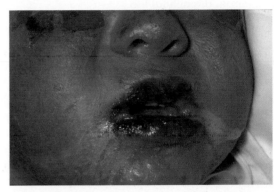

Figure 17.22 Stevens–Johnson syndrome

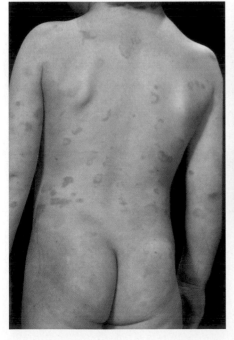

(a)

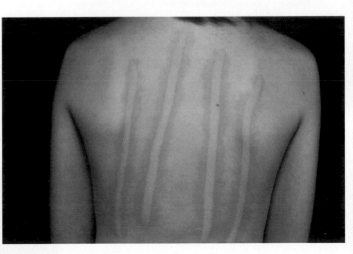

(b)

Figure 17.23 Urticaria. (a) Wheals. (b) Dermatographism on the back

- Child may exhibit **dermatographism**, i.e. a wheal at the site as a result of gently scratching the skin

Physical urticaria is due to agents such as pressure or cold.

Treatment
- Remove cause if identified
- Antihistamines orally

VASCULAR BIRTHMARKS

PORT-WINE STAIN

A port-wine stain (PWS) is a flat red area due to ectatic dermal capillaries, i.e. a vascular anomaly. These are present from birth and remain throughout life.

There may be associated eye and brain abnormalities:

Glaucoma	PWS of the face with eyelid involvement may be associated with glaucoma of the affected eye
Sturge–Weber syndrome	PWS of the face always including the area covered by the *ophthalmic branch of the trigeminal nerve*, and *Ipsilateral leptomeningeal vascular abnormality* with neurological symptoms, e.g. seizures, hemiplegia

The PWS may be treated with a course of pulsed-dye laser therapy which destroys the ectatic capillaries and fades the lesion.

SALMON PATCH

- Common pale pink vascular anomalies, present at birth on the face (eyelids, nose, forehead) or nape of the neck
- Generally fade during the first few weeks of life, except those on the nape of the neck (known popularly as a **stork bite** and present in around half of newborns) that usually persist for life

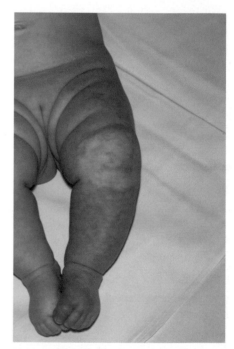

Figure 17.24 Port-wine stain of the left leg in an infant – there is some associated hypertrophy of the affected limb

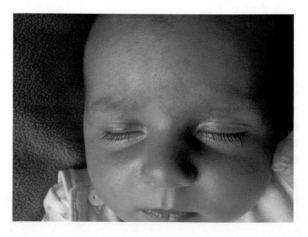

Figure 17.25 Salmon patch of the eyelids

Dermatology

INVOLUTING TUMOURS

INFANTILE HAEMANGIOMAS

- Raised red lesions which develop in the weeks after birth and are seen in 1 in 20 babies
- They are benign vascular tumours
- Enlarge over approximately 6 months and then slowly involute over a few years, usually leaving an insignificant mark
- May be *superficial* (bright red, known as 'strawberry haemangiomas'), *deep* (bluish) or *mixed*

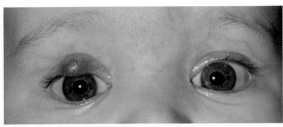

(b)

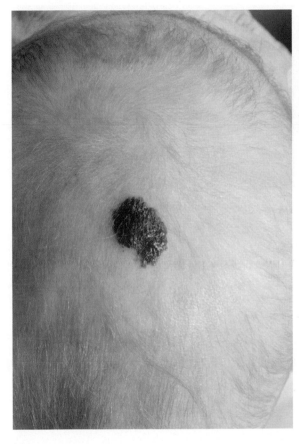

(a)

Figure 17.26 Haemangioma. (a) Involving the scalp in an infant – this requires no treatment.
(b) Involving the right eyelid – if this interferes with vision treatment is necessary (Courtesy of Dr J Uddin)

Treatment

No treatment is required unless they are *complicated* by:

- Interfering with **vision**
- Interfering with **feeding**
- Interfering with **breathing**
- **Bleeding**
- **Ulceration**

Treatment options include oral steroids to prevent enlargement, surgical excision and pulsed dye laser treatment (if ulcerated). Plastic surgery may sometimes be necessary for cosmetic reasons when the child is older.

PIGMENTED NAEVI

CONGENITAL MELANOCYTIC NAEVI

- Present at birth and may be small or very extensive (*'giant'*)
- Small increased risk of malignant transformation within the larger congenital melanocytic naevi
- May be associated with intracranial or intraspinal melanosis
- Treatment to improve the cosmetic appearance is possible but case specific. Treatment options include dermabrasion, laser therapy and full depth excision. Often they are left untreated

SPITZ NAEVUS

These are benign melanocytic naevi that usually develop during childhood on the face or limbs. They are usually round smooth pink or red lesions. The histology can sometimes be difficult to differentiate from a melanoma.

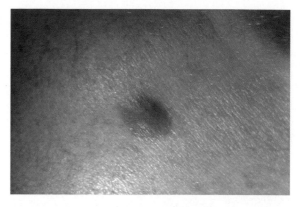

Figure 17.27 Spitz naevus

PYOGENIC GRANULOMA

- Common benign vascular tumour of the skin, made of proliferating capillaries
- Usually develops on the face or fingers after mild trauma
- Needs to be excised or treated with cauterization

The differential diagnosis includes melanoma (extremely rare in childhood) and therefore histology always needs to be obtained if there is any doubt about the diagnosis.

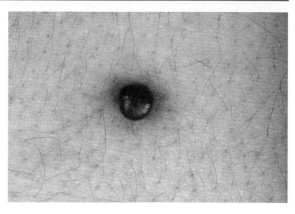

Figure 17.28 Pyogenic granuloma

PIGMENTARY DISTURBANCE

VITILIGO

Vitiligo is a common acquired disorder in which the melanocytes are destroyed, resulting in depigmented patches, which may be extensive. The disorder is not fully understood, but it is thought to be autoimmune and there is an association with other autoimmune disorders (especially thyroid). There is a positive family history in 40% of cases.

- Roughly *symmetrical* completely depigmented macules
- Peri-orbital and -oral, nipples, genitalia, knees and elbows are common sites
- 'Woods' ultraviolet light makes the depigmentation more obvious
- Spontaneous repigmentation in around 20%

Treatment is disappointing, but options include applying a topical steroid to affected areas for a few weeks or a course of narrow-band ultraviolet-B phototherapy to encourage repigmentation.

> **!** **NB: The depigmented areas of vitiligo are highly susceptible to sunburn, so full sun protection should be advised.**

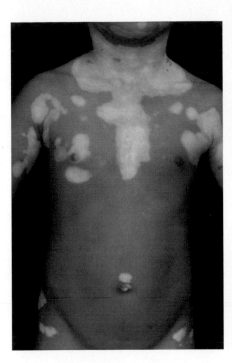

Figure 17.29 Vitiligo – note the symmetrical distribution

ALOPECIA

ALOPECIA AREATA

This is a condition in which gradual patchy hair loss occurs. It is thought to be autoimmune.

- Discoid areas of hair loss
- Lower occipital hairline only may be lost
- *Normal scalp* (not scaly)
- Short broken '*exclamation mark*' hairs
- Eyebrows, eyelashes, and body hair may also be affected

Alopecia areata totalis is total scalp hair loss; **alopecia universalis** is total scalp and body hair loss.

Hair usually regrows spontaneously within weeks–months, with 90% recovery if there is only one patch of alopecia, but worse prognosis if it is extensive. A short course of topical or systemic steroid can encourage regrowth.

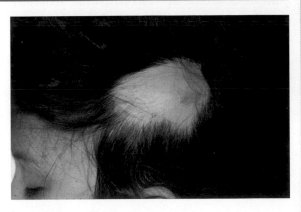

Figure 17.30 Alopecia areata

TRICHOTILLOMANIA

- Hair loss (usually patchy) due to the child pulling the hair
- Common in a mild form in young children in whom it may reflect anxiety
- Extensive disease (generally seen in adolescents) can be a sign of severe emotional disturbance, and associated with eating disorders and other psychopathology

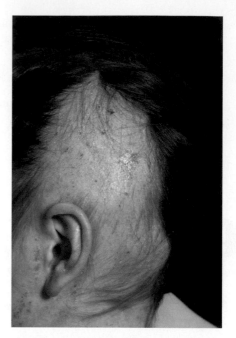

Figure 17.31 Trichotillomania

RARE INHERITED DISORDERS

ICHTHYOSES

This is a group of disorders with abnormal cornification resulting in *dry scaly skin*. There are several types including the following.

Ichthyosis vulgaris

- Common mild ichthyosis, incidence 1 in 300–500
- Dry rough skin, with hyperlinear palms
- Treated by regular moisturizing
- Associated with an increased incidence of atopic eczema

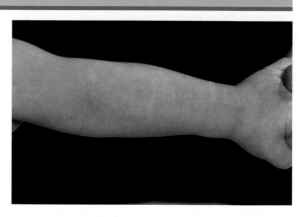

Figure 17.32 Ichthyosis vulgaris

Collodion baby

- Baby is born with a taut shiny membrane which slowly sheds to reveal the skin beneath
- Usually due to one of two rarer forms of ichthyosis (lamellar or ichthyosiform erythroderma), but in some cases the resulting ichthyosis is mild
- As the skin barrier is defective the baby is susceptible to infection, dehydration and hypothermia and needs to be managed on NICU with frequent application of emollients

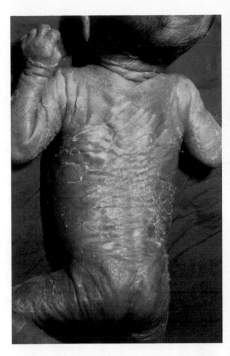

Figure 17.33 Collodian baby – taut shiny skin

Harlequin ichthyosis

- Severe type of ichthyosis where the baby is born with a hard membrane that cracks to produce a pattern like a harlequin. Similar to colloidion baby but more severe problems
- There is also **ectropion**, i.e. eyelids evert, and **eclabion**, i.e. lips evert, due to tightness of the skin
- Oral retinoids may be life-saving

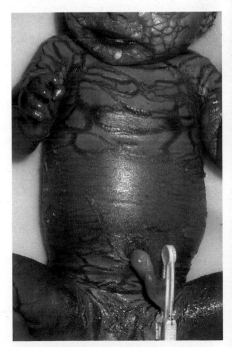

Figure 17.34 Harlequin ichthyosis

EPIDERMOLYSIS BULLOSA

Epidermolysis bullosa is a group of inherited skin disorders all characterized by **skin fragility**, resulting in **blister** formation. There are three main subgroups:

- **Epidermolysis bullosa simplex:**
  - Most common form. Autosomal dominant
  - Non-scarring intraepidermal blisters
  - Limits walking
- **Junctional epidermolysis bullosa:**
  - More severe form involving blisters in the lamina lucida of the epidermis
  - Internal blistering affects the larynx and gastrointestinal tract
- **Dystrophic epidermolysis bullosa:**
  - Autosomal dominant or recessive
  - Variably severe form involving blisters below the lamina densa of the epidermis
  - Blisters leave atrophic scars and milia
  - Oesophageal strictures affect nutrition
  - Fingers become enveloped 'mitten hands' due to scarring

Clinical scenario

A 6-year-old girl is seen by her family practitioner because of an itchy rash in the flexural creases of her joints.

1. The treatment which is most appropriate is prescribed. What would this be?

The rash continues to cause problems and it becomes thickened and painful.

2. What would the next step in treatment be?

It transpires that her family have a high incidence of atopy.

3. What are the three most important allergens to exclude from the diet? What might be two of the most important inhaled allergens to avoid?

Three days later she develops a vesicular rash which is painful and on discussion with her family it is apparent that she has had contact 14 days previously with a child with chicken pox.

4. What is your approach now?

ANSWERS

1. Topical steroids and an emollient
2. Stronger steroid creams or topical pibecrolimus
3. Diet: cow's milk protein; wheat; and either nuts or soya. Inhaled: grass pollen; animal dander (e.g. cat; dog)
4. Acyclovir for 14 days

FURTHER READING

Harper J, Oranje A, Prose N (eds.). *Textbook of Pediatric Dermatology*, 2nd edn. Oxford: Wiley-Blackwell, 2005.

Lewis–Jones S (ed.). *Paediatric Dermatology*. Oxford: Oxford University Press, 2010.

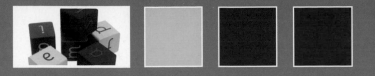

18 Haematology

- Haematopoietic physiology in the child
- Anaemia
- Haemoglobinopathies
- Polycythaemia and thrombocythaemia
- Haemostasis
- The spleen
- Further reading

HAEMATOPOIETIC PHYSIOLOGY IN THE CHILD

There are several important differences in the physiology of the haematopoietic system between the fetus, infant, child and adult:

- **Type** of haemoglobin
- Oxyhaemoglobin dissociation curve
- Location of haemoglobin **production** (haemopoiesis)
- **Normal level** of haemoglobin

Normal ranges of haemoglobin in childhood	
Age	Hb (g/dL)
Birth	14.9–23.7
2 weeks	13.4–19.8
2 months	9.4–13.0
6 months	11.1–14.1
1 year	11.3–14.1
2–6 years	11.5–13.5
6–18 years	11.5–16.0

Haemoglobin is the compound contained within red blood corpuscles which transports oxygen in the circulation. There are different types of haemoglobin, which have different affinities for oxygen and therefore are useful at different stages of development. Haemoglobin is composed of four polypeptide chains, each with a haem group attached, and it is a variation in the polypeptide chains that differentiates the types of haemoglobin. The switch from fetal haemoglobin to adult haemoglobin production occurs by 3–6 months of age.

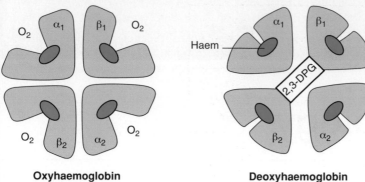

Oxyhaemoglobin

Deoxyhaemoglobin

Figure 18.1 Oxyhaemoglobin and deoxyhaemoglobin

Different types of haemoglobin produced from fetal to adult life

	Haemoglobin	Polypeptide chain
Fetal blood	HbF	$\alpha2\gamma2$
	HbA2	$\alpha2\delta2$
Adult blood	HbA	$\alpha2\beta2$ (96–98%)
	HbA2	$\alpha2\delta2$ (1.5–3%)
	HbF	$\alpha2\gamma2$ (0.5–0.8%)

Sites of haemopoiesis

Fetus	0–2 months	Yolk sac
	2–7 months	Liver and spleen
	5–9 months	Bone marrow (all bones)
Infant		Bone marrow (all bones)
Adult		Bone marrow (vertebrae, ribs, pelvis, skull, sternum and proximal end of femur)

RED BLOOD CELL TYPES

Several different types of red blood corpuscle are seen in various disorders (see Fig. 18.2).

ANAEMIA

Anaemia is an inadequate level of haemoglobin. There are several different types (see below):

- ■ Microcytic hypochromic anaemia — Iron deficiency, sideroblastic anaemia, thalassaemia, anaemia of chronic disease

- ■ Macrocytic anaemia
  - Megaloblastic anaemia — Vitamin B12 deficiency, folate deficiency, defects of DNA synthesis,
  - Macrocytic anaemia — Newborn, pregnancy, liver disease, reticulocytosis, hypothyroidism

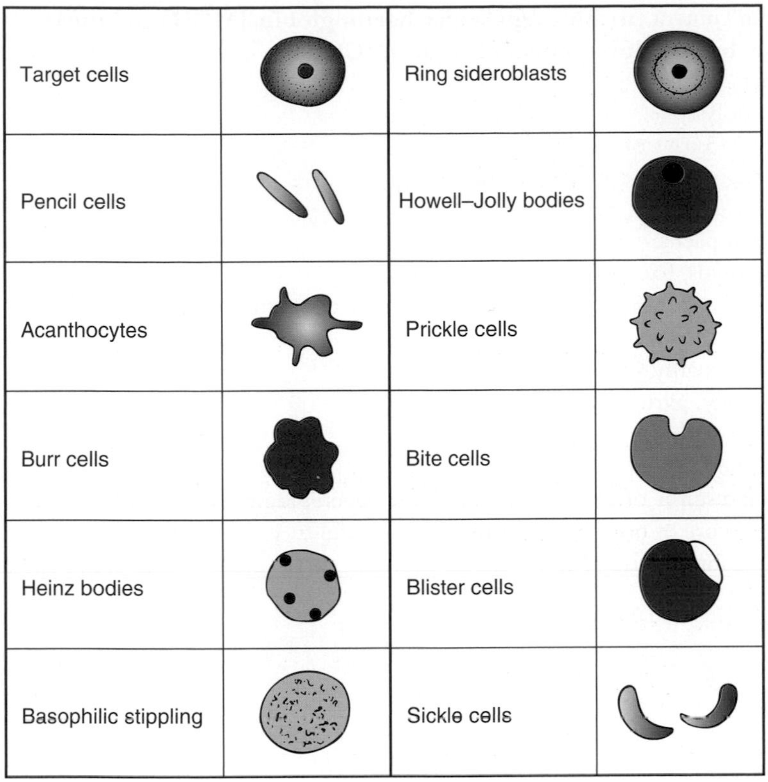

Target cells		Ring sideroblasts	
Pencil cells		Howell–Jolly bodies	
Acanthocytes		Prickle cells	
Burr cells		Bite cells	
Heinz bodies		Blister cells	
Basophilic stippling		Sickle cells	

Figure 18.2 Types of red blood cell

- Haemolytic anaemia
  - Hereditary   Spherocytosis, PK deficiency, G6PD deficiency, thalassaemia, sickle cell
  - Acquired   Autoimmune, haemolytic disease of the newborn, drug induced
- Aplastic anaemia
  - Primary   Fanconi anaemia, idiopathic
  - Secondary   Drugs, irradiation, infection (e.g. parvovirus), pregnancy

Clinical features

Symptoms	Tiredness, fainting
	Breathlessness
	Headaches
	Palpitations
General signs	Pallor
	Failure to thrive
	Tachycardia, cardiac failure, flow murmur (retinal haemorrhages if severe)
	Tachypnoea
	Hydrops fetalis (*in utero*)
Specific signs	E.g. koilonychia (iron), jaundice (haemolytic). See individual causes (below)

Investigations

Full blood count	To assess level of anaemia
Red cell indices	Size (**mean corpuscular volume [MCV]**) – can be normocytic, microcytic or macrocytic

	Haemoglobin content (**mean corpuscular haemoglobin [MCH]** and **mean corpuscular haemoglobin concentration [MCHC]**) – can be normocytic or hypochromic
Reticulocyte count	High in haemolysis
	Rises within 2–3 days of a bleed
	Low count suggests bone marrow failure
	Normal = 1.5–2%
Platelet and WCC	Low in pancytopaenia
	Rise in haemolysis, haemorrhage or infection
Blood film	Enables the red cell morphology to be studied under the microscope
Haematinics	Iron studies, B12, folate
Hb electrophoresis	If haemoglobinopathy suspected
Red cell enzymes	G6PD deficiency, pyruvate kinase deficiency
Coombs test or DAT	Haemolytic anaemia
Membrane studies	Hereditary spherocytosis
Bone marrow	**Aspiration** is a smear of bone marrow to view developing cells
	Trephine is a core of bone and marrow taken, useful to view marrow architecture, cellularity and abnormal infiltrates

MICROCYTIC HYPOCHROMIC ANAEMIA

Causes

- Iron-deficiency anaemia – commonest cause of anaemia in childhood and a very common finding in toddlers (see ch. 11)
- Thalassaemia
- Sideroblastic anaemia – due to impaired incorporation of iron into Hb
- Anaemia of chronic disease

Laboratory tests

	Iron deficiency	Chronic disease	Sideroblastic	Thalassaemia
MCV, MCH, MCHC	↓	↓ or N	↓ (congenital) ↑ (acquired)	↓↓
Serum iron	↓	↓	↑	N
Serum ferritin	↓	N or ↑	↑	N or ↑
TIBC	↑	↓	N	N
Marrow iron stores	Absent	Present	↑ in nucleated RBCs (ring sideroblasts)	Present/↑

MEGALOBLASTIC ANAEMIA

Causes

Megaloblastic anaemia	Vitamin B12 deficiency (most common)
	Folate deficiency (rare)
	Defects of DNA synthesis
Macrocytic anaemia	Newborn (fetal Hb)
	Reticulocytosis
	Hypothyroidism
	Liver disease
	Pregnancy

In children this is most commonly due to folate deficiency and very rarely due to B12 deficiency. There are erythroblasts with delayed maturation of the nucleus in the bone marrow due to defective DNA synthesis.

Causes of folate deficiency	
Inadequate intake	Coeliac disease, Crohn disease, special diets
Increased utilization	Prematurity, haemolysis, malignancy, inflammatory disease
Increased urine loss	Acute liver disease
Antifolate drugs	Trimethoprim, phenytoin, methotrexate

Causes of B12 deficiency	
Inadequate intake	Vegan diet
Impaired absorption	Ileal resection, bacterial overgrowth, Crohn disease (impaired ileal mucosa), ileal TB, congenital intrinsic factor impairment (pernicious anaemia)
Abnormal metabolism	Nitrous oxide, transcobalamin II deficiency

Specific clinical features

Mouth	Sore red glossitis, angular stomatitis
Skin	Pale yellow (mild jaundice), purpura, melanin pigmentation
Nervous system	Polyneuropathy and subacute combined degeneration of the cord (in B12 deficiency only)

Investigations

Blood film	Macrocytosis, hypersegmented polymorphs, WCC and platelets may be low
B12	Low in B_{12} deficiency
Serum and red cell folate	Low in folate deficiency
Bone marrow	Hypercellular marrow with megaloblastic changes
Chemistry	Unconjugated bilirubin ↑, LDH ↑
Iron and ferritin	Normal or ↑

Management

- Investigate underlying cause (dietary history, malabsorption tests, coeliac screen)
- Give supplements:
  - Folate given as oral daily supplements
  - B12 given as regular intramuscular injections

HAEMOLYTIC ANAEMIAS

Haemolytic anaemias result from an increased rate of red cell destruction. The clinical features are due to the anaemia, increased requirements and increase in red cell breakdown products (causing jaundice). Intravascular haemolysis (destruction of red cells within the circulation) occurs in some conditions and causes specific features.

Causes

Hereditary	Spherocytosis
	G6PD deficiency, PK deficiency★
Immune	Autoimmune★:
	■ Warm IgG Ab, e.g. SLE, dermatomyositis
	■ Cold IgM Ab, e.g. CMV, mycoplasma
	Alloimmune, e.g. haemolytic disease of the newborn
	Drugs, e.g. quinine
Red cell fragmentation syndromes★	Extracorporeal membrane oxygenation (ECMO)
	Prostheses, e.g. cardiac valves
	Microangiopathic:
	■ Haemolytic–uraemic syndrome
	■ Meningococcal septicaemia
	■ DIC
Systemic disease	Renal disease, liver disease
Infections	E.g. malaria★
Toxins	Burns, drugs, e.g. dapsone

★Intravascular haemolysis may occur.

Clinical features

- Features of anaemia (pallor, breathlessness, etc.)
- Fluctuating mild jaundice (unconjugated hyperbilirubinaemia)
- Folate deficiency (due to rapid turnover of RBCs)
- Splenomegaly
- Pigment gallstones
- Aplastic crises precipitated by parvovirus infection

Investigations

Increased RBC production	Reticulocytosis
	Erythroid hyperplasia of the bone marrow
Increased RBC breakdown	Unconjugated hyperbilirubinaemia
	Urine urobilinogen ↑, faecal stercobilinogen ↑
Damaged RBCs	Fragments, microspherocytes, eliptocytes
	Osmotic fragility ↑ and autohaemolysis
Autoimmune tests	Coombs test positive in immune haemolytic anaemia
Red cell enzymes	G6PD, PK
Membrane studies	Hereditary spherocytosis

Hereditary spherocytosis

An autosomal dominant condition. Incidence 1 in 3000 Caucasians. RBCs are spherical (not biconcave discs) due to a defect in a membrane protein (*spectrin*, *ankyrin* or *band 3*). This shape means they are unable to pass through the splenic microcirculation, and so die prematurely.

Clinical features

- Very variable even within families
- Neonatal jaundice
- Symptoms of mild haemolytic anaemia, especially splenomegaly, pigment gallstones and aplastic or anaemic crises with parvovirus infection
- May be asymptomatic

Investigations

Blood count	Anaemia (may be mild)
Film	Reticulocyte count 5–20%
	Microspherocytes
Membrane studies	Defect in membrane protein
Other	Autohaemolysis, bilirubin ↑

Management

- No treatment if mild
- Folic acid supplements for haemolysis
- Splenectomy after childhood if severe anaemia requiring regular transfusions or causing impaired growth

Glucose-6-phosphate dehydrogenase deficiency

X-linked recessive condition; females mildly affected. The gene is selected for because the carrier state protects against falciparum malaria.

Glucose-6-phosphate dehydrogenase (G6PD) is an enzyme in the hexose–monophosphate pathway of red cell metabolism, and is the only source of NADPH for the red cell, which prevents oxidant damage to the cell. Defective enzyme activity results in a susceptibility of the red cell to *acute haemolysis with oxidant stress*.

Millions are affected worldwide:

- Type A (African type) – milder. Young RBC have normal enzyme activity
- Type B (Mediterranean type) – severe. All RBCs affected

Clinical features

- Neonatal jaundice
- Haemolytic crises (rapidly developing intravascular haemolysis) induced by oxidant stress. Crises caused by:
  - Sepsis
  - Drugs, e.g. antimalarials, sulphonamides, chloramphenicol, aspirin
  - Fava (broad) beans (type B only)

Investigations

Diagnosis	G6PD levels in the red cell. (NB: these may be normal during a crisis)
During a crisis	Intravascular haemolysis, bite cells, blister cells, reticulocytes, Heinz bodies

Management of a crisis

Treat the cause (sepsis, stop suspected drug) and give IV fluids and transfuse as necessary.

Pyruvate kinase deficiency

Autosomal recessive condition. Less common than G6PD deficiency.

Pyruvate kinase is an enzyme in the Embden–Meyerhof pathway of red cell metabolism and its deficiency results in a reduction in ATP formation and rigid RBCs.

Clinical features

- Anaemia 4–10 g/dL (with relatively mild symptoms due to compensatory increase in 2,3-DPG levels)
- Splenomegaly, jaundice, gallstones

Investigations

Diagnosis	Direct assay of pyruvate kinase levels
Blood film	Prickle cells, poikilocytes, reticulocytes

Management

Repeated transfusions, and splenectomy if necessary.

APLASTIC ANAEMIA

Aplastic anaemia is an anaemia due to bone marrow aplasia and therefore all three cell lines are affected causing a **pancytopaenia** (anaemia, leucopaenia and thrombocytopaenia).

Causes

Primary	Fanconi anaemia
	Idiopathic (*most* cases)
Secondary	Drugs:

- Regular effect, e.g. cytotoxics
- Sporadic effect, e.g. chloramphenicol, penicillamine

Infections, e.g. viral hepatitis, measles, parvovirus, TB, EBV
Radiation, chemicals, e.g. solvents

Clinical features

These are of bone marrow suppression:

- Red cells – anaemia
- White cells – infection susceptibility
- Platelets – clotting deficiency (bruising, bleeding)

Investigations

Blood film	Anaemia (normochromic normocytic or macrocytic, low reticulocytes)
	Leucopaenia (particularly neutrophils)
	Thrombocytopaenia
Bone marrow	Trephine biopsy shows marrow hypoplasia with replacement by fat cells

Management

- Remove any cause
- Initial supportive therapy (blood and platelet transfusions, antibiotic therapy for infections)
- Specific therapy options:
  - Bone marrow transplant. This can offer a cure
  - Drugs, e.g. haemopoietic growth factors, methylprednisolone, immunosuppressants, e.g. antilymphocyte globulin and cyclosporin

Fanconi anaemia

This is an autosomal recessive condition that presents at 5–10 years of age.

Clinical features

There is increased chromosomal breakage with AML often developing. Stem cell transplant is the only chance of cure; most will die < 30 years from AML if not given a transplant.

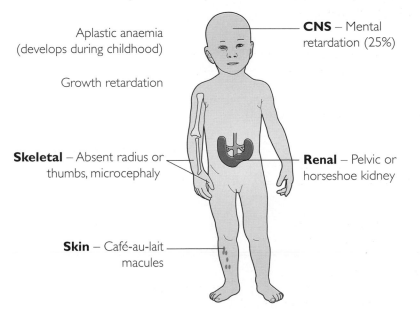

Aplastic anaemia
(develops during childhood)

Growth retardation

CNS – Mental retardation (25%)

Skeletal – Absent radius or thumbs, microcephaly

Renal – Pelvic or horseshoe kidney

Skin – Café-au-lait macules

Figure 18.3 Clinical features of Fanconi anaemia

Red cell aplasia

This is an isolated red cell aplasia due to absent or reduced erythroblasts in the bone marrow, causing anaemia only. It can be an acute transient disease lasting 2–3 months or a chronic problem.

Causes

Chronic disease   Congenital – Diamond–Blackfan syndrome
Acquired:

- Idiopathic
- Thymoma, SLE, leukaemia

Acute disease   Infections:

- Parvovirus infection in patients with shortened red cell survival, e.g. spherocytosis, sickle cell anaemia
- In infants following viral infection (transient erythroblastopaenia of infancy [TEC])

Drugs, e.g. co-trimoxazole, azathioprine

HAEMOGLOBINOPATHIES

SICKLE CELL HAEMOGLOBINOPATHIES

Sickle cell haemoglobin (HbS) is Hbα2βs2. Valine is substituted for glutamic acid on codon 6 in the β chain.

HbS is insoluble in low oxygen tensions and polymerizes as long fibres which result in the red cells becoming sickle shaped. They block areas of the microcirculation and result in microinfarcts. HbS releases oxygen in the tissues more readily than HbA, i.e. the oxyhaemoglobin dissociation curve is shifted to the right.

Sickle cell anaemia   HbSS (homozygous disease; 85–95% HbS, 5–15% HbF, no HbA)
Sickle cell trait   HbSA (heterozygous disease; 40% HbS, 60% HbA)

Sickle cell anaemia

This is HbSS disease, and is seen in Africans, Mediterraneans and Indians. Clinical features vary depending on any coexisting haemoglobinopathies, e.g. HbSβthalassaemia is mild. Clinical features are due to:

- *Anaemia* – Hb 6–9g/dL, reticulocytes 5–15%
- Intermittent *crises*

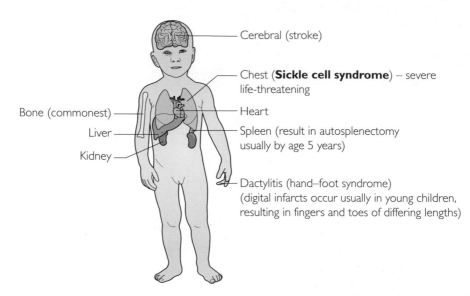

Cerebral (stroke)

Chest (**Sickle cell syndrome**) – severe life-threatening

Heart

Bone (commonest)

Liver

Kidney

Spleen (result in autosplenectomy usually by age 5 years)

Dactylitis (hand–foot syndrome) (digital infarcts occur usually in young children, resulting in fingers and toes of differing lengths)

Figure 18.4 Sites of painful (vaso-occlusive) crises in sickle cell anaemia

Sickle crises

- **Painful (vaso–occlusive) crises**. These are vascular-occlusive episodes precipitated by cold, hypoxia, infection or dehydration. They occur in (see Fig. 18.4):
- **Haemolytic crises**. This is haemolysis and it usually accompanies a painful crisis
- **Acute sequestration**. This is sickling within organs, resulting in blood pooling. It occurs in the spleen, chest and liver
- **Aplastic crises**. These occur in association with parvovirus infection. A sudden fall in the Hb and reticulocyte count is seen

Infection

These children are at high risk of infection with encapsulated bacteria such as *Streptococcus pneumoniae*, *Haemophilus influenzae B*, meningococcus and salmonella species. They are at risk of overwhelming infection, particularly if < 3 years of age, with meningitis, septicaemia and pneumonia.

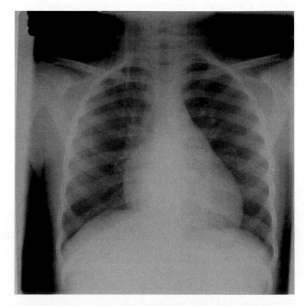

Figure 18.5 Chest X-ray of an 11-year-old girl admitted with sickle chest syndrome. Note the hyperinflated lung fields with lowered diaphragm, and the cardiomegaly secondary to chronic anaemia.

Long-term problems

- Failure to thrive (due to chronic disease)
- Pigment gallstones (due to haemolysis)
- Salmonella osteomyelitis
- Aseptic necrosis of the hip
- Priapism (pooling of blood within the corpora cavernosa)
- Renal failure
- Congestive heart failure
- Proliferative retinopathy
- Splenomegaly in infancy, with autosplenectomy (due to splenic crises) later
- Leg ulcers

Investigations

Blood film	Hb 6–8 g/dL usually
	Sickle cells, target cells and Howell–Jolly bodies present
Sickledex test	Specific test to identify sickle cells (HbS blood will sickle)
Hb electrophoresis	To detect the relative quantities of HbS, HbF and HbA

Management

General	Folic acid 5 mg daily
	Oral penicillin daily (because of autosplenectomy)
	Triple vaccination (pneumococcal, Hib and meningovax) essential (splenic protection)
	Regular influenza vaccination
	Avoid precipitants of crises
Crises	Admit to hospital
	Check FBC, film, reticulocytes, group and save, U&E, LFTs, CRP
	CXR if respiratory symptoms/signs, ECG if chest pain
	MSU and blood cultures if infection suspected
	Strong analgesia (usually IV opiates)
	Fluids (IV, 50% above usual formula)
	Oxygen (by CPAP if necessary, e.g. sickle chest syndrome)
	Bed rest and keep warm
	Monitor closely (saturations, pulse, blood pressure, respiratory rate, pain and nausea)
	Intravenous antibiotics if infection present or suspected
	Transfusion if necessary (multiple may be needed)
	Exchange transfusion if indicated (this decreases the proportion of sickle cells) (in severe painful crises, neurological damage, sequestration, sickle chest syndrome, priapism)
Surgery	Transfusions are performed preoperatively for major surgery to reduce the HbS fraction to < 30%
	Anaesthetic care is taken to keep the patient warm, well oxygenated and hydrated, pain free and acidosis avoided
New therapies	Bone marrow transplant (if an unaffected HLA-identical sibling and severe disease)
	Hydroxyurea (increases HbF and decreases the frequency of crises)

Sickle trait

Sickle trait is the heterozygote expression of the sickle Hb gene, i.e. HbSA. The HbS makes up 30–40% of the haemoglobin. This blood type appears to partially protect against falciparum malaria and is thus genetically selected for.

These children are usually asymptomatic with no anaemia. In severe hypoxia, however, sickling can occur with resulting ischaemic consequences. Haematuria is the commonest symptom. Care is needed with general anaesthetics and pregnancy. Diagnosis is made by the Sickledex test and Hb electrophoresis.

THALASSAEMIAS

Thalassaemia is derived from the Greek '*thalassa*' meaning 'sea', as the disease was first found in people on the shores of the Mediterranean. It is found in tropical and subtropical areas (Asia, North Africa and the Mediterranean).

This is a heterogeneous group of disorders in which there is a partial or complete deletion of globin chain genes, resulting in a *reduced rate of synthesis* of normal α- or β-chains, and *precipitation* of the other excess chains in the red cells, which causes *haemolysis*. Other haemoglobin types, e.g. HbA2, are also made with increased frequency.

β-thalassaemia   Due to reduced or absent **β-globin** chains (excess α-chains precipitate)
α-thalassaemia   Due to reduced or absent **α-globin** chains (excess β-chains precipitate)

Chromosome 16 codes for α-globin, Chromosome 11 codes for β-, δ- and γ-globins. In α-thalassaemias the entire α-globin genes are deleted, whereas in β-thalassaemia mainly point mutations within the β-globin genes occur.

Diagnosis

Thalassaemia may be suspected clinically and is diagnosed from the blood film, with specific identification of the type of thalassaemia from Hb electrophoresis and DNA analysis.

Haemoglobin types seen in thalassaemias

HbA	α2β2
HbA2	α2δ2
HbF	α2γ2
HbH	β4
HbBarts	γ4 (no oxygen carrying capacity)

Clinical types of thalassaemias

- α-thalassaemias
- β-thalassaemia major
- Thalassaemia intermedia
- Thalassaemia minor

β-Thalassaemia major

This is clinically the most significant form of thalassaemia. It is due to homozygous disease, and affected children have either no (βo) or very small amounts (β+) of β-chains.

Clinical features

The clinical features seen are a result of:

1. **Haemolytic anaemia**
2. Attempt by the body to make more haemoglobin (*medullary and extramedullary haemopoiesis*)
3. Effects of multiple transfusions (*iron overload, infections*)

- **Severe anaemia** from age 3–6 months (this begins when the switch from γ- to β-chain synthesis normally occurs)
- **Extramedullary and medullary haemopoiesis:**
  - Thalassaemic facies (frontal bossing, maxillary hyperplasia)
  - 'Hair on end' skull X-ray appearance
  - Cortical bone thinning with fractures
- **Hepatosplenomegaly** (due to haemolysis and haemopoiesis)
- **Iron overload** (due to multiple transfusions)
- **Infections:**
  - Hepatitis B and C (transfusions)
  - *Yersinia enterocolitica*
  - Encapsulated organisms (autosplenectomy)
- **Faltering growth**

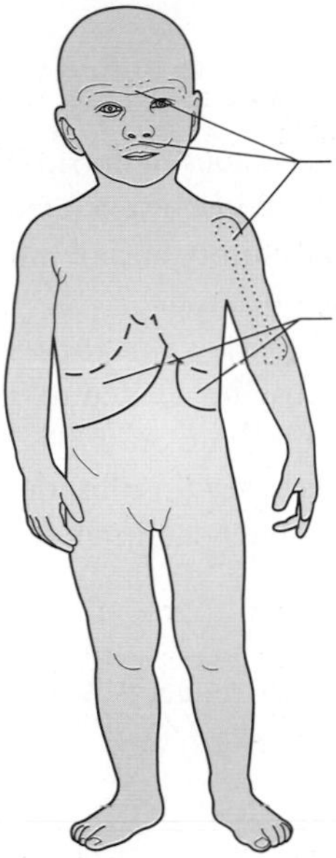

Severe anaemia

Extramedullary haemopoiesis

Hepatosplenomegaly

Iron overload

Infections

Faltering growth

Figure 18.6 Clinical features of β-thalassaemia major

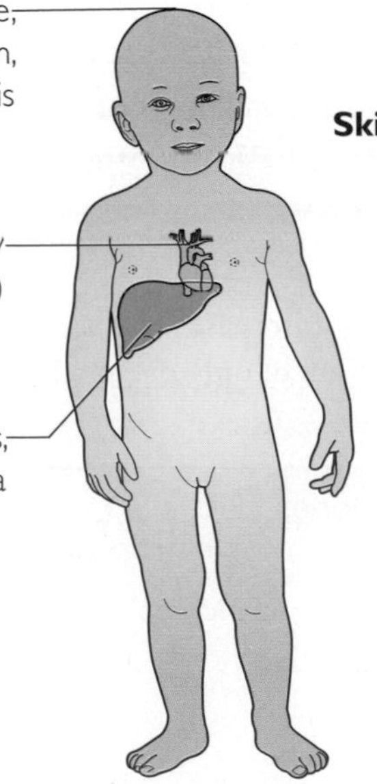

Endocrine – IDDM, growth failure, delayed puberty, hypothyroidism, hypoparathyroidism, osteoporosis

Skin – slate-grey appearance

Heart – Cardiomyopathy (arrhythmias, cardiac failure)

Liver – Fibrosis, cirrhosis, hepatoma

Figure 18.7 The effects of iron overload

Investigations

Hb electrophoresis	HbF 70–90% (↑ α-chains)
	HbA2 2% (↑ α-chains)
	± HbA 0–20%
Blood film	Microcytic hypochromic anaemia
	Target cells, basophilic stippling and nucleated red cells
DNA analysis	May be done to identify the mutation

Management

Transfusions	4–6 weekly (transfuse when the Hb < 10 g/dL)
Folic acid	5 mg daily
Iron chelation	Subcutaneous desferrioxamine for 8–12 h overnight, 5 days/week
	Chelated iron is excreted in the urine and stools
	NB: Auditory and ophthalmological assessments needed while on desferrioxamine
Vitamin C	200 mg/day. This increases iron excretion
Splenectomy	This may be needed to decrease blood transfusion requirements (Usually done only if > 6 years old) (see p. 330)
Endocrine therapy	As necessary (insulin, thyroid, parathyroid and pituitary hormones)
Bone marrow transplant	Recommended in childhood if an HLA-identical sibling is present

β-Thalassaemia minor (trait)

This is a heterozygous disease with reduced β-chains. It is asymptomatic, and picked up as an incidental finding.

Investigations

Blood film	Mild anaemia or normal Hb (Hb 10–15 g/dL)
	Microcytic hypochromic picture, target cells
Hb electrophoresis	HbA
	HbA2 > 3.5%
	HbF 1–3%

> **! NB: It is important to check the iron status to *exclude* iron deficiency as a cause of the blood film findings.**

α-Thalassaemias

These all involve decreased synthesis of α-chains. There are four genes for α-globin because the gene is duplicated on chromosome 16. Deletion of only one α-globin gene results in a silent carrier with only a mild microcytosis (α-thalassaemia trait).

Disease	α-Globin genes deleted	Hb electrophoresis	Blood film	Clinical features
α-Thalassaemia trait	1 or 2 α–/αα α–/α– αα/– –	Normal ± HbH	Hypochromic microcytic red cells Normal or mild anaemia	Asymptomatic iron deficiency
HbH disease	3 – –/α–	HbH, HbA, HbBarts	Hypochromic microcytic anaemia 'golf ball' cells (= aggregates of β-chains)	Thalassaemia intermedia syndrome
Hydrops fetalis (HbBarts)	4 – –/– –	HbBarts only		Hydrops fetalis with death *in utero* unless intrauterine transfusions

POLYCYTHAEMIA AND THROMBOCYTHAEMIA

POLYCYTHAEMIA

Polycythaemia is *Hb levels* increased above the upper limit of normal and increased *haematocrit*. It may be 'relative' due to decreased circulating volume.

Causes

Secondary
Appropriate:
- Congenital cyanotic heart disease
- Lung disease
- Central hypoventilation

Inappropriate:
- Renal disease, e.g. hydronephrosis, tumour
- Adrenal disease, e.g. CAH, Cushing syndrome
- Tumour, e.g. cerebellar haemangioblastoma
- Neonatal, e.g. IUGR, infant of diabetic mother, twin–twin transfusion

Relative
Dehydration, e.g. gastrointestinal losses, burns
Stress polycythaemia

Primary
Polycythaemia rubra vera (rare in children)

Clinical features

- Haemorrhage or thrombosis
- Headaches

Management

- Treat the cause
- Venesection if necessary (levels high)

THROMBOCYTHAEMIA

Thrombocythaemia is *platelet levels* increased to above the upper limit of normal.

Causes

Reactive
Haemorrhage
Postoperative
Kawasaki disease
Acute infections, e.g. URTI
Chronic infections, e.g. TB
Post-splenectomy
Iron-deficiency and haemolytic anaemia
Connective tissue disease
Chronic renal disease
Drugs, e.g. steroids
Malignancies

Endogenous
CML (very rare in childhood)

This is usually asymptomatic. The risk of thrombosis is low.

Treat the underlying cause. Often no treatment is necessary, but aspirin is occasionally required.

HAEMOSTASIS

Haemostasis involves:

- Normal *vasculature*
- *Platelets*
- *Coagulation factors*

Clinical features of a bleeding disorder

History	**Most likely cause (overlap considerable)**
Easy bruising (ecchymoses)	Coagulation defects, platelets or vascular

Petechiae (skin and mucous membranes)
Mucosal bleeding:
   Bleeding from gums
   Epistaxis
   Haematuria
   Menorrhagia
   Internal bleeding (gut, intracranial, intramuscular)
	Platelets

Bleeding into joints (haemarthroses) with minor injuries Bleeding into muscles Excessive bleeding after trauma, e.g. surgery, dental extractions	Coagulation defects

Examination

Skin	Ecchymoses and petechiae
Mucous membranes	Palatal petechiae, gum bleeding
Asymmetrical joint deformities (due to haemarthroses)	

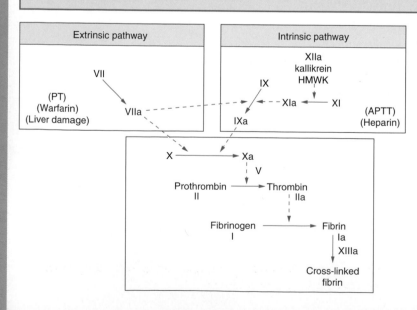

Figure 18.8 Coagulation cascade. HMWK, high molecular weight kininogen

Investigation of clotting disorders

Test	Mechanism	Abnormal in DIC
Blood count and film	Platelet morphology and count	
Bleeding time	Abnormalities of other blood cells measures platelet plug formation *in vitro*	Prolonged in thrombocytopaenia, platelet function disorders and von Willebrand disease
Prothrombin time (PT)	Measures factors VII, X, V, prothrombin and fibrinogen (extrinsic and common pathways) Normal = 10–14 s (INR = 1) May be expressed as the international normalized ratio (INR)	Prolonged in liver disease, vitamin K dependent clotting factors Used to monitor warfarin therapy
Activated partial thromboplastin time (APTT)	Measures factors V, VIII, IX, X, XI, XII, prothrombin and fibrinogen (intrinsic and common pathways) Normal = 30–40 s	Used to monitor heparin therapy
Thrombin clotting time (TT)	Normal = 14–16 s	Abnormal in fibrinogen deficiency or thrombin inhibition
Coagulation factors	Specific assays of individual clotting factors	Clotting factor deficiencies, e.g. haemophilia
Fibrinolysis tests	Detection of fibrinogen or fibrin degradation products (FDPs) Plasminogen and plasminogen activator (↑)	Abnormal in DIC (↓ in enhanced fibrinolysis)

DISORDERS OF THE VASCULATURE

The clinical features of these disorders are generally mild, with skin and mucous membrane bleeding (bruising, petechiae). All screening tests are normal including the bleeding time.

Causes

Inherited	Ehlers–Danlos syndrome
	Hereditary haemorrhagic telangiectasiae
Acquired	Easy bruising syndrome
	Henoch–Schönlein purpura (HSP) (see p. 236)
	Infections, e.g. meningitis
	Vitamin C deficiency (scurvy)
	Drugs, e.g. steroids

PLATELET DISORDERS

Platelet disorders include:

- Thrombocytopaenia
- Platelet function disorders

Thrombocytopaenia

Causes

Decreased platelet production	Megakaryocyte depression – infections, drugs, thrombocytopaenia and absent radii (TAR) syndrome

Increased platelet consumption	Abnormal megakaryocytes – Wiskott–Aldrich syndrome
	Bone marrow failure – aplastic anaemias
	Immune disease:

- ITP (see below)
- Drug induced, e.g. trimethoprim
- Post-infectious, e.g. malaria
- Neonatal isoimmune ITP (maternal antiplatelet antibodies)
- Post-transfusional (PlA1 antibodies)
- Heparin

Disseminated intravascular coagulation (DIC)
Haemolytic–uraemic syndrome

| Abnormal platelet distribution | Splenomegaly |

Immune thrombocytopaenia

This is common in children, and the mechanism is thought to be mediated via immune complex platelet destruction.

Clinical features

- 1–4 weeks following viral infection, e.g. chicken pox, measles, EBV, or vaccination
- Bleeding, bruising, petechiae, mucosal bleeding if platelets $< 20 \times 10^9/\text{L}$
- Intracranial bleeds may rarely occur
- Most cases will spontaneously go into remission after 1–3 months. Chronic disease lasting 2–3 years occurs in 5–10% in childhood

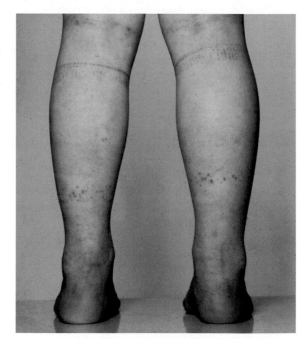

Figure 18.9 Purpura along the sock line in immune thrombocytopaenia

Investigations

Blood film	Platelets ↓ (< 10–$12 \times 10^9/\text{L}$)
	Hb and WCC normal
Bone marrow	Increased megakaryocytes (to make more platelets). May be normal
Antibodies	Antiplatelet IgG, antiplatelet IgM

Management options

- Monitoring only – platelet count and clinically (most children)
- Oral steroids for 2–3 weeks ⎫ If bleeding
- IV immunoglobulin ⎭
- Platelet transfusions (used only in emergencies as they are quickly destroyed by the antibodies)
- Immunosuppression and/or splenectomy if no response to above treatments and chronic disease
- Avoid aspirin and contact sports

Platelet function disorders

In platelet function disorders the platelet count is normal but the *bleeding time* is prolonged and specific platelet function tests are abnormal. They may be inherited or acquired.

Causes of acquired disease

- Drugs – aspirin (inhibition of cyclo-oxygenase), heparin (platelet segregation and secretion inhibited)
- Myeloproliferative disease
- Uraemia

CLOTTING FACTOR DISORDERS
Haemophilia A

This is an X-linked recessive disorder due to a mutation in the gene at Xq2.8 (one-third are spontaneous mutations). Incidence 30–100 in 100 000 males. Disease results from absent or reduced **factor VIII**.

Clinical features

- Spontaneous bleeding
- Excessive traumatic bleeding – surgery, e.g. post-circumcision, dental extractions
- Infection (transfusion related) – hepatitis B and C, HIV (now all screened for)

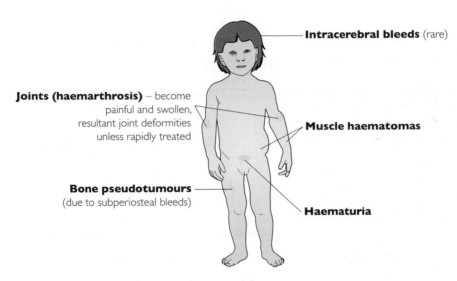

Figure 18.10 Clinical features of Haemophilia A

Boys with this disease have *varying levels* of factor VIII and the level determines the severity of their disease:

< 1% of normal	Severe disease with frequent spontaneous bleeds
1–5% of normal	Moderate disease, severe bleeds with injury, occasional spontaneous bleeds
> 5% of normal	Mild disease. Bleed a lot after surgery

Investigations

- Factor VIII activity (reduced or absent)
- APTT ↑

Management

- Prophylactic recombinant factor VIII infusions (aim to keep > 2% of normal, usually given 2–3 times/week)
- Recombinant factor VIII infusions after injury
- Prior to surgery give recombinant factor VIII infusion to elevate factor VIII level
- Desmopressin (DDAVP) infusion. Used in mild disease and causes a rise in the patient's own factor VIII levels
- Fibrinolytic inhibitor, e.g. tranexamic acid. Can be given with DDAVP
- Advice – these children should avoid contact sports and have good oral hygiene

Factor VIII infusions after injury

Injury	Factor VIII levels aimed for (% of normal)
Minor bleed	> 30%
Severe bleed	> 50%
Pre major surgery	100%

Factor VIII antibodies

These develop in 10% of haemophiliacs as a result of their frequent factor VIII transfusions, and are troublesome as they inhibit the factor VIII treatment. Options for management are:

- Give very large doses of factor VIII
- Immunosuppression therapy
- Give factor IX concentrate, which bypasses the factor VIII, or recombinant factor VIII, or porcine factor VIII

Antenatal and carrier detection

In at-risk couples, i.e. family history of haemophilia or father is a haemophiliac, the status of the mother can be detected antenatally, and the fetus can be checked for the disease:

Carrier female detection	Analyse plasma factor VIII activity (usually half normal in carrier females)
	DNA analysis (more accurate method)
Antenatal fetal screening	Chorionic villous sampling (at 8–10 weeks)
	Fetal blood sampling for factor VIII activity (18–20 weeks)

Haemophilia B (Christmas disease)

This is an X-linked recessive disorder due gene mutation at Xq2.6. Incidence 1 in 30 000 males. Disease results from a deficiency of **factor IX**. The *clinical features* are identical to haemophilia A. *Management* is with infusions of factor IX concentrate.

von Willebrand disease

This is an autosomal dominant disorder with variable expression but worse in females due to menstruation. Incidence 3–10 in 100 000. It is a disorder of low **von Willebrand factor (vWF)** (carrier protein for factor VIII and promotes platelet adhesion, thus deficiency causes low factor VIII activity) and **platelet adhesion** abnormalities.

Clinical features

These are variable.

- Excessive traumatic bleeding – from cuts and operative and mucous membranes (epistaxis, gums, menorrhagia)
- Spontaneous bleeding (rare except in homozygotes) – haemarthroses and muscle bleeds

Investigations

- Bleeding time prolonged (as platelet adhesion ↓)
- Factor VIII activity ↓
- vWF levels ↓
- Platelet aggregation with ristocetin ↓

Management

Acute bleeds are treated with infusions of factor VIII concentrate containing vWF (severe disease), or DDAVP and fibrinogen inhibitors (milder disease).

Disseminated intravascular coagulation

This is a state of consumption of platelets and clotting factors with widespread intravascular fibrin deposition due to uncontrolled activation of the clotting cascade. It may be acute or, more rarely, a chronic milder form.

Causes

- Sepsis, e.g. meningococcaemia, Gram-negative sepsis, viral (purpura fulminans)
- Widespread tissue damage – trauma, burns, surgery
- Hypersensitivity reactions – anaphylaxis
- Malignancy – acute promyelocytic leukaemia
- Other – hypoxia, hypothermia

Clinical features

The child is severely unwell with generalized bleeding, petechiae and bruising (in acute disease).

Investigations

- Blood count and film – platelets ↓, microangiopathic anaemia
- TT ↑
- APTT ↑
- PT ↑
- FDPs ↑, fibrinogen ↓
- Factors V and VIII ↓

Management

- Treat the underlying cause
- Supportive therapy on ICU (blood, fresh frozen plasma, fibrinogen, platelets)
- Protein C concentrates given in meningococcal sepsis DIC

Table 18.1 Haemostasis tests

	BT	Platelet	PT	APTT	TT	FVIIIc	FIX	vWFAg
Haemophilia A	N	N	N	↑	N	↓	N	N
Haemophilia B	N	N	N	↑	N	N	↓	N
vW disease	↑	N	N	↑ or N	N	↓	N	↓
Liver disease	N or ↑	↓	↑	↑	N or ↑	N	↓	N
DIC	N or ↑	↓	↑	↑	↑↑	↓	↓	↓

APTT, activated partial thromboplastin time; BT, bleeding time; PT, prothrombin time; TT, thrombin time

Congenital prothrombotic conditions

Factor V Leiden deficiency	These children have an abnormal factor V protein (1% in Caucasian population)
Protein C deficiency	Protein C inactivates factor V and VIII and stimulates fibrinolysis
Protein S deficiency	Cofactor for protein C
Antithrombin III deficiency	Involved in inhibition of thrombin and factor X

THE SPLEEN

SPLENECTOMY

Splenectomy may occur naturally (autosplenectomy, e.g. in sickle cell disease) or as a result of therapeutic surgical removal of the spleen, e.g. ITP, or secondary to trauma.

Blood count and film findings

- High platelets
- Monocytosis, lymphocytosis
- Howell–Jolly bodies, target cells, irregular contracted red cells

Consequences

Immediate	Marked thrombocytosis (platelets > 1000×10^9/L) for 2–3 weeks, then only moderately elevated
Long term	Susceptibility to encapsulated organisms, e.g. pneumococcus, and malaria infection
	Young infants in particular at risk of infection with *Streptococcus pneumoniae*, *Haemophilus influenzae* and *Neisseria meningitidis*
	Splenectomy is avoided if possible in children < 6 years old due to the increased infection risk

> ❗ **Children with no spleen need:**
> - **Prophylactic penicillin for life**
> - **Triple vaccination (pneumococcal, *Haemophilus influenzae* and meningococcal C) > 2 weeks prior to splenectomy if not already done**
> - **Malaria prophylaxis when travelling to endemic areas**

SPLENOMEGALY

This can result in abdominal discomfort and a pancytopaenia because the spleen sequesters and destroys red cells.

Causes

- Infections – bacterial endocarditis, septicaemia, TB, brucellosis, schistosomiasis
- Extramedullary haemopoiesis – haemolytic anaemias, haemoglobinopathies
- Neoplasms – leukaemia, lymphoma, haemangioma
- Portal hypertension
- Storage diseases – mucopolysaccharidoses, Neimann–Pick disease, Langerhans' cell histiocytosis
- Systemic disease – SLE, JCA, amyloidosis
- Massive splenomegaly – malaria, CML

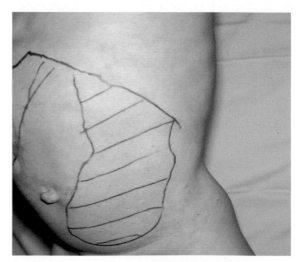

Figure 18.11 Massive splenomegaly (as well as hepatomegaly) in a child

Clinical scenario

An 8-year-old girl is admitted to her local District General Hospital with apparent anaemia, mouth ulcers, and apparently extreme pain emanating from her knee.

1. What diagnoses go through your mind?

It transpires that she is from mid-Africa and therefore determined by the local medical representatives to be potentially HIV-positive.

Her pain is extreme and decisions need to be made regarding urgent treatment.

2. What is your initial management?
3. What would you do after her pain treatment and initial management were completed?

ANSWERS

1. Acute leukaemia; connective tissue diseases such as juvenile chronic arthritis; infection such as salmonella, TB, etc.; inflammatory bowel disease
2. Oxygen; adequate pain relief – including parenteral morphine if needed; broad-spectrum intravenous antibiotics; intravenous hydration; blood transfusion if necessary
3. Ensure good haematology follow-up; sort out her immigration status and involve relevant care authorities as necessary; orthopaedic opinion re aspiration of any knee effusion

FURTHER READING

Bailey S, Skinner R (eds.). *Paediatric Haematology and Oncology*. Oxford: Oxford University Press, 2009.

Hann I, Smith O (eds.). *Essential Paediatric Haematology*. London: Informa Healthcare, 2002.

Hann I, Gibson B. *Paediatric Haematology*. Oxford: Bailliere Tindall, 1991.

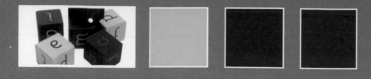

19 Oncology

- Childhood cancers
- Neuroblastoma
- Nephroblastoma (Wilms tumour)
- Rhabdomyosarcoma
- Bone tumours
- Retinoblastoma
- Germ cell tumours
- Liver tumours
- Brain tumours
- Leukaemias
- Lymphomas
- Childhood histiocytosis syndromes
- Further reading

CHILDHOOD CANCERS

AETIOLOGY

Cancer occurs when the normal control over growth and differentiation of a cell alters such that the cell is capable of inappropriate proliferation. Cells of a tumour are usually *monoclonal*, i.e. they all derive from one ancestral cell.

Definitions	
Cancer	Disorder involving uncontrolled cell growth
Carcinogenesis	Cellular events leading to cancer
Neoplasm (tumour)	Mass of cells
Malignant neoplasm	Can invade local tissues, may also form distant metastases

Tumour types	
Carcinoma	Epithelial
Sarcoma	Connective tissue
Lymphoma	Lymphatic tissue
Glioma	CNS glial cells
Leukaemia	Haematopoietic cells

Mechanisms of carcinogenesis

- Cancer develops when there is genetic alteration of the normal *cell regulatory system* (growth and development) via mutation(s)
- *Cancer causing genes* fall into three types (see below)
- Mutations activating the cancer genes can be *germline* (familial/inherited), *somatic* (most) or both
- The environment can increase the *frequency* of genetic mutations (see below)

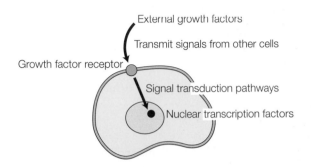

Figure 19.1 Normal regulation of cell growth and differentiation

1. External **growth factors** (steroid hormones and proteins, e.g. PDGF) transmit signals from other cells via specific *growth factor receptors* on the cell surface
2. These send messages to the cell nucleus via *signal transduction* pathways, e.g. protein kinases, which regulate/interact with
3. **Nuclear transcription factors** (genes, e.g. *myc*) that alter DNA transcription in the nucleus of specific genes whose protein products affect cell growth and differentiation

Mutations anywhere along the pathway of cell regulation can result in cancer. Mutations in the regulatory genes are rare. The **multi-hit concept of carcinogenesis** is that several mutations are needed to produce a malignant neoplasm.

Types of cancer genes

There are three major categories of cancer genes.

Tumour suppressor genes	Involved in restricting cell proliferation *Inactivation* can result in tumours Examples: ■ RB1 gene (ch 13q14) – retinoblastoma, osteosarcoma ■ WT1 gene (ch 11p13) – Wilms tumour
Oncogenes	Genes whose product can lead to unregulated cell growth Most arise from mutations in *proto-oncogenes* Examples: ■ *Bcr-abl* gene – ALL, CLL ■ MYCN amplification – neuroblastoma
DNA repair genes	DNA repair and replication continually occur throughout life Some inherited disorders involve defective DNA repair mechanisms, thus the chance of cancers developing secondary to somatic mutations is increased Examples: ataxia telangiectasia, xeroderma pigmentosum

Mechanism of activation

Cancer genes may be altered by:

- Single gene germline mutations – sporadic or inherited, e.g. retinoblastoma, and/or
- Somatic mutations

Two-hit theory of carcinogenesis is that a tumour will develop only when both copies of a gene are damaged. In many inherited cancers, the first allele is a germline mutation and the second a somatic mutation. This would explain why not all children who inherit the retinoblastoma mutation develop the tumour, and that they develop it at different ages.

Environmental factors can increase the risk of mutations:

- Carcinogens – environmental cancer-causing agents, i.e. increase the frequency of genetic cancer-causing events
- Ionizing radiation, e.g. leukaemia
- Ultraviolet radiation, e.g. skin cancers
- Viruses, e.g. Epstein–Barr virus (Hodgkin lymphoma and Burkitt lymphoma)
- Drugs, e.g. immunosuppressive drugs (non-Hodgkin lymphoma)

Many cancers are inherited in a multifactorial fashion, e.g. breast and colon cancers.

INCIDENCE

1 in 650 children develop cancer by age 16 years.

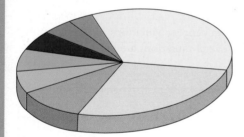

Leukaemia	31%
Brain tumour	24%
Lymphomas	10%
Neuroblastoma	6%
Wilms tumour	6%
Bone tumours	5%
Rhabdomyosarcoma	4%
Retinoblastoma	3%

Figure 19.2 Relative frequencies of childhood cancers

TREATMENT

Cancer management is multifactorial involving many specialists and therapists, and includes:

- Chemotherapy
- Immunotherapy and small molecule inhibitors
- Radiotherapy
- Surgery
- Stem cell transplantation (which acts by either high dose therapy or immunological means)

Chemotherapy

Many different drugs and regimens are used, and new developments are continually being made in this area, so that many children are treated as part of continually evolving drug trials. These drugs preferentially target rapidly dividing cells, e.g. cancer cells, but also affect normal cells that rapidly divide, e.g. bone marrow progenitors, gut epithelium.

Chemotherapeutic drug groups

Drug group	Example	Action
Antimetabolite	Methotrexate	Folic acid antagonist
Alkylating agents	Cyclophosphamide	Inhibits DNA synthesis
Vinca alkaloids	Vincristine	Inhibits microtubule formation
Antibiotics	Doxorubicin	Binds to DNA
Enzymes	L-Asparaginase	Depletes L-asparagine

Side effects

Bone marrow suppression	Anaemia
	Thrombocytopaenia
	Immunosuppression (neutropaenia, most marked 10 days after chemotherapy commenced). Infections treated with broad–spectrum antibiotics
Nausea and vomiting	Many agents
Mouth ulcers	Many agents
Tumour lysis syndrome	Any agent (see below)
Hair loss	Many agents
Liver damage	Certain drugs, e.g. methotrexate
Cardiotoxicity	Certain drugs, e.g. doxorubicin
Lung fibrosis	Certain drugs, e.g. bleomycin
Neurotoxicity	Certain drugs, e.g. vincristine
Secondary malignancy	Many agents, especially alkylating agents

Tumour lysis syndrome

The high rate of cellular breakdown in fast-growing tumours after chemotherapy can cause this potentially life-threatening syndrome of:

- Rise in urate levels
- Hypocalcaemia and hyperphosphataemia with renal failure
- Hyperkalaemia

Prevention with hyperhydration, allopurinol and rasburicase is essential. If the syndrome develops, treatment is with dialysis or haemofiltration.

Radiotherapy

This is often used as an adjunct to chemotherapy, e.g. cranial irradiation in ALL.

Side effects

Early	Nausea and fatigue, inflammation of skin, gut and bladder
Late	Organ damage dependent on location of treatment:

- Brain – cognitive impairment
- Skin – radiation damage, skin malignancies
- Gonads – infertility
- Other organs – secondary malignancy

Surgery

Direct initial surgical excision may be done, or the tumour may be 'pre-shrunk' using chemo- or radio-therapy, and then excised. Regional lymph nodes are generally also excised if affected or for disease staging.

Immunotherapy

Immunotherapy is being developed with both non-specific mediators of immune defence, e.g. interferon-α, and cancer-targeted therapies using monoclonal antibodies and T-cell based tumour vaccines.

Small molecule inhibitors

A new class of drugs that target signal transduction pathways, e.g. Glivac, is being used in CML.

Stem cell transplantation

Haematopoietic stem cells replace the diseased marrow with normal marrow cells.

- Child's diseased marrow is initially ablated with high-dose chemotherapy ± radiotherapy
- **Autologous** – child's own marrow is harvested before ablation, purged of malignant cells and then re-infused into the child after marrow ablation. *Peripheral blood stem cells* may be used. Residual cancer cells may cause relapse
- **Allogeneic** – marrow from a matched donor (HLA screened, preferably an HLA-identical sibling) is used. Marrow rejection and GVHD may occur

Graft-versus-host-disease

This is due to a reaction of the *donor T cells* mounting an immune response to the host major histocompatibility complex (MHC) antigens. It may be acute or chronic, though the former can transform into the latter.

Acute GVHD	< 100 days of BMT (usually 10–14 days post BMT)
	Fever, skin rash (fine maculopapular), enteritis
Chronic GVHD	> 100 days of BMT
	Skin rash (pigmentary changes, lichen planus, sclerosis), arthritis, malabsorption, obstructive jaundice, autoimmune diseases, e.g. SLE

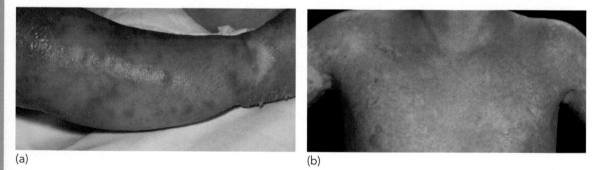

(a)   (b)

Figure 19.3 Graft-versus-host disease. (a) Acute rash in an infant. (b) Chronic disease

A beneficial graft-versus-leukaemia effect also occurs in the process and this helps eliminate any remaining cancer cells.

FAMILY CARE, LONG TERM CONSEQUENCES AND TERMINAL CARE

Having a child with cancer puts a lot of strain on the family, and they need help coping with all the many issues involved:

Parents	Emotional (guilt, fear, anxiety), treatment dilemmas, financial issues
Child	Understanding the diagnosis, coping with symptoms of the cancer
	Coping with treatments and side effects
	Issues surrounding mortality

Oncology

Continuing education whilst unwell

Being 'different', isolation

Siblings   Fear, jealousy, lack of attention

A team is involved in the holistic care of the child and family, including the oncology team (oncologist, oncology nurses, radiotherapist, palliative care), surgeons and pain team, educational team (teachers, educational psychologist) and psychiatric team (psychiatrist, psychologist).

Long term sequelae of childhood cancer

- Permanent deformity or disability, e.g. limb resection, post brain tumour
- Impaired growth due to endocrinopathy or spinal irradiation
- Psychiatric – depression, issues of mortality, fear of death
- Secondary malignancy – risk increased (post chemotherapy, SCT, radiotherapy or genetic factors)
- Endocrine – hypothyroidism, growth hormone and sex hormone deficiency (especially after total body irradiation)
- Neurocognitive problems – post cranial irradiation for brain tumours or leukaemia (only done for CNS disease)
- Infertility – post-irradiation in gonadal area (SCT) or high-dose chemotherapy

Terminal care

Some children will not survive their cancer. They and their families must be supported, emotionally and physically, through this time. The palliative care team coordinates this. Physical comforts include adequate analgesia and attention to alleviate all other symptoms. The child is managed at home if possible or in hospices (who provide respite and terminal care if the child cannot be managed at home).

NEUROBLASTOMA

Neuroblastoma is a tumour arising from the *neural crest cells* of the *sympathetic nervous system*. It may develop in the:

- Adrenal medulla (50%)
- Sympathetic chain (50%) (anywhere from the cranial fossa to the coccyx)

Clinical features

- Usually < 5 years old
- Abdominal mass
- Metastatic symptoms (70%):
  - Bone pain
  - Proptosis, periorbital bruising
  - Massive hepatosplenomegaly
  - Skin nodules, lymphadenopathy
  - Weight loss, pallor, malaise

Investigations

The tumour can be detected by:

- Urinary catecholamine metabolites – ↑ vanillylmandelic acid (VMA) and homovanillic acid (HVA)
- CT or MRI scan
- Meta-iodobenzylguanidine (MIBG) scan (a catecholamine precursor, will also outline metastases)
- Tissue biopsy (or positive bone marrow) is necessary to confirm diagnosis and define molecular features that determine prognosis and therapy

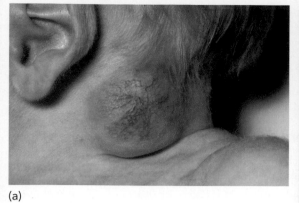

(a)

Figure 19.4 Neuroblastoma. (a) Skin nodule in an infant. (b) T1-weighted coronal MRI scan showing a left adrenal neuroblastoma (courtesy of Dr Anthony Michalski)

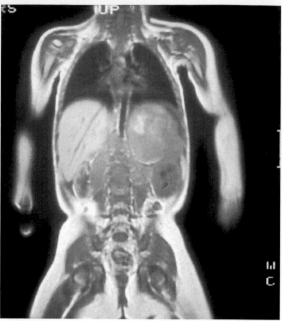

(b)

Management

Treatment is dependent on the child's age, and the tumour stage and biology (presence or absence of amplification of the *MYCN* oncogene).

Low-risk tumours	Managed with surgical resection ± chemotherapy
	Sub-type (stage 4S) resolves with no therapy
High-risk disease	More aggressive chemotherapy, surgery, high-dose chemotherapy with stem cell rescue, local radiotherapy and differentiation treatment

Differentiation therapy is the use of retinoic acid derivatives to force cells to differentiate past a point of development so that they lose the capacity to grow quickly or spread.

New therapies using targeted radiation therapy with ^{131}I-MIBG monoclonal antibodies are being trialled.

Prognosis

Low-risk tumours cure rate is > 90%; high-risk tumours cure rate is 10–40%.

> **! NB: Neonates with a small adrenal tumour and metastases in the skin, liver or bone marrow only can undergo spontaneous remission (stage 4S).**

NEPHROBLASTOMA (WILMS TUMOUR)

Nephroblastoma is a tumour of *embryonic renal precursor cells*. Incidence is 7.8 per million.

Clinical features

- Mean age 3 years

- Abdominal mass (most common presentation)
- Abdominal pain and vomiting
- Hypertension
- Haematuria
- 5% have bilateral disease at presentation

Associations

- Genitourinary abnormalities
- Overgrowth disorders (hemihypertrophy, Beckwith–Wiedemann syndrome)
- Aniridia
- Chromosome 11 short arm deletions involving one of two Wilms genes, e.g. W1T gene (11p13)

Investigations

Imaging	Abdominal USS, CT or MRI scan, AXR and CXR (? metastases)
Urinalysis	Haematuria

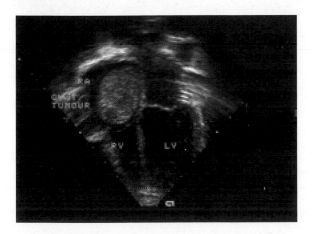

Figure 19.5 Echocardiogram showing right atrial cardiac metastasis in a child with Wilms tumour (courtesy of Robert Yates)

Staging (determined after definitive resection of the tumour)

I	Completely resected disease of kidney only
II	Disease beyond the kidney but completely resected
III	Residual disease post surgery or nodal involvement
IV	Metastatic disease (usually lung)

Management

Dependent on the stage.

- Primary nephrectomy then chemotherapy is still used in the USA
- Initial chemotherapy, then nephrectomy is now standard in the UK and Europe
- Radiotherapy is used as part of a combined strategy for local residual disease post surgery and for pulmonary metastatic disease

Prognosis

This is related to histology and disease stage, tumour size and child's age:

Favourable histology	89–98% 2-year survival
Poor histology	17–70% 4-year survival (variation secondary predominantly to precise histology of tumour)

RHABDOMYOSARCOMA

Rhabdomyosarcoma is a tumour of *primitive mesenchymal tissue* (which striated muscle arises from). These tumours may occur anywhere, but the commonest sites are:

- Head and neck
- Genitourinary tract
- Extremities

Clinical features

Head and neck tumour	Proptosis
	Facial swelling
	Nasal obstruction, blood-stained nasal discharge
	Cranial nerve palsies
Genitourinary tract tumour	Urinary tract obstruction
	Dysuria
	Blood-stained vaginal discharge

Associations

- Neurofibromatosis type 1
- Beckwith–Wiedemann syndrome

Management

Treatment depends on the site, resectability, stage, location, histology and presence of metastases:

- Initial surgical resection then chemotherapy
- If unresectable initially, chemotherapy, second look surgery ± radiotherapy

Prognosis

Localized standard risk histology disease has a 70% 5-year survival.

BONE TUMOURS

Incidence of bone tumours is 5.6 per million (whites > blacks, male > female). They most commonly present in *adolescents*. The two most common bone tumours are **osteosarcoma** (the most common) and **Ewing sarcoma**.

	Osteosarcoma	Ewing sarcoma
Site	Proximal end (metaphysis) of long bones Knee, proximal humerus	Diaphysis of long bones Flat bones, e.g. ribs, pelvis
Presentation	Bone pain and mass	Bone pain and mass and soft tissue component
X-ray findings	Sclerotic with 'skip lesions'	Lytic lesions 'Onion skinning' periosteal reaction
Tumour cells	Spindle cells	Small round cells
Metastases	Lung and bones	Lung and bones
Treatment	Surgery and chemotherapy	Surgery or radiotherapy to the primary, then chemotherapy
Prognosis	50% survival if non-metastatic < 20% survival if metastatic	65–70% survival if non-metastatic 25–30% survival if metastatic

RETINOBLASTOMA

A retinoblastoma is a tumour arising in the *retina*. Annual incidence is approximately 4 per million children.

Both   *hereditary* (40%) (retinoblastoma [*RB1*] gene on chromosome 13q [tumour suppressor gene]; autosomal dominant inheritance, incomplete penetrance) and
sporadic (60%) forms exist

May be *unilateral* (75%) or *bilateral* (the latter is always hereditary).

Clinical features

- White pupillary reflex (leucoria) – may be picked up on the developmental checks
- Squint (any *new* squint in a child should be investigated, though retinoblastoma will be an unusual finding in these children. Ophthalmological problems and brain tumours will be more common pathologies)
- Decreased vision
- If advanced disease – proptosis, raised intracranial pressure, orbital pain

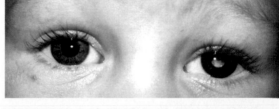

Figure 19.6 Leucoria (white pupillary reflex) of the left eye due to retinoblastoma (courtesy of Moorfields Eye Hospital, London)

Management

- Local therapy (radiotherapy, photocoagulation or cryotherapy)
- Enucleation of the eye if unavoidable
- Chemotherapy to reduce tumour volume prior to local therapy or if residual or metastatic disease

Treatment that minimizes radiotherapy to improve visual sparing and reduce the incidence of future secondary tumours is being optimized.

Prognosis

Overall survival is > 90%. Poor survival if extensive or metastatic disease. Familial cases have an increased incidence of secondary malignancies (osteosarcomas, soft tissue sarcomas and melanomas).

GERM CELL TUMOURS

Germ cell tumours are tumours arising from *primitive pluripotent germ cells* which migrate from the fetal yolk sac to form the gonads. They are mostly benign and include sacrococcygeal teratoma, choriocarcinoma, seminoma and dysgerminoma.

SACROCOCCYGEAL TERATOMA

This is the most common neonatal tumour.

Clinical features

- Rectum and urinary tract may be involved, and 90% have an external component
- 10% are malignant at birth, but if benign teratomas are left unresected malignant transformation can occur. (Malignancy is defined by a tumour that secretes alpha-fetoprotein or β–hCG, or has a particular histological appearance [yolk sac tumour])

Investigations

Imaging	CT or MRI scan of affected area, bone scan, chest CT
Biological markers	↑ AFP and β–hCG
Histology of lesion	Biopsy or resection specimen

Management

This involves surgical resection wherever possible for benign tumours. Malignant tumours should be treated with chemotherapy before surgery to minimize morbidity.

Prognosis

This is excellent if benign, and 60–90% 5-year survival if malignant.

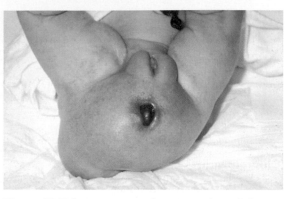

Figure 19.7 Sacrococcygeal teratoma in an infant (courtesy of Dr Anthony Michalski)

LIVER TUMOURS

Liver tumours may be:

- Primary:
  - Benign, e.g. haemangioma
  - Malignant, e.g. hepatoblastoma (see Fig. 16.2), hepatocellular carcinoma
- Metastatic, e.g. Wilms tumours, neuroblastoma

	Hepatoblastoma (65%)	Hepatocellular carcinoma (35%)
Age	< 3 years	12–15 years
Clinical features	Abdominal mass	Abdominal mass, systemic features more common
Tumour cells	Immature hepatic epithelium	Abnormal hepatocytes
Markers	AFP ↑ in 60% of patients	AFP ↑ in 50% of patients
Metastases	Lung, lymph nodes	Lung, lymph nodes
Prognosis	3-year survival: ■ 75% if resectable ■ 65% if unresectable (only if successful liver transplant fully removes tumour) ■ 10–20% if metastatic	Very poor survival figures. Recurrence common

Treatment: Surgical resection ± chemotherapy

BRAIN TUMOURS

In children, brain tumours are almost always primary. They can be divided into *supratentorial* and *posterior fossa (infratentorial)*.

Infants < 2 years	Equal frequencies of posterior fossa and supratentorial tumours
2–12 years	Two-thirds are posterior fossa (infratentorial)

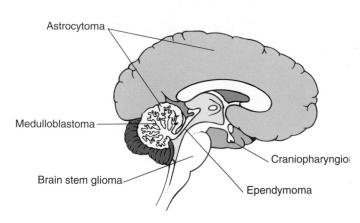

Astrocytoma

Medulloblastoma

Brain stem glioma

Craniopharyngioma

Ependymoma

Figure 19.8 Location of brain tumours

Clinical features

Signs of raised intracranial pressure	Morning headache, drowsiness, vomiting
	Diplopia, strabismus, papilloedema (a late sign in young children)
	Nystagmus (horizontal, vertical or rotatory)
	Bulging fontanelle, macrocephaly
	Head tilting and nuchal rigidity
	Cranial nerve palsies (IV and VI)
Focal neurological signs	Complex partial seizures
	Ataxia (cerebellar tumours)
	Hemiparesis
	Endocrinopathies such as diabetes insipidus

INFRATENTORIAL (POSTERIOR FOSSA) TUMOURS
Medulloblastoma

- Usually midline, cause truncal ataxia and ↑ ICP signs
- Treatment is surgical resection followed by chemotherapy and radiotherapy
- Standard risk tumours have 80% long term disease control; poor risk 20% long term disease control
- Neurocognitive sequelae are problematical secondary to tumours, raised ICP, radiotherapy and probably chemotherapy

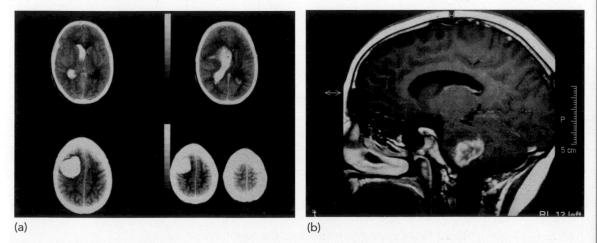

(a) (b)

Figure 19.9 Brain tumours. (a) Transverse CT scan showing a large intracranial tumour. (b) Sagittal section on MRI scan showing a craniopharyngioma

Brain tumours

343

Brain stem glioma

- These may be:
  - Diffusely infiltrating the pons (most cases; very poor outlook)
  - Low grade focal midbrain or cervico-medullary tumours (good outlook if resectable)
- Present with ataxia, cranial nerve palsies and long tract signs

Astrocytoma

- Usually slow growing
- ↑ ICP by blocking the aqueduct of Sylvius or the fourth ventricle
- Treatment is surgical resection ± chemotherapy and radiotherapy
- 5-year survival > 90–95%

SUPRATENTORIAL TUMOURS

Craniopharyngioma (see p. 246)

- Develop from a remnant of Rathke's pouch in the sella turcica
- Present with bitemporal hemianopia, endocrine abnormalities, e.g. diabetes insipidus, and ↑ ICP
- Investigations include visual field and cranial nerve examination, and hormonal investigation
- Treatment is surgical resection (± radiotherapy)

LEUKAEMIAS

Leukaemias are the most common form of childhood cancer. They include:

- **Acute lymphoblastic leukaemia (ALL)** (75%) – peak incidence age 4 years
- **Acute myeloid leukaemia (AML)** (20%) – stable incidence < 10 years, increase in adolescence
- **Chronic myeloid leukaemia (CML)** (3%)
- **Juvenile CML** and the **myelodysplastic syndromes** (2–3%)

They are classified according to morphology and cytochemistry.

ACUTE LYMPHOBLASTIC LEUKAEMIA

This is the most common form of childhood leukaemia. It arises from early cells in the *lymphoid series*.

There are certain genetic associations including:

- Down syndrome
- Hyperdiploidy
- Translocations, e.g. t(9:22) Philadelphia chromosome (poor risk)

Types/classification of ALL

Immunophenotype classification

Precursor B-ALL	75% (includes c-ALL [common], null-ALL and pre-B-ALL)
T-ALL	20%
B-ALL	5%

French–American–British (FAB) classification

L1	Small lymphoblasts, little cytoplasm (good prognosis)
L2	Larger and pleomorphic lymphoblasts, more cytoplasm
L3	Cytoplasmic vacuoles, finely stippled nuclear chromatin

Clinical features

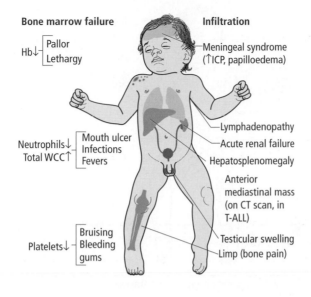

Bone marrow failure

Hb↓ ⎡ Pallor
⎣ Lethargy

Neutrophils↓ ⎡ Mouth ulcer
Total WCC↑ ⎢ Infections
⎣ Fevers

Platelets↓ ⎡ Bruising
⎢ Bleeding
⎣ gums

Infiltration

Meningeal syndrome
(↑ICP, papilloedema)

Lymphadenopathy
Acute renal failure
Hepatosplenomegaly

Anterior
mediastinal mass
(on CT scan, in
T-ALL)

Testicular swelling
Limp (bone pain)

Figure 19.10 Clinical features of acute lymphoblastic leukaemia

Investigations

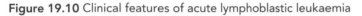

FBC and film	Anaemia (normochromic, normocytic)
	Blasts present (these are normally only found in the bone marrow)
	WCC ↓, normal or ↑ (blasts)
	Platelets ↓
Bone marrow (aspirate or biopsy)	> 30% leukaemic blast cells
CXR	Mediastinal mass (in T-ALL)
CSF	Blasts seen if CSF involvement
Renal function and uric acid	Impaired renal function with raised uric acid (if renal infiltration or tumour lysis syndrome)
Special classification tests	Chromosomal analysis, immunocytochemistry, immunophenotyping
	Immunoglobulin and T-cell receptor gene rearrangement studies

Management

- **Induction of remission** Multiagent chemotherapy – vincristine, danorubicin, asparagine, steroid
- **Consolidation of remission** Intensive multiagent chemotherapy – Ara-c, cyclophosphamide, etoposide
  CNS prophylaxis (treatment that crosses the blood–brain barrier), e.g. high-dose IV methotrexate, intrathecal chemotherapy, CNS radiotherapy
- **Intensification** 2–3 blocks of intensive multiagent chemotherapy to clear submicroscopic or minimal residual disease
- **Maintenance chemotherapy** 2 years chemotherapy (outpatient treatment) usually with oral 6-MP, methotrexate, vincristine and prednisolone or dexamethasone

Relapse

Intensive chemotherapy (and cranial irradiation in CNS relapse). BMT may offer the best chance of cure.

Common sites for *relapse* are:

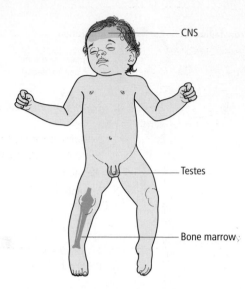

Figure 19.11 Common sites for relapse

Prognosis

This is dependent on the type and other factors (see below). Overall 5-year survival is 70–80%.

Prognostic indicators	
Good prognosis	**Poor prognosis**
Low initial WCC	High initial WCC
Female	Male
2–10 years	< 2 years or > 10 years
< 4 weeks to remission	> 4 weeks to remission
t(12:21)	t(9:22), t(4:11)
Hyperdiploidy	Hypoploidy
c-ALL or L1	CNS involvement

ACUTE MYELOID LEUKAEMIA

AML arises from a pluripotent cell or myeloid progenitor committed to erythroid, granulocyte–monocytic or megakaryocyte lines.

Associations

- Down syndrome
- Aplastic anaemia
- Fanconi anaemia (see p. 316)
- Previous chemotherapy

Clinical features

- Bone marrow failure   As in ALL. NB: WCC may be ↑, ↓ or normal
- Other   Gum hypertrophy (especially M4 and M5)
                          DIC (M3)
                          Chloroma (localized mass of leukaemic cells, e.g. skin, retro-orbital epidural)
                          Bone pain less common than in ALL

Classification of AML

French–American–British (FAB) system

M0	Undifferentiated	No Auer rods
M1	Myeloblastic, no maturation	Few Auer rods
M2	Myeloblastic, some maturation	Good prognosis, Auer rods common, chloroma common
M3	Acute promyelocytic	Good prognosis, many Auer rods, DIC common, retinoic acid as initial therapy
M4	Myelomonocytic	Good prognosis
M5	Monocytic	Renal damage, gum hypertrophy, meningeal involvement
M6	Erythroleukaemia	Poor prognosis
M7	Megakaryoblastic	Marrow fibrosis

Investigations

As for ALL. The bone marrow must contain at least 30% blast cells (the blasts may contain Auer rods).

Management

- Induction of remission   Chemotherapy, e.g. danorubicin, cytosine arabinoside, thioguanine or etoposide
  > 80% achieve remission. If not achieved then BMT is necessary
- Consolidation   e.g. danorubicin, cytosine arabinoside, thioguanine or etoposide
  Intrathecal chemotherapy (± cranial irradiation) if CNS leukaemia at diagnosis or CNS relapse
- Further consolidation   Total of 4–5 courses of multiagent chemotherapy, e.g. etoposide, cytosine arabinoside, m-amascrine
  BMT is usually only considered after relapse of AML in children

Relapse

Relapse is treated with intensive chemotherapy (and intrathecal chemotherapy and cranial irradiation in CNS relapse). BMT offers the best chance of cure.

A common site for *relapse* is the bone marrow (CNS rarely).

Prognosis

Overall cure rate is 60–70%. Cure rates depend on the type (highest for M3 AML), and decrease with increasing age.

MYELODYSPLASTIC SYNDROMES

Juvenile myelomonocytic leukaemia

- Generally occurs in young children
- Blood:
  - Abnormal monocytes
  - Leukocytosis
  - Elevated HbF
  - Platelets ↓
- Hepatosplenomegaly, lymphadenopathy
- Desquamative maculopapular rash
- Allogeneic bone marrow transplant needed as resistant to other treatment.

LYMPHOMAS

These malignancies of *lymphoid tissue* are classified into:

- Hodgkin lymphoma
- Non-Hodgkin lymphoma

HODGKIN LYMPHOMA

Hodgkin lymphoma is a malignancy of lymphoid tissue, with Reed–Sternberg (RS) cells and Hodgkin cells seen on histology. It is a B-cell malignancy, but the exact origin of the malignant cells is unclear. It has a bimodal age distribution (adolescents and > 50 years) and a male preponderance (2:1).

Histological classification of Hodgkin lymphoma		
Nodular sclerosing	50%	Good prognosis. Mediastinal mass common
Mixed cellularity	40%	Generally present with more advanced disease
Lymphocyte predominant	10%	Best prognosis
Lymphocyte depleted	V. rare	Present with disseminated disease, poor prognosis

Clinical features

- Lymphadenopathy
  Painless, firm lymph nodes
  Cervical, supraclavicular, axillary, inguinal
  Mediastinal (cough, airway compression), retroperitoneal
- 'B' symptoms
  Fever '*Pel-Epstein*'
  Night sweats
  Weight loss
- Other constitutional symptoms
  Fatigue, pruritis, anorexia
- Extranodal involvement
  Hepatosplenomegaly, bone pain, skin deposits, SVC obstruction
  Bone marrow failure (rare)

Investigations

Careful clinical examination is essential.

Bloods
FBC:
- Anaemia (normochromic, normocytic)
- Neutrophils ↑, eosinophils ↑
- Platelets initially high, then low in advanced disease
ESR ↑ (used to monitor disease progress)
LDH ↑, LFTs ↑ (both indicate poor prognosis)

Lymph node biopsy
For diagnosis and histological classification

CT chest/abdomen/pelvis
For staging

Other (if necessary)
Bone marrow aspirate
Bone scan, MRI scan
Liver biopsy

Management

Stages IA and IIA
Radiotherapy only or chemotherapy (ABVD)

Advanced disease
Chemotherapy, e.g. adriamycin (doxorubicin), bleomycin, vinblastine, dacarbazine (ABVD)
± Radiotherapy

> **Stages of disease**
>
> **I** Single lymph node region (LNR)
> **II** ≥ 2 LNR same side of the diaphragm
> **III** LNR both sides of the diaphragm
> ± spleen
> **IV** Disseminated involvement of extralymphatic organs, e.g. liver, bone marrow
>
> The stage is also: **A** (absence of 'B' symptoms) or
> **B** (presence of 'B' symptoms)

Relapse	Alternative combination chemotherapy, e.g. MOPP, and autologous stem cell transplant

Prognosis

Stage I and II	> 90% 5-year survival
Stage IIIA	> 80% 5-year survival
Stage IIIB and IV	> 70% 5-year survival

NON-HODGKIN LYMPHOMA

Non-Hodgkin lymphoma arises from abnormal T or B lymphocytes. Children have high-grade diffuse disease and it is associated with congenital immunodeficiency disorders. There are several classifications.

Clinical features

These vary depending on the site of the primary.

Systemic symptoms	Fever, night sweats, weight loss
Organ involvement	Abdomen (31%) – abdominal distension, nausea, vomiting, acute abdomen, hepatosplenomegaly
	Mediastinum (26%) – dyspnoea, pleural effusions, SVC obstruction
	Oropharyngeal – stridor, sore throat
	Lymph nodes – painless hard lymph nodes. Most commonly cervical
	Bone marrow – bone marrow failure features
	CNS – headache, cranial nerve palsies, raised ICP
	Other organ – skin deposits, testes mass

Investigations

Excision biopsy or fine needle aspirate	Of lymph node or other mass
Bloods	FBC (anaemia, neutropaenia, lymphoma cells, platelets ↓)
	U&E (↑), uric acid (↑), bone profile
	LDH ↑ (prognostic indicator)
Bone marrow aspirate or trephine	Involvement in around 20%
CSF	? CNS involvement
Imaging	CT scan chest/abdomen/pelvis and bone scan
Special tests	Chromosome analysis, immunological markers

Staging is the same as for Hodgkin lymphoma, although it is less clearly related to prognosis than is the histological type.

Management

This depends on the grade of malignancy. The high-grade T cell malignancy seen in children is usually treated with multiagent chemotherapy, like the ALL protocols. *Relapses* are treated with intensive chemotherapy, radiotherapy and autologous or allogeneic SCT.

Prognosis

- Limited stage disease > 90% cure
- Stage III and IV 70% cure

BURKITT LYMPHOMA

This is an unusual B-cell lymphoma that is related to Epstein–Barr virus infection. It is endemic in Africa (jaw involvement classically seen) and sporadic in developed countries (abdominal involvement seen).

Clinical features

- Massive jaw lesions
- Abdominal extranodal involvement
- Ovarian involvement

Specific investigations

- Lymph node biopsy – few histiocytes among masses of lymphocytes ('**Starry sky**')
- Cell culture for EBV
- Chromosome analysis – t(8:14) is usually present

Management

Intensive chemotherapy (four cycles), with SCT if relapse. Recently good results to treatment have been obtained (70% cure).

CHILDHOOD HISTIOCYTOSIS SYNDROMES

The histiocytoses are a group of disorders involving proliferation of histiocytic cells in the bone marrow of the *dendritic cell* or *monocyte–macrophage* systems. Many are benign proliferations, though some are malignant. They are classified on the basis of histology.

CLASS I: DENDRITIC CELL DISORDERS

Langerhans' cell histiocytosis (LCH)

Langerhans' cells are skin histiocytes with antigen-presenting function (part of the antigen-specific immune response). They are CD1a positive and are identified on EM with the cytoplasmic organelles *Birbeck granules* – look like tennis rackets.

The cause of Langerhans' cell histiocytosis (LCH) is unknown. Incidence is 2–5 cases per million children annually, peak age 1–3 years, boys > girls.

Clinical features

The features are a result of *infiltration* with Langerhans' cells and the subsequent immunological reaction to these cells. The presentation and extent of involvement *vary widely*, and LCH may be single system or disseminated.

- Bone pain and swelling
  Due to isolated or multiple lytic lesions:
  - Punched-out skull lesions, mastoid necrosis with middle ear involvement
  - Jaw (floating teeth), orbit (proptosis), vertebral fractures, long bone lesions
  - Bone marrow infiltration seen

  A skeletal survey should be performed at diagnosis

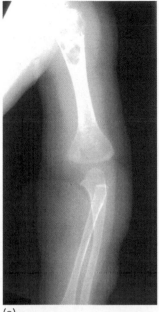

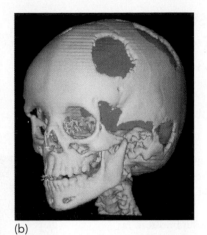

(b)

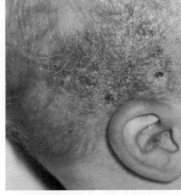

(c)

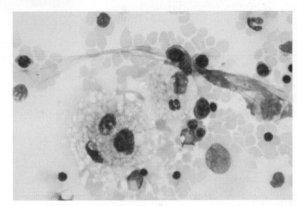

(a)

(d)

Figure 19.12 Langerhans' cell histiocytosis.
(a) X-ray showing lytic lesions in the humerus.
(b) Multiple classical 'punched out' lesions on
3D MRI scan of the skull. (c) Eczematous scaly
rash behind the ears in an infant. (d) Foamy
histiocytes with erythrophagocytosis

- Skin rash   Pink or brown papules becoming eczematous, scaly and pruritic
  Involving face, scalp, behind ears, axillary and inguinal folds, back and nappy area
- Ear discharge
- Lymphadenopathy
- Hepatosplenomegaly
- Lung infiltration   Causing cough, tachypnoea, chest pain
  CXR – diffuse micronodules, later reticulonodular pattern
- Endocrine   Especially diabetes insipidus

Management

Single system disease   Observation alone
                        Topical treatment (rash), analgesia, steroids and chemotherapy if necessary
Multisystem disease   Chemotherapy then BMT if necessary, i.e. non-responders with bone marrow
                        disease

Prognosis

May regress spontaneously or progress to life-threatening disease. The prognosis is worse if multisystem, > 1
year old and with active disease.

CLASS II: MACROPHAGE DISORDERS

These are proliferations involving **macrophages**. There are many different types, divided into:

- Systemic forms, e.g. haemophagocytic lymphohistiocytosis (HLH)
- Cutaneous forms, e.g. juvenile xanthogranuloma (JXG)

Haemophagocytic lymphohistiocytosis

This may be:

- **Primary** (familial or sporadic). Mutations in the *perforin gene* found (10q21–22) in some cases (with absent perforin granules in cytotoxic lymphocytes). Future pregnancy risk is 1 in 4, or
- **Secondary** (to infections, immunosuppression, fat infusions or malignancy)

It is a disorder involving *immune dysregulation*.

Diagnostic criteria

- Fevers
- Splenomegaly
- Pancytopaenia
- High triglyceride or low fibrinogen
- Typical histology (with haemophagocytosis)
- Other features – lymphadenopathy, skin rash, LFT ↑, ferritin ↑

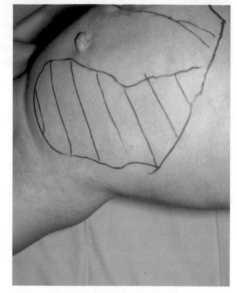

Figure 19.13 Massive hepatosplenomegaly in a patient with haemophagocytic lymphohistiocytosis

Treatment

Primary disease	Chemotherapy, then BMT if needed (persistent or familial disease)
	Primary HLH is generally fatal without BMT
Secondary disease	May resolve with treatment of the precipitating factor

Juvenile xanthogranuloma

- Single or multiple yellow–orange papules
- Lipid-laden macrophages seen on histology
- Usually regresses over a few years
- Systemic involvement (most commonly ocular) is rare

CLASS III

These are *malignant histiocytoses* of lymphoid origin.

Examples	Acute monocytic leukaemia (M5)
	Acute myelomonocytic leukaemia (M4)

Treatment is with chemotherapy or BMT.

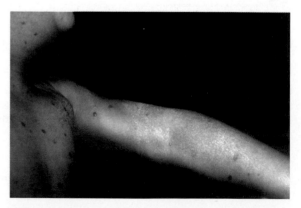

Figure 19.14 Juvenile xanthogranulomatosis in an 18-month-old infant

Clinical scenario

A 7-year-old girl is seen by her family practitioner with lethargy and an occasional mouth ulcer. She is told that a viral illness is 'going round' and the parents are told to give paracetamol and return in one week if she is not better.

One week later she re-presents with some discomfort in her right knee and the GP examines her, finding her to have pale conjunctivae, a few non-blanching punctate lesions on her abdomen and legs, and apathetic to examination, allowing the doctor to press her abdomen on palpation with no upset, whereupon the GP surprisingly feels masses in her upper right and upper left abdomen.

1. What three diagnoses are possible?
2. What first test would you arrange?

The full blood count reveals the following:

Hb 7.6 g/dL

White cell count 56.3 x 10^6/L

Platelets 35 x 10^6/L

3. What subsequent investigation is most likely to be helpful in the diagnosis?
4. What is the most likely diagnosis?
5. How would you approach this with the parents?

ANSWERS

1. Acute leukaemia; neuroblastoma; lymphoma
2. FBC
3. Bone marrow aspirate. (Possibly abdominal ultrasound as well)
4. Acute lymphoblastic leukaemia
5. Quiet room with both parents present; honesty; compassion; provide repetition of all conversations and written information as the shock of the initial diagnosis will prevent much being taken in initially; indicate that 5-year survival rates are in excess of 80% nowadays but that the type of the disease needs further elucidation before predictions can be made. White cell count above 50 x 10^6/L is not a good prognostic factor.

FURTHER READING

Coppes M, Dome J. *Pediatric Oncology: An Issue of Pediatric Clinics of North America* London: Saunders, 2008.

Pizzo P, Poplack D (eds.). *Principles and Practice of Paediatric Oncology*, 5th edn. London: Lippincott Williams & Wilkins, 2005.

Lanzkowsky P. *Manual of Pediatric Hematology and Oncology*, 3rd edn. California: Academic Press, 2000.

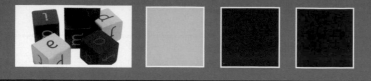

20 Neurology

- Neurological examination in a child
- Structural brain anomalies
- Raised intracranial pressure
- Seizures
- Headaches
- Ataxia
- Cerebral palsy
- Stroke
- Neuroectodermal disorders
- Neurodegenerative disorders
- Further reading

NEUROLOGICAL EXAMINATION IN A CHILD

- Neurological examination of a child can be a challenge, particularly of a young child
- Examination needs to be adapted to suit the *child's age*, and it need *not* be done in the textbook order – examine parts as they present themselves
- In a child with a neurological problem, a *full examination* must be done and, with practice, can be done in a few minutes
- Always check *vision and hearing*, as problems with these will cause an expected delay in development
- Much of the examination can be done by *observation* of the child, e.g. at play, whilst taking the history. Specific points to remember in the history are listed below

Points to remember in the history

Pregnancy	Teratogenic drugs? Exposure to infection? Were fetal movements normal?
Delivery	? Difficult birth (forceps, delay, fetal distress, resuscitation required)
Neonatal period	? In NICU ? Feeding difficulties, respiratory difficulties, seizures, severe jaundice
Family history	e.g. epilepsy, neural tube defects, deafness
Medications	
Seizures	
Vision and hearing	Visual impairment? Squint? Deafness?
Speech	Delay? Stutter?

Intellectual abilities	Developmental milestones achieved?
	Schooling
Feeding	
Continence	(Urinary and faecal), urinary retention, constipation
Daily living activities	
Mobility	Wheelchair, sticks?
Social interactions	Friends and family

Neurological examination summary

General	Growth parameters (height, weight, head circumference)
	Dysmorphic features, resting posture and any obvious neurological problems
Senses	Vision and hearing
Development	Language, speech and social interaction (observe during examination)
	Fine motor
	Gross motor (infant – 180° ['*flip over*'] examination; older child – gait)
Limbs	Including primitive reflexes and responses (infants), and movement and coordination
Cranial nerves	

NB: Always measure the blood pressure

NEUROLOGICAL ASSESSMENT

	Infant or disabled child	Older child
1. General		
Growth parameters	Weight, height, head circumference	As for infant/disabled child
Dysmorphic features	Head size, shape and fontanelle, ? ex-prem appearance (dolicocephalic i.e. 'narrow tall' head)	Head size ? Dysmorphic appearance
Resting posture	Obvious neurological problems, e.g. floppy, hemiplegic posturing, involuntary movements	As for infant/disabled child
2. Development		
Vision		
Acuity	Fixing and following	Reading ability
	Pick up raisin or hundreds and thousands	
	Formal testing if necessary (see p. 409)	
Squint testing	See p. 414	
Hearing	Enquire of parents	As for infant/disabled child
	Formal testing if necessary (see p. 112)	
Language and speech	Ask parents, observe	As for infant/disabled child, talk to child

	Infant or disabled child	**Older child**
Social interaction	Ask parents, observe	As for infant/disabled child, observe interaction
Fine motor control	? Milestones achieved on time	As for infant/disabled child
Gross motor control	**180° examination (flip over)**	**Gait examination**
	1. Lying down – posture and movement	Walking – normally, heel– toe – on toes, on heels, on outsides of feet Running, hopping

2. Pull to sitting (look for head control)

Standing – with feet together, on each foot
Touching toes

3. Ability to sit unaided

Squatting and rising again
Lying on floor and rising again
(children < 3 years roll onto tummy first. If this continues, suggests weakness [Gower's sign, see p. 386–7])

Abnormalities:
■ **Knee locking gait** (weak knees)
■ **Trendelenburg gait** (weak hip muscles)
■ **Wide base** (weakness or ataxia)
■ **Toe–heel walk** (pyramidal dysfunction, e.g. cerebral palsy)
■ **Foot drop** (superficial peroneal nerve lesion)
NB: If unsure of gait, look at shoe soles to see if worn unevenly

4. Up to weight bearing (lower limb scissoring, stiffness, weakness)

5. In ventral suspension (head, trunk and limb posture)

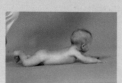

6. Lay prone (ability to raise head and extend limbs)

Ask child to run and this may unveil a mild hemiplegia as the affected leg will go into flexion at knee and plantar flexion at ankle, and arm will flex at elbow and wrist

	Infant or disabled child	Older child
3. Limbs		
Inspection	Resting **posture**, e.g. floppy, or scissoring of legs in cerebral palsy **Muscle wasting**, e.g. cerebral palsy, or **hypertrophy** (muscular dystrophy) **Involuntary movements** Limb length discrepancies, growth arrest Scars, skin changes, e.g. port-wine stain **Check neck and back for scars**, scoliosis, stigmata of spina bifida, flat buttocks (sacral agenesis)	As for infant/disabled child
Palpation	Muscle bulk, tenderness, ? peripheral nerve hypertrophy	As for infant/disabled child
Tone	Truncal tone and head lag Limb tone **Hypotonia** (floppy baby) **Spasticity, rigidity** (hip adductors in cerebral palsy)	Take weight of leg or arm in hand and bend it to assess tone
Power	Difficult in babies Observe antigravity movement motor function, and mobility **If weakness:** ■ Symmetrical? Proximal or distal? ■ A specific nerve root or muscle group? ■ Upper or lower motor neurone pattern?	Formal testing > 4 years: Graded out of 5 (see below) **If weakness**: as for infant/ disabled child
Reflexes	Deep tendon reflexes Primitive reflexes NB: Plantars unreliable < 1 year **Brisk – ? UMN dysfunction**, *? Anxiety* **Absent- ? Lower motor neurone**	Deep tendon reflexes **Brisk/absent**: as for infant/ disabled child
Coordination	Build pile of bricks Finger–nose to teddy's nose (eyes open = **cerebellar**; eyes closed = **proprioception**)	Finger–nose test Dysdiadokinesis Hold arms out in front (? **Drifting** – seen in weakness, proprioception loss and cerebellar hypotonia)
Sensation	Difficult in infants Withdraw if tickled	Proprioception Vibration (has the buzzing stopped?) Light touch (cotton wool) ⎫ Pain (with blunt pin) ⎭ In dermatomal distribution

	Infant or disabled child	Older child
4. Cranial nerve assessment	Cannot be tested formally in young infants	Formal testing is possible > 4 years
I Smell	Not possible in infants	Ask parents can they smell things?
II Visual acuity	Fixing and following Pick up hundreds and thousands	Read a paragraph See p. 409 for formal test
Direct and consensual, pupillary reflexes to light, and accommodation	With pen torch	As for infant/disabled child
Visual fields		Directly facing child, both index fingers out: wiggle each finger in high, low and halfway positions
III, IV, VI Voluntary eye movements Squint testing Nystagmus?	Get child to follow a face or toy (up, down, left, right, figure of 8)	Follow a pen (as for infant/disabled child)
V Motor function	Bite	Clench teeth, move jaw side to side
VII Motor function	Smiles symmetrically Face symmetrical Closes both eyes normally	Smile, close eyes tightly
VIII Hearing	Ask parents (see p. 111 formal testing)	As for infant/disabled child
IX Levator palate	Observe crying	Say 'ahh'
X Recurrent laryngeal nerve	? Hoarse cough/voice	? Hoarse voice
XI Trapezius and sternomastoid	Turns head to both sides	Shrug shoulders
XII Hypoglossal	Tongue moves symmetrically	Stick out tongue and move side-to-side

Grading of power

	Memory guide
0 – Complete paralysis	(*None*)
1 – Flicker of contraction	(*Minuscule*)
2 – Movement possible but not against gravity	(*V. little*)
3 – Antigravity movement, but not against resistance	(***Antigravity***)
4 – Movement against some resistance	(*Antiresistance, not quite normal*)
5 – Normal power	(*Normal*)

NEUROLOGICAL INVESTIGATIONS

	Indications
Electroencephalogram (EEG)	Brain activity assessment, seizure investigation
Neuroimaging:	
CT or MRI brain scan	Soft tissue imaging
Skull X-ray	Bony defects, pituitary fossa outline
Cranial USS	Soft tissue imaging (infants with patent fontanelle only)
Angiography, MRA scan	Intracranial vessel outline
Lumbar puncture	Possible meningeal infection
	Metabolic disorders

Lumbar puncture

Indications

- Severely sick child if cause unapparent
- First febrile convulsion in a child < 12 months age
- Investigation of metabolic disorder

Technique

1. Good positioning imperative:
   - Restraint needed for young children
   - Curled tightly, back at right angles to bed
2. Sterile technique:
   - Hands well scrubbed; sterile surgical gloves and gown
3. Point of entry (skin markings):
   - Skin overlying lower lumbar spine
   - Highest points of iliac crests line passes over 4th lumbar spine
   - Introduce needle just below or just above 4th lumbar spine
4. Anaesthetic:
   - Skin and tissues to the dura where needle to be introduced
5. Spinal needle introduction – at *right angles* to the skin
6. Obtain CSF samples:
   - Take fluid and measure pressure
   - Send for: microscopy, bacterial and viral culture (± PCR); glucose and protein

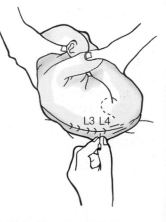

Figure 20.1 Surface markings and position for lumbar puncture in an infant

359

NB: Also send serum glucose, U&Es and FBC (and blood cultures and viral titres if infection suspected).

Complications

Bloody tap (hit vascular plexus surrounding the cord) – attempt space above. Send off bloody sample if only one obtained.

Contraindications

↑ICP (may result in cerebral herniation – very rare if fontanelle still open), cardiopulmonary compromise, local skin infection overlying site of LP, coagulopathy, thrombocytopaenia, see p. 84.

Findings

CSF colour	**Clear** – normal
	Bright red blood – damage to a blood vessel during LP or recent subarachnoid haemorrhage (SAH)
	Yellow (xanthochromia):
	■ Altered haemoglobin (after sub-arachnoid haemorrhage [SAH])
	■ Pus, jaundice or very high protein levels
CSF turbidity	If high indicates high WCC in infection
CSF pressure	**Normal:**
	■ 0–80 mmH$_2$O, mean 3 cmH$_2$O (neonate)
	■ 60–200 mmH$_2$O (older child)
	High in raised intracranial pressure
CSF glucose	**Normal CSF glucose** = ⅔ blood glucose
	Low:
	■ Bacterial or TB meningitis (NB: May be normal)
	■ Hypoglycaemia (NB: therefore compare to blood glucose)
	■ Widespread malignant infiltration of meninges
	■ *After SAH*
CSF protein	(Albumin and immunoglobulins)
	High in neonates (1.2 g/L), and falls by 6 months of age to adult levels (0.25–0.4 g/L)
	High:
	■ Blood or pus in CSF
	■ Non-purulent cerebral inflammation, e.g. Guillain–Barré syndrome
	■ Blockage of spinal canal, e.g. tumour, TB (very high levels)

! NB: Spinal cord extends to third lumbar vertebra in an infant. It gradually shortens relative to the vertebrae, to extend to the first lumbar vertebra in an adult.

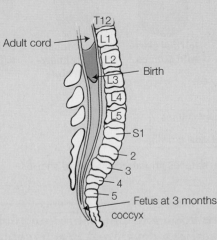

Figure 20.2 Termination of the spinal cord in a 3-month old fetus, a newborn infant and an adult

STRUCTURAL BRAIN ANOMALIES

ABNORMAL HEAD SHAPE AND SIZE

The head may be large or small, or abnormal in shape (symmetrical or asymmetrical).

Causes

Large (macrocephaly) > 98th centile	Familial, i.e. normal
	Neurofibromatosis
	Raised intracranial pressure, e.g. hydrocephalus, subdural haematoma
	Sotos syndrome (~ macrosomia)
	Metabolic storage disorder, e.g. Hunter syndrome
Small (microcephaly) < 2nd centile	Familial, i.e. normal
	Autosomal recessive
	Craniosynostosis (affecting all sutures)
	Prenatal/delivery cerebral insult, e.g. cerebral palsy, congenital infection
	Postnatal cerebral insult, e.g. meningitis
Abnormal shape (symmetrical or asymmetrical)	Positional moulding, e.g. premature babies – head lying on side a lot (dolicocephaly), floppy babies – head remains stationary for prolonged time, normal babies – always put on back (brachycephaly) or preferring one side only (plagiocepahly)
	Premature suture closure (craniosynostosis)
	Differential growth rate at the sutures

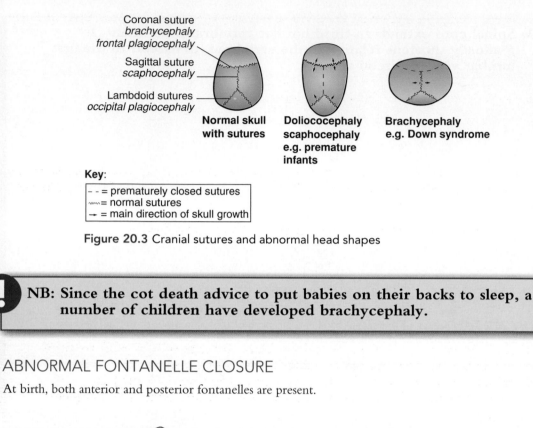

Figure 20.3 Cranial sutures and abnormal head shapes

! **NB: Since the cot death advice to put babies on their backs to sleep, a number of children have developed brachycephaly.**

ABNORMAL FONTANELLE CLOSURE

At birth, both anterior and posterior fontanelles are present.

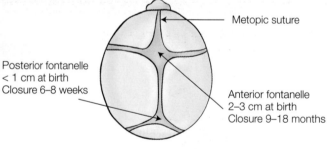

Figure 20.4 Anterior and posterior fontanelles

Causes

Delayed closure	Hypothyroidism
	Malnutrition
	Rickets
	Hydrocephalus
	Osteogenesis imperfecta
	Alpert syndrome
	Chromosomal abnormality, e.g. Down syndrome
Premature closure	Microcephaly
	Craniosynostosis
	Hyperthyroidism

Craniosynostosis

This is premature closure of the cranial sutures, which results in cranial deformities dependent on the particular sutures involved (see Fig. 20.3). It can be an isolated defect affecting one suture, causing an asymmetrical scalp, or affect all sutures, causing microcephaly. It can also be associated with a syndrome, e.g. Alpert syndrome, Crouzon syndrome.

These children may develop:

- Hydrocephalus, raised intracranial pressure and optic atrophy
- Deafness, deviated nasal septum and speech disorders

Craniofacial surgery may be necessary.

NEURAL TUBE DEFECTS

Neural tube defects (NTDs) result from failure of the neural tube to close on day 21–26 of intrauterine life and may involve the spinal cord and/or the brain. If compatible with survival, these defects may be closed surgically soon after birth.

Antenatal detection – direct view on ultrasound scan, raised α-FP in amniotic fluid.

Associations

- Folate deficiency
- Sodium valproate
- Previous neural tube defect (*recurrence risk* – one previous NTD 4%, two previous NTD 10%)

> **!** **NB: Daily folic acid (400 μg) is advised preconceptually for all women trying to become pregnant, and to be continued for the first trimester to prevent NTDs. High dose folic acid (5 mg) is recommended for those with a previous infant with a NTD (see p. 42).**

Normal spine

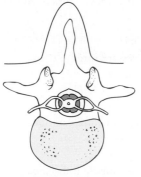

Normal spine

May be normal with surgical repair

Spina bifida occulta (see below)
(failure of vertebral arch fusion)

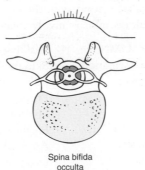

Spina bifida
occulta

Up to 5% of the population affected
Overlying hair tuft or lipoma
Mostly asymptomatic
Neural tethering may cause bladder and lower limb problems (**cauda equina syndrome**) but not until around 10–12 yrs of age
Neuropathic bladder and bowel
Hydronephrosis, renal failure
Hip dislocation, talipes, scoliosis
± Hydrocephalus (Arnold–Chiari malformation)

Encephalocoele
(*midline defect of skull with brain protrusion*)

Developmental delay, visual defects
Hydrocephalus, seizures
Operative excision and repair of defect

Anencephaly
(*failure of closure of rostral neuropore, rudimentary brain, large defect of skull and meninges*)

Incompatible with survival

Meningocoele
(*protrusion of meninges only*)

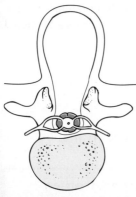

Meningocoele

Meningomyelocoele
(*protrusion of meninges and spinal cord/nerves*)

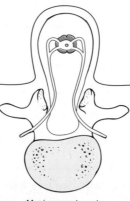

Meningomyelocoele

1 in 1000 live births
Paralysis (UMN) and sensory loss in legs

Figure 20.5 Neural tube defects

Spina bifida

The problems of spina bifida are secondary to the neural damage with subsequent underdevelopment of the lower body, and require multidisciplinary involvement:

Lower limb paralysis (spastic, UMN)	Walking aids, physiotherapy, wheelchair
Lower body absent/abnormal sensation	Skin care to prevent trauma, burns, pressure sores
Bladder and bowel incontinence	Indwelling or intermittent urinary catheter
	Prophylactic antibiotics to prevent recurrent UTIs
	Hydronephrosis may be present
	Regular BP and renal function tests (renal failure can develop)
	Artificial sphincter insertion in some cases
	Laxatives, suppositories, low roughage diet
Orthopaedic	Hip dislocation, talipes, scoliosis (due to muscle imbalances)
Brain	Hydrocephalus (if Arnold–Chiari malformation, see below)

HYDROCEPHALUS

Hydrocephalus is a dilatation of the CSF spaces.

Causes

■ Obstruction to CSF pathways   Intraventricular block:
■ Meningitis
■ Congenital aqueduct stenosis

- **Dandy–Walker syndrome** (occlusion of exit to 4th ventricle, large 4th ventricle and cerebellar hypoplasia)
- **Arnold–Chiari malformation** (downward displacement of cerebellar tonsils and brain stem ± spina bifida)
- Neoplasm or vascular malformation

Extraventricular block:
- Posthaemorrhagic, e.g. SAH in premature infants
- Infection, e.g. TB meningitis
- Leukaemic infiltrates

↓ CSF reabsorption	Venous hypertension from dural sinus thrombosis (from severe dehydration)
↑ CSF production	Choroid plexus tumour (very rare)

Clinical features

These will vary depending on the *duration* and *rate of increase* of the CSF pressure.

Infant	Head circumference increasing and crossing centiles
	Bulging fontanelle and distended scalp veins
	'Setting-sun' eye sign
	Developmental delay
	Ataxia
Older child	Signs of raised intracranial pressure (see below)

Management
- Underlying cause is treated if possible
- Surgical shunt is inserted to drain the excess CSF either to the peritoneum (VP shunt) or the right atrium (VA shunt)

Complications – shunt blockage, shunt infection, traction of line with growth

RAISED INTRACRANIAL PRESSURE

This may be an acute emergency or a chronic disorder, and their presentation is different.

Causes

- Infection – meningitis, encephalitis
- Trauma – intracranial haemorrhage, stroke
- Intracranial mass – brain tumour
- Cerebral oedema – stroke, hepatic encephalopathy, infection
- Disorder of CSF – causes of hydrocephalus, blocked VP or VA shunt
- Benign intracranial hypertension (BIH)

Clinical features of acute raised ICP

Vital signs	BP ↑ and pulse ↓ (the 'Cushing reflex') due to medullary brain ischaemia
	Pupillary dilatation
False localizing signs	III and VI nerve palsies (because these nerves undergo traction injury or compression due to their long pathway)
Coning	i.e. herniation of brain contents
	Bradycardia, hypertension, respiratory depression, bilateral papillary dilatation, decerebrate posturing and then death

Emergency management of acute raised ICP

1. Mannitol 0.25 g/kg over 30 min on 2–3 occasions maximum
2. Hyperventilation (low end of normal range CO_2 causes vasoconstriction)
3. Minimize cerebral metabolism – low–normal temperature, sedation, analgesia, muscle paralysis
4. Treat the cause, e.g. surgery for blocked shunt or acute bleed, steroids for cerebral oedema

Clinical features of chronic raised ICP

- Headache (early morning, worse on lying down and with crying and coughing)
- Drowsiness, diplopia, vomiting
- Papilloedema
- In an infant – bulging fontanelle, macrocephaly and failure to thrive

Features of papilloedema (see p. 409)

Symptoms	Blurred vision and enlarged blind spot
Disc	Blurring of edges, redness and heaping up of the margins, and loss of physiological cup
Retina	Retinal vein dilatation with loss of pulsation and retinal haemorrhages

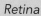

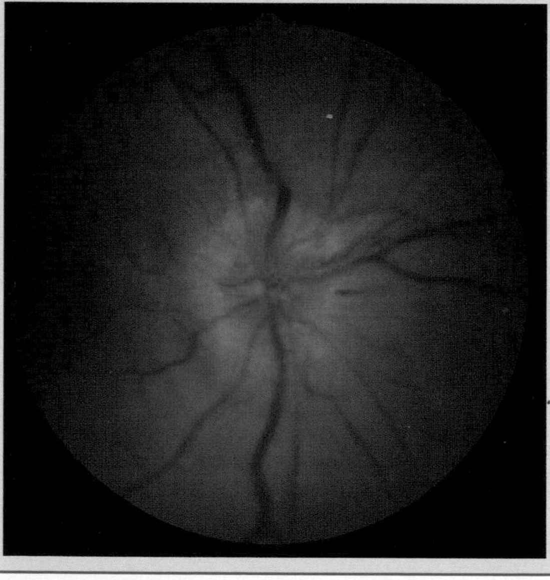

Figure 20.6 Papilloedema. Note the blurring of the disc margins and loss of the physiological cupping (courtesy of Moorfields Eye Hospital, London)

Treatment

- Drugs – acetazolamide, steroids
- Surgical – shunt insertion

SEIZURES

FEBRILE CONVULSIONS

These are convulsions secondary to a fever (often *during rapid temperature rise*) caused by an infection (not directly involving the CNS). They are common (2–4% of children < 5 years will have at least one) and occur because the developing brain cannot withstand rapid and large increases in temperature.

- Males > females
- Positive family history in up to one third
- Normal prior development

Features

Typical febrile convulsion	Age 6 months–5 years
	Generalized tonic–clonic seizure
	< 15 min duration
Complex febrile convulsion	< 6 months or > 5 years
	Focal seizure
	> 15 min duration
	Recurrent episodes within same febrile illness

Investigations

The specific investigations looking for the source of infection depend on the clinical examination and age of the child. A urine specimen for microscopy and culture should be sent, and further tests depend on the clinical findings and any developments in the situation (FBC, CRP, blood cultures, CXR and LP if < 1 year old or unwell and not contraindicated).

Management

- Admit child if it is his/her first fit, if complex or child unwell
- Management of the ABC and seizure control if still fitting (give rectal diazepam if the fit lasts > 5 min, then follow seizure protocol)
- Control the fever with paracetamol or ibuprofen and tepid, i.e. warm, sponging
- If infectious bacterial focus or sepsis suspected, give antibiotics. If herpetic lesions or contact, give aciclovir
- Give parental advice for the future on fever control and management of a fit

> **!** **NB: Tepid sponging means *warm* sponging. If the sponge or cloth becomes cold this has the effect of increasing the infant's core temperature as a compensatory measure to the cold stimulus, with peripheral vasoconstriction.**

Risk of later development of epilepsy

General population risk	0.5%
History of febrile convulsions	1% if typical
	5–10% if risk factors, i.e. complex, family history of epilepsy, delayed milestones, febrile fit < 9 months age

EPILEPSY

A **seizure** is an abnormal burst of electrical activity in the brain. **Epilepsy** is recurrent seizures unrelated to fever or acute brain insult.

Seizures may be:

- **Generalized seizures** (whole cortex involved, always impaired consciousness)
- **Partial seizures** (one area of cortex involved; these may become generalized)

The seizure type is defined by the International Classification of Epileptic Seizures. The EEG shows distinct features with particular seizure types, and specific drugs are used to treat different types.

International Classification of Epileptic Seizures

Generalized seizures	Partial seizures
Absence:	Simple partial (remain conscious):
■ Typical	■ Motor
■ Atypical	■ Sensory
Myoclonic (involuntary jerks)	■ Autonomic
Tonic	■ Physic
Tonic–clonic	Complex partial (impaired consciousness):
Atonic (loss of muscle tone)	■ Simple partial extended
	■ Initial complex partial, e.g. temporal lobe epilepsy
	Partial with secondary generalization

Investigation

It is necessary to do:

- Full history
- Clinical examination, including *developmental check*

For a first convulsion, investigation is necessary only if there are abnormal findings on the examination or the child is < 1 year of age. Further investigations are:

EEG	Demonstrate baseline activity and seizure if occurs during recording
Blood tests	Glucose (peri-ictal)
	Electrolytes, metabolic screen and congenital infection screen
Neuroimaging	USS (infants with patent fontanelle)
	Skull X-ray (shows intracranial calcification and trauma)
	CT brain (do this urgently if unwell)
	MRI brain (?intracranial lesion)

Common seizure types

Absence seizures

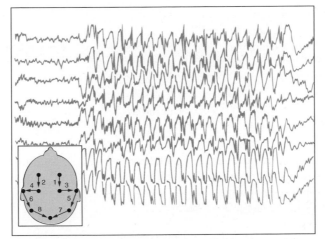

Figure 20.7 EEG pattern in absence seizure

Seizure features	Sudden loss of awareness with eyelid fluttering, last a few seconds, no post–ictal phase
	EEG – 3/s generalized spike and wave
Treatment	Ethosuximide, sodium valproate or lamotrigine

Generalized tonic–clonic seizures

These may be present as idiopathic epilepsy or induced by infection, drugs or stress. An 'aura' preceding them suggests a focal origin.

Seizure features	1. **Tonic phase** – sudden loss of consciousness with a tonic contraction, apnoea, cyanosis and eyes roll backwards
	2. **Clonic phase** – rhythmic contractions of all muscle groups, tongue-biting, loss of sphincter control
	3. **Post-ictal phase** – semiconscious for 30 min–2 h
Treatment	Sodium valproate, carbamazepine or lamotrigine.

Simple partial seizures

These are usually motor seizures, where one limb will have asynchronous tonic or clonic movements and the child is conscious. They can be confused with tics, but the latter can be suppressed temporarily, unlike seizures.

Epilepsy syndromes

There are several syndromes involving one or more types of seizure with associated features. Some of the more well-known epilepsy syndromes are outlined below.

Infantile spasms

This is a rare but devastating epilepsy syndrome in which, at 4–6 months of age, distinctive seizures begin, and development of the child stops. Most have an underlying pathology:

Aetiology not identified (20%)	Normal prior development, examination and brain scan
Aetiology identified (80%)	Structural brain disease, e.g. tuberous sclerosis
	Metabolic disease
	Birth injury, e.g. birth asphyxia
	Postnatal injury, e.g. trauma, meningitis

Epilepsy syndrome	Special features	Seizure types	EEG	Treatment
Childhood absence epilepsy	3–10 years Induced by emotion, hunger, hyperventilation	Absence seizures, typical or atypical	3/s spike and wave	As for absence seizures
Infantile spasms	Onset 4–6 months Associated with arrested development	Symmetrical contractions, extensor, flexor (Salaam spasms) or mixed	Hypsarrhythmia	See below
Temporal lobe epilepsy	May manifest as outbursts of emotions, e.g. laughing or crying Aura, e.g. dysphoria, fear or GI symptoms Due to focal temporal lobe brain injury	Complex partial originating in the temporal lobe	Anterior temporal lobe spikes or waves	Carbamazepine Lamotrigine
Benign Rolandic epilepsy	Peak onset 9–10 years Good prognosis Drooling, abnormal sensations in mouth 25% occur on waking 75% occur in sleep	Partial epilepsy *Complex ?*	Repetitive spikes in Rolandic (centrotemporal) area	Carbamazepine Spontaneous resolution usual by mid-teens
Juvenile myoclonic epilepsy	Onset 12–16 years 25% family history Worse in morning 25% develop absences 90% develop generalized tonic–clonic	Myoclonic jerks, conscious	4–6/s irregular polyspike and wave	Sodium valproate Lamotrigine

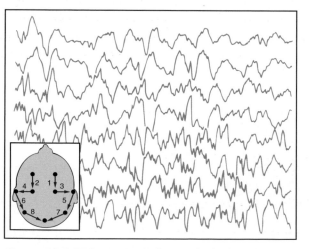

Figure 20.8 EEG pattern in hypsarrhythmia

Seizure features   Bursts of symmetrical contractions of whole body, which may be flexor, extensor or mixed

EEG – hypsarrhythmia (a chaotic EEG with high amplitude activity)

Management	First investigate the cause with:

- MRI brain scan
- Metabolic screen (see ch. 4)
- Chromosome analysis
- If tuberous sclerosis is suspected do a renal USS and echocardiogram

Treatment is with vigabatrin or ACTH

Status epilepticus

See p. 493.

NON-EPILEPTIC FUNNY TURNS

Several conditions mimic epilepsy and must be distinguished from it.

Syncope	Due to cerebral hypoperfusion and hypoxia. There is bradycardia, pallor and collapse. There are different forms:

- **Vasovagal syncope** – precipitated by stress, emotions, confined spaces
- **Reflex anoxic seizures** – due to sensitive vago-cardiac reflex, seen in toddlers after trauma
- **Orthostatic hypotension** – seen in adolescents on standing.
- **Cardiac syncope** – rare in children. Secondary to arrhythmias

Breath-holding attacks	Age 6 months–3 years
	Child holds his/her breath in expiration causing cyanosis, then limpness, unconsciousness, and then tonic stiffening if severe. Rapid recovery
	Precipitated by anger, fear and pain
Night terrors	18 months–7 years
	Child partially wakes upset from deep sleep and is difficult to calm down
Benign paroxysmal vertigo	1–5 years
	Sudden onset of unsteadiness, pallor, horizontal nystagmus and vomiting
	Consciousness is maintained. May be related to migraine

HEADACHES

Headaches are a common problem and are rarely due to serious underlying pathology. A full history and examination should be performed and further investigations done only if there are concerning findings in the history or abnormal examination.

Concerning features in the history

Increase in frequency or severity of headaches
Developmental deterioration
Behavioural change
Features of ↑ ICP, i.e. diffuse, frontal, worse on coughing, on sneezing or lying down, and in the mornings

---

Examination

- Full neurological examination, especially visual fields (? intracranial mass), squint and pupil examination
- Fundoscopy (?ICP↑) and visual acuity
- Head size (? crossing centiles) and growth

- Blood pressure (? high)
- Teeth (? dental caries)
- Face (? sinus pain)
- Cranial bruits examination (? AV malformation)

TENSION HEADACHE

- Common
- Dull ache or sharp pain at the vertex or unclear location
- May occur daily for weeks or be continuous
- Medication often ineffective
- No aura, no precipitants, no neurological signs
- Associated with difficulty sleeping, family or school problems and dizziness

MIGRAINE

These are recurrent headaches of uncertain pathology thought to involve both neurogenic and cerebrovascular mechanisms.

Clinical features

- Throbbing, bifrontal, central, photophobia, better in a dark room, phonophobia
- May wake child from sleep
- Transient hemiplegia or ataxia
- Last 1–72 h
- Headache must be accompanied by at least two of:
  - Nausea
  - Vomiting
  - Abdominal pain
  - Visual aura
  - Family history of migraine

Treatment

General measures	Regular bedtimes, regular meals, sufficient sleep, relaxing after a stressful situation
Avoid stimuli	Stress, insufficient food, some foods (e.g. chocolate, cheese), dehydration, bright lights, sunshine, lack of sleep
Acute episode	Bed rest/sleep in a quiet dark room

Causes of headaches and other underlying pathology

Neurological	Post-ictal
	Post-concussion
	Meningitis or encephalitis
	Hydrocephalus (VP shunt blockage)
	Intracranial haemorrhage
	Benign intracranial hypertension
	Brain tumour
Other	Other infective illness (commonly URTI or viral illness)
	Dental malocclusion (Costen's syndrome), dental caries, e.g. tooth abscess
	Myopia, hypermetropia
	Sinusitis

Drugs:
- Analgesics, e.g. paracetamol, and antiemetic if nausea
- If severe and > 12 years old can give selective 5-HT agonist

Prophylaxis Pizotifen (histamine [H1] and serotonin receptor antagonist licensed in children > 2 years old)

ATAXIA

Ataxia is due to:

- Cerebellar disease (*most common cause in children*), or
- Sensory loss (proprioception)

It is useful to divide cerebellar ataxia into **acute** or **chronic**, **intermittent** or **progressive** causes (see below).

Causes

Acute	**Chronic**
Cerebral infections (encephalitis):	Cerebral palsy (ataxic)
During infection, e.g. coxsackie, echovirus, EBV	Congenital anomalies – Dandy–Walker malformation (see p. 365)
Post-infectious, e.g. varicella	
Toxic – phenytoin, alcohol	
Tumour – posterior fossa/brain stem	
Acute intermittent	**Progressive**
Seizures	Cerebellar tumour
Migraine	Cerebellar abscess
	Subdural haematoma
	Friedreich ataxia
	Ataxia telangiectasia

Examination of cerebellar function

General	Nystagmus, tremor
Speech	Dysarthria?
Eyes	Horizontal nystagmus (goes towards the side of the lesion)
Upper arms out	? Drifting (with eyes open) (a drift only with eyes closed = proprioception defect)
Truncal ataxia	Sit from lying with arms folded
Finger–nose	Intention tremor and past-pointing
Dysdiadokinesis	Rapid pronation and supination of the hand
Lower limbs	Hypotonia ?, heel–shin test, toe–finger test, tap feet rapidly
Knee jerks	? Pendular (severe cerebellar dysfunction)
Walk	Normally, then heel–toe (staggering to affected side)

FRIEDREICH ATAXIA

Autosomal recessive disorder of progressive degeneration of cerebellar tracts and dorsal columns. Gene on chromosome 9q13.21.1, encodes for the protein frataxin.

Clinical features

- Progressive ataxia and dysarthria
- Lower limb weakness (present with difficulty walking around 10–12 years of age)
- Loss of position and vibration sense
- Loss of deep tendon reflexes
- Pes cavus and scoliosis
- Cardiomyopathy, diabetes mellitus, optic atrophy, nystagmus
- Death around age 40 years

CEREBRAL PALSY

Cerebral palsy is a disorder of movement and posture due to a *non-progressive* lesion in the developing brain. Prevalence 2 in 1000 population.

Several additional impairments accompany the above definition:

- Learning impairment
- Visual impairment and squint
- Hearing loss
- Speech and language difficulties
- Behavioural problems
- Epilepsy

Causes

Antenatal (80%)	Cerebral malformation, cerebral dysgenesis, congenital infection
Intrapartum (10%)	Hypoxic–ischaemic encephalopathy (birth asphyxia)
Postnatal (10%)	Cerebral ischaemia, intraventricular haemorrhage, head trauma, Hydrocephalus, non-accidental injury, hyperbilirubinaemia (severe neonatal)

Classification of types

Spastic	Initial hypotonia progressing to spasticity with UMN signs. It may be:
	- **Hemiplegia** – unilateral involvement, e.g. meningitis
	- **Diplegia** – legs > arms, e.g. hypoxic ischaemic encephalopathy (HIE)
	- **Quadriplegia** (whole body), e.g. HIE
Ataxic hypotonic	Hypotonia, poor balance, tremor, incoordinate movements
Dyskinetic	Involuntary movements, fluctuating muscle tone (dyskinesia), poor postural tone

---

Presentations of cerebral palsy

Delayed motor milestones
Abnormal tone in infancy
Persistence of primitive reflexes
Abnormal gait
Feeding difficulties
Other developmental delay, e.g. language, social

Investigations

It is necessary to do:

- Brain imaging (USS in neonates, CT or MRI scan)
- Metabolic screen (see p. 279)
- Congenital infection screen

Management

Cerebral palsy can be very mild, requiring little input, or if severe, huge resources and multidisciplinary involvement from:

- Occupational therapist, physiotherapist, speech therapist,
- Social worker, teacher, developmental psychologist
- Paediatrician, orthopaedic surgeon, neurologist, ophthalmologist and audiologist

STROKE

A *focal* neurological deficit with an *underlying vascular pathology* is defined as:

- **Stroke** – lasting > 24 h
- **Transient ischaemic attack (TIA)** – lasting < 24 h
- **Reversible ischaemic neurological deficit (RIND)** – lasting > 24 h but with full recovery

There are also 'stroke-like episodes', in which there is a focal neurological deficit lasting > 24 h, but no obvious vascular pathology, e.g. brain tumour, brain abscess.

Causes

Stroke is due to **haemorrhage** or **ischaemia**. Ischaemia is caused by vessel spasm, stenosis, dissection, or vessel occlusion (by thrombosis or embolism).

Ischaemia	Thrombosis:
	■ Sickle cell disease
	■ Severe dehydration (venous sinus thrombosis)
	■ Meningitis
	■ Clotting disorder, e.g. protein S or C deficiency, factor V Leiden
	■ Leukaemia, thrombocytosis
	Embolism – cyanotic congenital heart disease, endocarditis
	Vessel spasm – meningitis
	Large vessel stenosis:
	■ Sickle cell disease
	■ Varicella
	■ Homocystinuria
	Vessel dissection:
	■ Trauma
	■ Congenital heart disease
Haemorrhage	Thrombocytopaenia – immune thrombocytopaenia (ITP)
	Bleeding disorder – haemophilia
	Vessel disorder – cerebral aneurysm, A-V malformation
	Trauma

Clinical features

- Seizures (common in neonates)
- Deterioration in level of consciousness (in extension of bleed)
- Hemiparesis, hemisensory loss, visual field defect
- ↑ ICP

Investigations

These will be led by any underlying disease. A good history and examination are essential to elucidate the cause.

Imaging

MRI brain scan	To outline affected area (thrombosis, bleed, abscess, tumour, etc.)
CT scan	(If MRI unavailable) to exclude haemorrhage
Magnetic resonance angiography (MRA)	For a vascular outline
Transcranial Doppler USS	Large vessel disease
Cerebral angiogram	For more detailed vascular outline
	If MRA is normal in ischaemia
	After haemorrhage to look, e.g., for AV malformation

Other investigations

ECG and echocardiogram	To check for cardiac anomaly or arrhythmia
Infection screen	
Haematological screen	Including sickle screen, FBC and clotting defects
Metabolic screen	If metabolic disease suspected

Management

The acute management is dependent on the cause, e.g. surgery in cerebral aneurysm. Aspirin therapy is commenced in ischaemic stroke.

Extensive rehabilitation, depending on the severity of the stroke, with a multidisciplinary input will be required for recovery, including involvement from a paediatrician, physiotherapist, neurologist, neurosurgeon, occupational therapist, educational psychologist and speech therapist.

NEUROECTODERMAL DISORDERS

The neuroectodermal disorders involve a defect in the differentiation of the primitive ectoderm (which makes both the *skin* and *nervous system*), and include:

- Neurofibromatosis
- Tuberous sclerosis
- Sturge–Weber syndrome (see p. 302)
- von Hippel–Lindau disease
- Ataxia telangiectasia (see p. 106)

NEUROFIBROMATOSIS (VON RECKLINGHAUSEN DISEASE)

This relatively common condition (incidence 1 in 4000) is autosomal dominant or a result of a new mutation (in 50% of cases). It is extremely variable in its severity, and there are two distinct types.

Neurofibromatosis type 1 (NF1)

Gene on chromosome 17q.

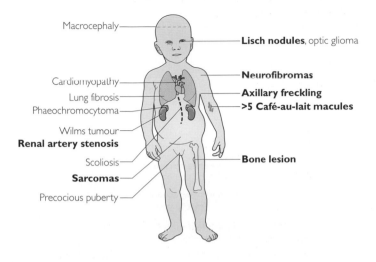

Macrocephaly

Lisch nodules, optic glioma

Cardiomyopathy

Neurofibromas

Lung fibrosis

Axillary freckling

Phaeochromocytoma

>5 Café-au-lait macules

Wilms tumour

Renal artery stenosis

Scoliosis

Bone lesion

Sarcomas

Precocious puberty

Figure 20.9 Clinical features of neurofibromatosis type 1 (NF1). Pathognomonic features are in bold

Diagnosis of NF1

Made if two or more of:

- Six or more café-au-lait macules (prepubertal 5 mm size; postpubertal 15 mm size)
- Axillary freckles
- At least two neurofibromas or one plexiform (large) neurofibroma
- At least two Lisch nodules (hamartomas) in the iris
- Bone lesion – osseous dysplasia of the sphenoid or cortex of a long bone
- Optic glioma
- First-degree relative with NF

Neurofibromatosis type 2 (NF2)

Gene on chromosome 22q. This is rarer than NF1 and the features are:

- VIIIth nerve acoustic neuromas (unilateral or bilateral)
- Other brain or spinal tumours, e.g. meningioma, glioma, Schwannoma
- Neurofibromas, café-au-lait macules

Investigations

These are led by clinical examination:

- MRI brain and optic nerves (optic glioma?)
- Ophthalmological assessment
- Skeletal survey
- EEG
- Audiogram
- Psychometric testing

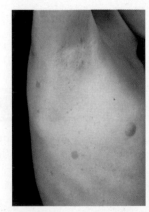

Figure 20.10 Axillary freckling and café-au-lait macules in a 10-year-old boy with neurofibromatosis type 1

Management

Genetic counselling to the family. Yearly assessment including:

- Neurological examination
- Auditory and visual screening
- Blood pressure check

TUBEROUS SCLEROSIS COMPLEX

This autosomal dominant condition is very variable in its clinical severity. Genes on chromosome 9q and 16p. Autosomal dominant 80% new mutations.

Clinical features

Three major features (in bold) are required for diagnosis.

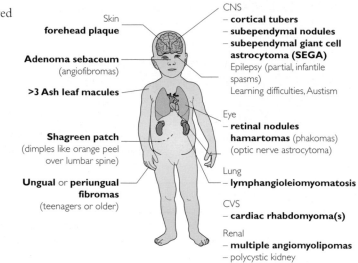

Skin
forehead plaque

Adenoma sebaceum
(angiofibromas)

>3 Ash leaf macules

Shagreen patch
(dimples like orange peel
over lumbar spine)

Ungual or **periungual
fibromas**
(teenagers or older)

CNS
– **cortical tubers**
– **subependymal nodules**
– **subependymal giant cell
astrocytoma (SEGA)**
Epilepsy (partial, infantile
spasms)
Learning difficulties, Austism

Eye
– **retinal nodules
hamartomas** (phakomas)
(optic nerve astrocytoma)

Lung
– **lymphangioleiomyomatosis**

CVS
– **cardiac rhabdomyoma(s)**

Renal
– **multiple angiomyolipomas**
– polycystic kidney

Figure 20.11 Clinical features of tuberous sclerosis complex

Investigations

Baseline investigations to look for associated features.

Management

- Seizure control
- Genetic counselling
- Regular follow-up – renal USS, BP check, echocardiogram, CXR, eye examination, neuroimaging (CT/MRI brain scan)

NEURODEGENERATIVE DISORDERS

Neurodegenerative disorders are diseases with a *progressive deterioration in neurological function*, with loss of speech, vision, hearing or locomotion, and often associated with seizures, feeding difficulties and intellectual impairment.

Features

- Usually rare neurometabolic autosomal recessive disorders due to a specific enzyme defect, but may be due to chronic viral infection, e.g. subacute sclerosing panencephalitis (SSPE), prion infection, e.g. Creutzfeldt–Jakob disease (CJD) or other unknown cause

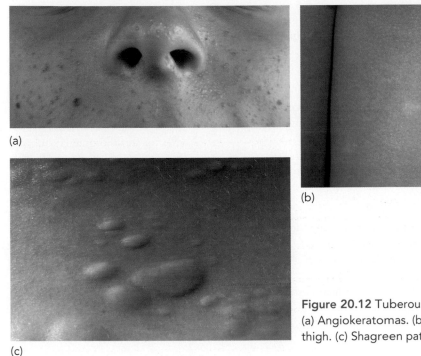

(a)

(b)

(c)

Figure 20.12 Tuberous sclerosis complex.
(a) Angiokeratomas. (b) Ash leaf macule on the
thigh. (c) Shagreen patches on the lower back

- In the metabolic conditions, neuronal degeneration occurs as a result of a build-up of the product preceding the missing enzyme, which is toxic to the nervous system, or lack of an essential metabolite. The excess product will also cause other effects and result in the characteristic disease findings. Some of these diseases are termed 'storage disorders' referring to the storage of the accumulated substance
- Subdivided into predominantly grey matter or white matter disorders:
  - White matter disease – UMN signs early on
  - Grey matter disease – convulsions, intellectual and visual impairment
- May present congenitally or in early or late childhood, adolescence or adulthood
- Generally progress relentlessly until death occurs months or years from onset

Types

Neurometabolic disorders	
Lysosomal storage disorders	Mucopolysaccharidosis, e.g. Hunter disease (see p. 274)
	Sphingolipidosis, e.g. Tay–Sachs disease (see p. 274)
Peroxisomal disorders	Peroxisomal biogenesis disorders (see p. 279)
Organic acidaemias	Methylmalonic acidaemia (see p. 275)
Amino acidopathies	Homocystinuria (see p. 274)
Metal overload disorders	Wilson disease (see p. 207)
Infections	
Slow virus	SSPE (due to altered host response to measles), HIV dementia
Prion infection	Creutzfeldt–Jakob disease
Other	Rett syndrome

Investigations

These should be led by the clinical features, especially MRI findings. Often there will be features strongly suggesting a certain group of diagnoses.

All patients

Radiology	MRI brain scan
Blood	Blood tests for metabolic disorders
	Copper and caeruloplasmin (Wilson disease)
	HIV status
	Karyotype
Urine	Urine tests as for metabolic disorders

Consider

DNA	E.g. Rett, fragile X
	(Molecular tests are becoming more first-line in the investigation of neurodegenerative conditions)
CSF	Tests as for metabolic disorders
	Measles antibody (SSPE)
Neurophysiology	EMG, EEG, nerve conduction studies
Histology	Muscle biopsy (mitochondrial disorders [see p. 286])

RETT SYNDROME

A rare neurodegenerative disease. The gene is *McCP2* on chromosome Xq28. Only females are affected.

Presentation is generally after 1 year of age with:

- Developmental regression (language and motor milestones)
- Characteristic 'hand wringing' repetitious movements and loss of hand function
- Ataxic gait
- Acquired microcephaly
- Autistic features
- Apnoeas, sighing respirations
- Seizures (generalized tonic–clonic)
- Death between 10 and 30 years (often from cardiac arrhythmias)

SUBACUTE SCLEROSING PANENCEPHALITIS

This is a neurodegenerative disease secondary to an altered host response to the measles virus. Incidence 1 in 100 000.

Usually develops 5–7 years after measles infection with:

- Insidious onset of intellectual deterioration, abnormal behaviour
- Rapid progression with intractable myoclonus, dementia and death
- EEG shows characteristic periodic complexes
- CSF may contain intrathecal antimeasles antibody

There is no effective treatment.

Clinical scenario

An 8-year-old girl starts complaining of headaches in the morning and has a strong family history of migraines. The headaches are accompanied by nausea and are worsening, exacerbated by coughing and lying down.

She is examined by her GP who notes a lack of meningism and delivers a diagnosis of school-related stress which is indeed occurring with a degree of bullying.

1. What is your differential diagnosis?

She then develops a squint and diplopia. On examination she has blurred disc margins and a degree of double vision especially on looking upwards.

2. What management and investigations are most appropriate now?

ANSWERS

1. Causes of raised intracranial pressure, e.g. space-occupying lesion; encephalitis; benign intracranial pressure; less likely congenital structural block to flow of CSF
2. Consider reduction of intracranial pressure with agents such as intravenous mannitol. Assisted ventilation to induce hypocapnia can provide temporary fall in intracranial pressure. Close and frequent neuro-observations. Urgent CT or MRI scan

FURTHER READING

David R (ed.). *Clinical Pediatric Neurology*, 3rd edn. New York: Demos Medical Publishing, 2009.

Fenichel G. *Clinical Pediatric Neurology: A Signs and Symptoms Approach*, 5th edn. London: Saunders, 2005.

Cohen M, Duffner P. *Weiner & Levitt's Pediatric neurology*, 4th edn. London: Lippincott Williams & Wilkins, 2003.

21 Neuromuscular Disorders

- Floppy baby
- Hereditary motor–sensory neuropathies (Charcot–Marie–Tooth)
- Myasthenia gravis
- Guillain–Barré disease
- Muscular dystrophies
- Congenital myopathies
- Further reading

Neuromuscular disorders are diseases in which the main pathology is peripheral. They can be remembered and classified according to where along the motor pathway the pathology exists.

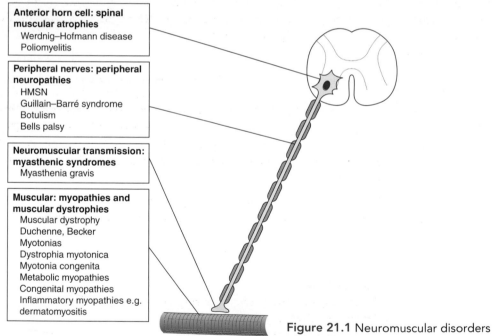

Anterior horn cell: spinal muscular atrophies
  Werdnig–Hofmann disease
  Poliomyelitis

Peripheral nerves: peripheral neuropathies
  HMSN
  Guillain–Barré syndrome
  Botulism
  Bells palsy

Neuromuscular transmission: myasthenic syndromes
  Myasthenia gravis

Muscular: myopathies and muscular dystrophies
  Muscular dystrophy
  Duchenne, Becker
  Myotonias
  Dystrophia myotonica
  Myotonia congenita
  Metabolic myopathies
  Congenital myopathies
  Inflammatory myopathies e.g. dermatomyositis

Figure 21.1 Neuromuscular disorders

They result in muscular weakness, often progressive.

CLINICAL FEATURES

Neonatal presentation

In utero:
- Polyhydramnios
- Reduced fetal movements

	Arthrogryphosis
	Hypotonia (floppy baby)
	Feeding difficulties
	Breathing difficulties (may need respiratory support)
Older children	Motor delay
	Gait abnormalities
	Muscle weakness
	Muscle fatiguability

SPECIFIC INVESTIGATIONS

These are tailored to the clinical features.

EMG	Specific features may be seen, e.g. muscular dystrophy, myotonic dystrophy
Muscle imaging (USS, MRI)	Myopathies, muscular dystrophies
Muscle biopsy	Spinal muscular atrophy (SMA), Duchenne muscular dystrophy, myotonic dystrophy, congenital myopathies
Nerve stimulation test	Myasthenia gravis
Nerve conduction studies	Hereditary motor–sensory neuropathy (HMSN), SMA, Guillain–Barré disease
Sural nerve biopsy	HMSN
Creatine phosphokinase	↑ in myotonic dystrophy and Duchenne muscular dystrophy
DNA analysis	Specific disorders, e.g. muscular dystrophy, myotonic dystrophy
Tensilon test	Myasthenia gravis
Acetylcholine receptor antibodies	Myasthenia gravis

FLOPPY BABY

The congenital neuromuscular disorders present as a neonatal hypotonia ('floppy baby'). The many causes of a floppy baby can be divided into *central* (brain and spinal cord) and *peripheral* (neuromuscular). The latter are identified by the additional presence of *weakness* (limb movement absent or decreased), although in practice they can be difficult to differentiate:

- *Central causes* – floppy only (*limb antigravity movement present*)
- Neuromuscular causes – *floppy and weak* (*no/reduced limb antigravity movement*)

Causes

Central	Neonatal sepsis
	Drugs, e.g. maternal pethidine during delivery
	Hypoxic–ischaemic encephalopathy
	Metabolic disease, e.g. hypothyroidism
	Syndromic, e.g. Down syndrome, fetal alcohol syndrome
Neuromuscular	Anterior horn cell disorder, e.g. SMA
	Neuromuscular junction disorder, e.g. transient neonatal myasthenia
	Skeletal muscle disorder, e.g. congenital myopathy, congenital myotonic dystrophy

Clinical features of a floppy baby with a neuromuscular disorder

In utero:
- Polyhydramnios
- Reduced fetal movements

Arthrogryphosis

Hypotonia:
- **Frog-like** position while resting
- **Head lag** (little or no head control)
- Neurological 'flip-over' examination
- demonstrates weakness in all positions (see p. 356)

Feeding difficulties

Breathing difficulties

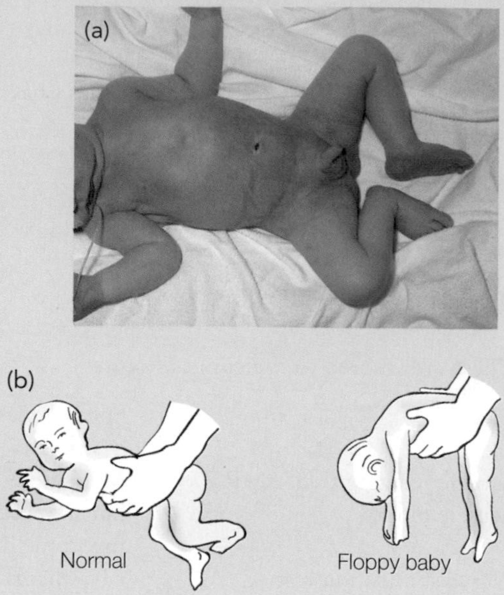

Figure 21.2 Floppy baby. (a) Frog-like position (b) Poor head control in ventral suspension.

Normal   Floppy baby

SPINAL MUSCULAR ATROPHY TYPE 1 (WERDNIG–HOFFMAN DISEASE)

This is an autosomal recessive, severe disease due to *progressive degeneration of the anterior horn cells.* Deletion in *SMN1* gene 5q11–13. Incidence approximately 4 in 100 000.

Clinical features

- **Severely affected** – *floppy and weak*
- **Decreased fetal movements *in utero***
- Respiratory distress (death in infancy from respiratory failure)
- Tongue and other muscle **fasciculation**
- Absent reflexes
- Progressive weakness

DNA testing is possible to confirm diagnosis and management is supportive only.

HEREDITARY MOTOR–SENSORY NEUROPATHIES (CHARCOT–MARIE–TOOTH)

This is a group of many disorders in which there is *progressive disease of the peripheral nerves* involving demyelination and/or axonal degeneration. Treatment is supportive only.

HMSN Type 1 (CMT 1)

Autosomal dominant disorder with different genes underlying different subtypes. Peripheral myelin protein 22 (PMP-22) gene mutations in CMT 1A. Prevalence 15 in 100 000.

Clinical features

- Presentation in late childhood
- Progressive distal weakness:
  - Weakness of dorsiflexion (foot drop), pes cavus
  - Gait disturbance

- Absent tendon reflexes
- Milder involvement of hands
- Distal sensory loss:
  – Paraesthesias
  – Loss of proprioception and vibration

Investigations

DNA testing	
Nerve conduction studies	Reduced motor and sensory velocities; differentiate demyelinating from axonal
Sural nerve biopsy	'Onion bulb' formations of Schwann cell cytoplasm (due to de- and re-myelination. Not necessary for diagnosis)

MYASTHENIA GRAVIS

This is a disease of immunological neuromuscular blockade in which there are *IgG antibodies to acetylcholine receptors (AchR)*. Incidence approximately 15 in 100 000.

Clinical features

- External ocular muscle weakness, diplopia, ptosis
- Dysphagia (bulbar muscle involvement)
- Sad facial expression (facial muscle weakness)
- Proximal muscle weakness
- **Muscle fatiguability**, i.e. progressive weakness with *use* (a cardinal feature)
- Reflexes fatiguable

Investigations

Tensilon test	Anticholinesterase given intravenously – causes transient relief
Serum	AChR antibodies present (in 90%)
Nerve stimulation	Fibrillation and decreased muscle response with repetition

Management

- Regular anticholinesterase drugs, e.g. neostigmine, given 4–6 hourly
- Antibodies can be removed using thymectomy, steroids or plasmapheresis

---

Transient neonatal myasthenia gravis

In a pregnant mother suffering from myasthenia gravis, AChR antibodies will cross the placenta (they are IgG antibodies) and cause a transient neonatal disease, generally lasting 2–3 weeks.

GUILLAIN–BARRÉ DISEASE

This is a *postinfectious demyelinating neuropathy*, developing 1–3 weeks after an often trivial viral infection.

Clinical features

- Distal limb weakness which is ascending and symmetrical
- Areflexia

385

- Muscle pain and paraesthesia
- Urinary retention or incontinence
- Respiratory muscle and facial weakness (20%)

Investigations

This is a clinical diagnosis.

Lumbar puncture	Very high CSF protein (twice normal), oligoclonal bands
	Normal WCC and normal glucose
Nerve conduction studies	Delay in both motor and sensory conduction

Management

This is essentially supportive, with ventilation in severe cases. Spontaneous recovery after 2–3 weeks is usual, although there may be some residual weakness. Intravenous gamma-globulin reduces the duration and severity. Plasmapheresis is occasionally used.

MUSCULAR DYSTROPHIES

These are genetic myopathies involving *progressive disease and death of muscle fibres*.

	Inheritance	Features
Duchenne MD	XR (dsytrophin absent)	See below
Becker MD	XR (dystrophin reduced)	Similar but less severe then Duchenne MD
Emery–Dreifuss MD	XR	Scapulohumeral weakness, contractures
Facioscapulohumoral MD	AD	Face and shoulder weakness
Limb girdle MD	AD, AR	Proximal limb weakness

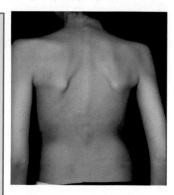

Figure 21.3 Scapulohumeral dystrophy – note winging of the scapula

DUCHENNE MUSCULAR DYSTROPHY

This is an X-linked recessive disorder, i.e. only boys affected, caused by mutation in the dystrophin gene (chromosome Xp21.3), leading to absence of this muscle protein.

Clinical features

Normal early motor development	
Proximal limb weakness	Evident from 3 years of age
	Gower's sign present – a manoeuvre to stand from lying down involving rolling over, then using the hands to 'climb up' the knees
	Waddling (**Trendelenburg**) gait
Calf muscle pseudohypertrophy	As a toddler
Progressive deterioration	Eventually wheelchair bound (usually by teenage) with scoliosis
	Pharyngeal weakness and respiratory failure develop

| Cardiac muscle | Dilated cardiomyopathy |
| Learning disability | In one-third |

Investigations

Creatinine phosphokinase (CK)	Extremely elevated (↑ × 10 normal)
Muscle biopsy	Fibre necrosis, fat infiltration, no dystrophin on staining
EMG	Myopathic pattern
Cardiac investigations	ECG and CXR

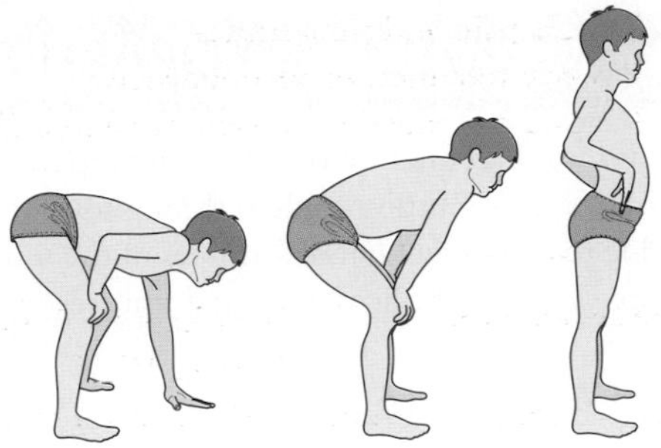

Figure 21.4 Gower's sign

Management

This is supportive only, with physiotherapy, nutritional support, orthopaedic involvement and occupational therapy.

The *prognosis* is poor with eventual death from respiratory complications.

> **!** **NB: Antenatal detection of Duchenne muscular dystrophy is possible on CVS sampling using DNA probes. Female carriers have CK ↑ in 70% of cases.**

MYOTONIC DYSTROPHY

This is an autosomal dominant condition of progressive distal muscle weakness in which the cardinal feature is a *failure of muscle relaxation (myotonia)*. Chromosome 19q13 expansion with numerous trinucleotide CTG repeats. **Anticipation** occurs, i.e. more severe with each generation (see p. 26).

Clinical features

May present in the neonatal period or later.

Face	**Fish mouth** (inverted 'V' shape to upper lip)
	Facial muscle weakness
Eyes	Ptosis, cataracts
Other muscles	Weakness of distal limbs and respiratory muscles
Cardiac	Cardiomyopathy, conduction defects
Mental	Learning disabilities (50%)
Hair	Frontal baldness in males
Endocrine	Hypogonadism, glucose intolerance
Immunity	IgG ↓
Gastrointestinal	Constipation

Investigations

■ Diagnosis is clinical. Shake hands with the child (if old enough) and the parent and they *cannot* quickly let go
■ Muscle biopsy – prognostic value in neonates
■ EMG – classic findings seen after infancy
■ Endocrine, immunoglobulin and cardiac assessment is necessary

Management

Phenytoin or carbamazepine can help with the myotonia.

CONGENITAL MYOPATHIES

The term congenital myopathies encompasses many unrelated congenital diseases of the muscles. These may be mild, causing little problem throughout life, or severe; they may also be either static or progressive. Some are due to ultrastructural deformities of the muscles, and some to abnormalities within the mitochondrial DNA and involve metabolic defects and features in other organs. Muscle biopsy is usually involved in diagnosis.

Clinical features

- Those of neuromuscular causes of a floppy baby, i.e. neonatal hypotonia with *weakness* (see p. 383)
- Distinctive appearance with a thin muscle mass at birth and undescended testicles
- Features may be mild at birth but are often progressive

Examples

	Underlying problem	Features in addition to myopathy
Myotubular myopathy	Disorder of muscle ultrastructure Possibly due to developmental arrest Usually X-linked recessive	Features of severe myopathy at birth – ptosis prominent Most die within few weeks of birth
Nemaline rod myopathy	Abnormal rod-shaped inclusions within muscle fibres (mostly α-actinin) Autosomal dominant or recessive	Dolicocephalic, high arched palate May die in infancy or survive with severe weakness

Clinical scenario

A 4-year-old boy, who was only walking at 2 years of age, is noted by his parents to have a strange way of getting up from the floor when sitting, using his upper limbs to 'climb' up his legs, and when lying down he would roll over then perform the same manoeuvre. On examination, his calves are noted to be quite large and he walks with his hips dropping down on the side on which his leg bears weight.

He is examined by his GP, who notes a lack of meningism and delivers a diagnosis of school-related stress, which is indeed occurring with a degree of bullying.

1. What is the likeliest diagnosis?
2. What three investigations would you perform?
3. What treatment regime would you organise?

ANSWERS

1. Duchenne muscular dystrophy
2. Any three of: creatine phosphokinase, muscle biopsy, electromyography, *dystrophin* gene testing; possibly ECG and echocardiogram for cardiomyopathy
3. Physiotherapy. Occupational therapy. Later nutritional support e.g. gastrostomy feeding, and prevention of chest infections. Orthopaedic involvement for splints and orthotic devices to aid in mobility. Financial support with Childcare Disability Allowance

FURTHER READING

Benson M, Fixsen J, Parsch K, Macnicol M (eds.). *Children's Neuromuscular Disorders*. Berlin: Springer Verlag, 2011.

Royden Jones H, De Vivo D, Darras B. *Neuromuscular Disorders of Infancy, Childhood and Adolescence: A Clinician's Approach*. Oxford: Butterworth-Heinemann, 2002.

Further reading

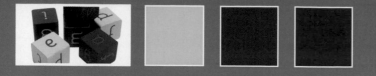

22 Rheumatological and Musculoskeletal Disorders

- History and examination
- Juvenile idiopathic arthritis
- Systemic lupus erythematosus
- Juvenile dermatomyositis
- Scleroderma
- Ehlers–Danlos syndromes
- Vasculitis
- Non-inflammatory pain syndromes
- Osteogenesis imperfecta
- Osteochondrodysplasias
- Back disorders
- Infections
- Further reading

HISTORY AND EXAMINATION

HISTORY/COMMON SYMPTOMS OF JOINT DYSFUNCTION

Joint	Stiffness (early morning)
	Swelling
	Pain
	Restricted joint movement
	Reduced activities of daily living
	Limp, abnormal gait
	Growth deformity
General	Trauma
	Fevers, malaise, weight loss
	Rashes
	Infection (preceding, concurrent or contact)
	Sore mouth
	Hair loss, nail changes
	Visual disturbance
	Bowel symptoms
	Family history
	Travel history

! **NB: Knee pain may be referred hip pain.**

JOINT EXAMINATION

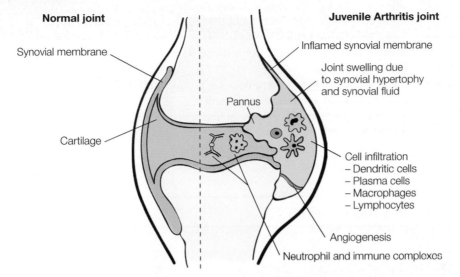

Figure 22.1 Joint – normal and in juvenile arthritis. In response to chemical and cytokine mediators released by inflammatory cells, the synovial membrane hypertrophies to form pannus and, with time, this erodes into the articular surface of the joint

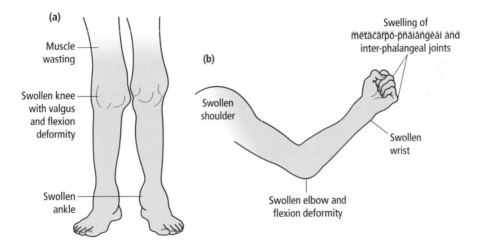

Figure 22.2 Arthritis. (a) Effects on the lower limb. (b) Effects on the upper limb (courtesy of Dr Nick Wilkinson)

Examine with child facing so that movements to be copied can be demonstrated to the child.

Inspection   Limbs fully exposed
                       Swelling, loss of normal contours, erythema, scars
                       Resting position, deformity
                       Muscle wasting, protective muscle spasm
                       Distribution and symmetry of joint involvement

Palpation	Warmth, tenderness (percuss spine for tenderness)
	Effusion, synovial thickening (boggy swelling)
	Enthesitis (swelling of insertion of tendon/ligament/capsule to bone)
	Tendonitis, contractures
Movement	**Active** (describe the angle from neutral. Use your own joints or compare to normal limb)
	Passive (if active movement does not produce full range. Note excess movement)
	Pain during and at limits of movement
	Test ligaments (hypermobile, tight/shortened or tender)
	Muscle power
Measurements	Limb length, muscle wasting (circumference)
Function	Gait, undressing and dressing, combing hair, shaking hands, writing, scratching back

Joint-dependent movements

Flexion and extension, e.g. elbow
Pronation and supination, e.g. elbow
Radial deviation and ulnar deviation, e.g. wrist
Abduction and adduction, e.g. hips, shoulders
Internal rotation and external rotation, e.g. hips
Rotation, e.g. neck

Order of joint examination

Assess the **normal joint first** (for comparison), then the abnormal.

Upper limbs	Fingers, wrists, elbows, shoulders
Spine	Jaw, cervical spine, thoracolumbar spine, sacroiliac joints
Lower limbs	Hips, knees, ankles, feet

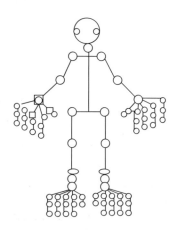

Figure 22.3 Joints assessed in rheumatological examination

RHEUMATOLOGICAL INVESTIGATIONS

Full blood count	Hb – anaemia of chronic disease, haemolytic anaemia (SLE)
	Platelets – thrombocytosis (JIA, vasculitis, e.g. Kawasaki disease), thrombocytopaenia (SLE)
	WCC – lymphopaenia (SLE), neutropaenia (SLE, drugs), leukocytosis (JIA)

Autoantibodies   None is diagnostic!
Imaging   X-rays
                  Bone scans
                  USS bone/joints
                  MRI and CT scans

JUVENILE IDIOPATHIC ARTHRITIS

Juvenile idiopathic arthritis (JIA) is a group of disorders defined as:

- *Chronic synovitis > 6 weeks* ± extra-articular features
- Occurring *before 16 years* of age
- Sub-classified at 6 months since onset according to the sum of features:
  - **Oligoarticular JIA** (≤ 4 large joints)
  - **Polyarticular JIA** (> 4 joints involved)
  - **Systemic-onset JIA**
  - **Spondyloarthropathies**

The cause is unknown, although genetic, immunological and infective mechanisms are contributory.

Clinical features of involved joints

- Early morning joint stiffness
- Joint swelling, warm (not hot), occasionally red and tender
- Limited painful joint movement
- Joint contractures may develop rapidly

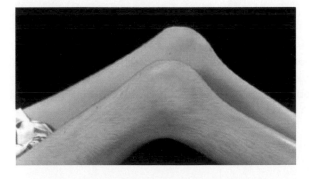

Figure 22.4 Fixed flexion deformity in the knee of a child with JIA (courtesy of Dr Nick Wilkinson)

Distortion of bone growth by chronic synovitis

	TMJ (temperomandibular joint)	micrognathia, dental and anaesthetic problems
	Cervical spine	fusion or subluxation (anaesthetic difficulties)
	Wrist	subluxation and ankylosis
	Hips	destruction (avascular necrosis) and limb shortening
	Knees	bony overgrowth, increased leg length, valgus deformity

X-ray changes

Early — Soft tissue swelling
Osteopaenia
Periosteal new bone
formation

Late — Bony overgrowth
Osteoporosis
Subchondral bone
erosions
Joint space narrowing
Collapse, deformity,
subluxation, fusion

Osteopaenia

Carpal crowding

No specific
evidence of
erosions

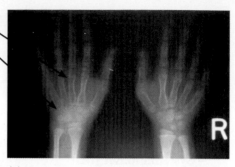

(a)

Osteopaenia
and
overgrowth of
medial condyle
resulting in valgus
deformity and
likely leg length
discrepancy

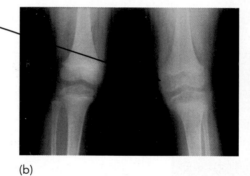

(b)

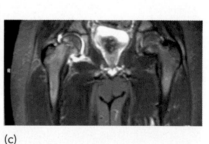

(c)

Figure 22.5 JIA. (a) Hand X-ray in early disease. Note osteopaenia and carpal crowding. There is no specific evidence of erosions. (b) Knee X-ray in more advanced disease. Note osteopaenia and overgrowth of the medial condyle resulting in valgus deformity and likely leg length discrepancy. (c) MRI of the hips (STIR sequence) showing increased signal around the right femoral head consistent with synovial hypertrophy and/or fluid (courtesy of Dr Nick Wilkinson)

Management

Early intervention improves prognosis and may delay or prevent irreversible bony changes and loss of function.

- Physiotherapy, occupational therapy, podiatry (for stretching, increasing strength, improving function, joint splinting, foot orthoses)
- NSAIDs
- Intra-articular steroid injections
- Disease-modifying drugs (DMARDs) if polyarticular or uncontrolled oligoarticular or systemic, e.g. methotrexate; etanercept (anti–TNF therapy); monoclonal anti–TNF antibody therapy
- Sulphasalazine for enthesitis–related arthropathy (ERA)
- Steroids – oral prednisolone or pulsed intravenous methylprednisolone if rapid control required, but aim to withdraw as soon as possible

(a)
(b)

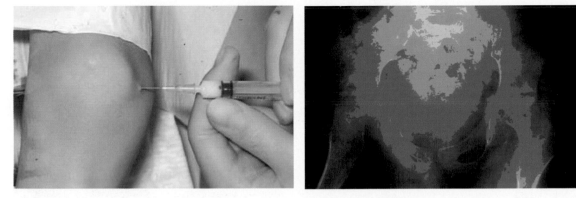

Figure 22.6 (a) Injection of a knee joint with corticosteroid. (b) Bilateral avascular necrosis of the femoral head secondary to uncontrolled synovitis and chronic steroid usage. Both femoral heads are flattened and sclerotic (and the right femur is internally rotated) (courtesy of Dr Nick Wilkinson)

OLIGOARTICULAR JUVENILE IDIOPATHIC ARTHRITIS

< 4 large joints in the first 6 months of disease. Female > male.

- Under 4 years of age
- Typically ankles, knees and elbows
- Leg length discrepancy and valgus deformity important features
- One-fifth will go on to have > 4 joints affected beyond 6 months (extended oligoarticular JIA)
- One-third develop **chronic iridocyclitis (uveitis).** Silent progression to possible blindness, therefore slit lamp examination 3 monthly
- ANA positive – increased risk eye disease
- RhF and HLA-B27 negative

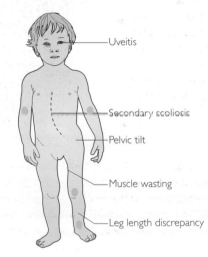

Uveitis

Secondary scoliosis

Pelvic tilt

Muscle wasting

Leg length discrepancy

Figure 22.7 Clinical features of oligoarticular juvenile idiopathic arthritis

POLYARTICULAR JUVENILE IDIOPATHIC ARTHRITIS

> 4 joints involved by 6 months of onset. Subdivided according to presence of rheumatoid factor checked on at least two occasions:

RhF negative   Moderate to severe disease
                Asymmetrical
                Small and large joints, cervical spine and TMJ especially
                Typically < 8 years old
RhF positive   Often severe disease
                Symmetrical
                Hands, feet and hips
                > 8 years old
                Rheumatoid nodules, tenosynovitis and vasculitis may develop

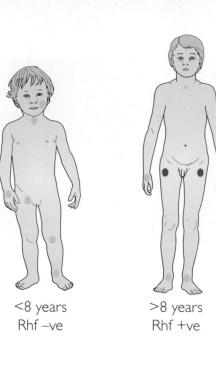

<8 years
Rhf −ve

>8 years
Rhf +ve

Figure 22.8 Clinical features of polyarticular juvenile idiopathic arthritis

(b)

(a)

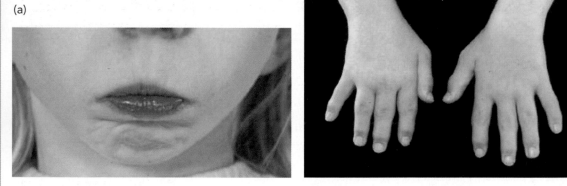

Figure 22.9 Polyarticular JIA. (a) Micrognathia due to TMJ disease. (b) Polyarthropathy of the hands (courtesy of Dr Nick Wilkinson)

SYSTEMIC-ONSET JUVENILE IDIOPATHIC ARTHRITIS

All ages affected. Male = female.

- **Diagnosis of exclusion** (see below)
- Defined by:
  - *Arthritis and characteristic fever* – quotidian fever (39–40°C × 1–2/day returning to baseline)
  - Plus one of:
    - Evanescent rash – classically heat/fever-induced salmon pink macules
    - Lymphadenopathy
    - Hepatosplenomegaly
    - Serositis (typically pericarditis)

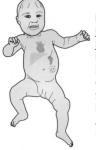

Misery
Joint swelling
Joint deformity
Hepatosplenomegaly
Rash
Quotidian fever
Serositis, e.g. pericarditis
Lymphadenopathy
Amyloidosis
Macrophage activation syndrome

Figure 22.10 Clinical features of systemic-onset juvenile idiopathic arthritis

- Also myalgia, arthralgia, abdominal pain, pleuritis
- Child often appears unwell while febrile
- Polyarthritis may be delayed and is severely destructive in approximately half of patients. The other half have uniphasic or mild disease
- Anaemia of chronic disease, neutrophilia, thrombocytosis
- ESR ↑↑, CRP ↑

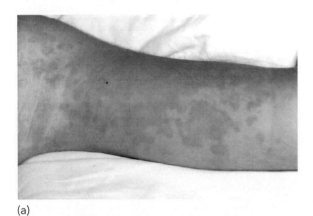

(a)

Figure 22.11 (a) Systemic JIA rash (courtesy of Dr Nick Wilkinson). (b) Quotidian fever seen in systemic-onset JIA

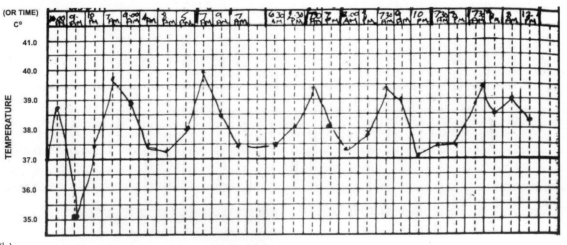

(b)

❗ **NB: Remember systemic–onset JIA is a diagnosis of exclusion.**

Differential diagnosis:
- **Infection**
- **Malignancy, e.g. leukaemia, neuroblastoma**
- **Vasculitis**
- **Other connective tissue disease**

Spondyloarthropathies

Enthesitis-related arthropathy (ERA)	Arthritis and/or enthesitis with other features
Reactive arthritis/Reiter syndrome	Sterile arthritis following infection
Arthritis of inflammatory bowel disease	Arthritis associated with Crohn disease or ulcerative colitis
Juvenile psoriatic arthropathy	Arthritis associated with psoriasis. Often destructive. Rare in childhood

Causes of acute monoarthritis and polyarthritis

Monoarthritis	**Polyarthritis**
Septic arthritis	JIA, ERA, psoriatic arthropathy, IBD, sarcoid
Reactive arthritis	Connective tissue disease, e.g. SLE, JDM, mixed connective tissue disease
Early oligoarticular JIA or ERA	Vasculitis, e.g. HSP, Kawasaki disease
Haemarthrosis	Reactive arthritis
Malignancy (leukaemia, neuroblastoma, osteogenic sarcoma)	Infection:
Perthes disease	– disseminated bacterial infective arthritis, Lyme disease
Trauma (including pulled elbow and NAI)	– Viral infection, e.g. parvovirus, rubella
	Malignancy (as for monoarthritis)
	Haematological disorder, e.g. haemophilia and sickle cell disease

SYSTEMIC LUPUS ERYTHEMATOSUS

This is a multisystem autoimmune disease associated with serum antibodies against nuclear components. It is rare in childhood.

A transient neonatal form (**neonatal lupus**) exists secondary to placental transfer of antigen:

■ Infants of mothers with anti-Ro or –La antibodies

■ Congenital heart block (permanent)

■ Skin rash, blood and liver involvement (self-limiting)

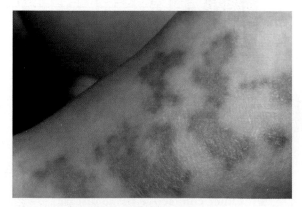

Figure 22.12 Neonatal lupus rash

JUVENILE DERMATOMYOSITIS

This is a multisystem disease involving *inflammation of striated muscle and skin*.

Clinical features

Muscle	Symmetrical proximal muscle weakness and pain (Gower's sign positive)
	Respiratory muscle weakness
	Palatal regurgitation, dysphagia, dysphonia
Skin	Classic **heliotrope violaceous rash** over upper eyelids
	Gottron's papules (red rash overlying dorsal interphalangeal joints and knees)
	Nailfold capillaritis and photosensitive rash
	Subcutaneous calcium deposits (calcinosis cutis)
Joints	Arthralgia and arthritis with contractures
Gastrointestinal	Vasculopathy (ulcerations and bleeding), hepatosplenomegaly
Cardiac	Myocarditis (arrhythmias)
Other	Interstitial lung disease, nephritis, retinitis, CNS involvement

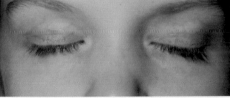

Figure 22.13 Clinical features of juvenile dermatomyositis

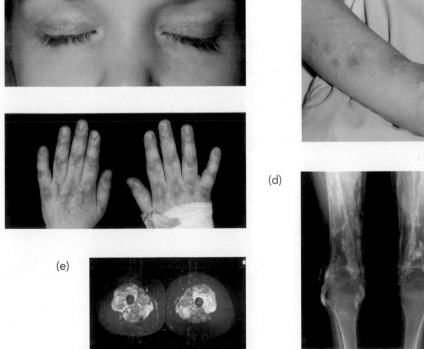

Figure 22.14 Juvenile dermatomyositis. (a) Heliotrope rash on the eyelids. (b) Calcinosis cutis (some lesions are red and infected). (c) Gottron's papules. (d) Complication of juvenile dermatomyositis showing extensive sheet-like calcinosis that occupies fascial and intermuscular planes. (e) MRI of thighs (STIR sequence) demonstrating widespread symmetrical polymyositis (courtesy of Dr Nick Wilkinson)

Differential diagnosis

■ Polymyositis/SLE
■ Viral/post-infection myopathy
■ Congenital and genetic myopathies

Investigations

Diagnosis is based on clinical picture plus:

MRI	Confirms inflammation of thigh muscles
Muscle biopsy	Vasculopathy and then muscle fibre necrosis, may be helpful
Muscle enzymes	**LDH**↑, also ↑CK, AST, ALT – may be deceptively normal
EMG	Rarely performed
Autoantibodies	ANA may be positive, RhF usually negative

Management

■ Physiotherapy and splinting
■ Systemic steroids (oral or intravenous)
■ Methotrexate
■ Cyclophosphamide in severe disease
■ Other treatments include intravenous immunoglobulin therapy and plasmapharesis

SCLERODERMA

Scleroderma is a multisystem connective tissue disease characterized by *fibrosis* and *occlusive vasculitis*. It may be:

■ Diffuse (systemic sclerosis or CREST syndrome, rare in childhood with high morbidity and mortality)
■ Localized to skin (morphoea)

EHLERS–DANLOS SYNDROMES

These are a group of inherited disorders of connective tissue in which there is *hyperextensibility* and increased *fragility of the skin.* The underlying defect varies with the subtype, but some involve defects in collagen synthesis. Each subtype has individual features.

Clinical features

Joints	Hypermobile joints, delayed walking in childhood, scoliosis, backache
Skin	Hyperextensibility, soft velvety skin
	Fragile skin, thin 'tissue paper' scars, poor healing
	Easy bruising

(a)

(b)

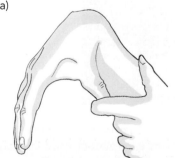
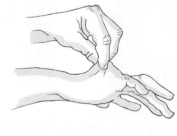

Figure 22.15 Ehlers–Danlos syndrome. (a) Wrist joint hypermobility. (b) Hyperelastic skin (courtesy of Dr Nick Wilkinson)

| Cardiovascular | Mitral valve incompetence, aortic rupture (type IV) |
| Pregnancy | Premature delivery of infants secondary to premature rupture of membranes, uterine rupture (type IV) |

VASCULITIS

Vasculitis refers to inflammation of the blood vessel wall. **Kawasaki disease** and **Henoch–Schönlein purpura** account for 70–80% of childhood vasculitides with 10–20% unclassified. There are several classifications, but none is totally satisfactory.

Classification of vasculitis

Polyarteritis	Polyarteritis nodosa (PAN)
	Microscopic polyangiitis
	Kawasaki disease
Granulomatous vasculitis	Churg–Strauss syndrome, Wegener granulomatosis
Leukocytoclastic vasculitis	Henoch–Schönlein purpura (see p. 235)
	Hypersensitivity arteritis
Cutaneous polyarteritis	Post-streptococcal arteritis
Giant cell arteritis	Takayasu disease
Secondary to connective tissue disease	JDM, SLE, JIA, scleroderma
Miscellaneous vasculitides	Behçet disease, familial Mediterranean fever

Features suggestive of vasculitis

General	Weight loss, fever, fatigue
Skin	Levido reticularis, palpable purpura, fixed vasculitic urticaria, nodules, ulcers
CNS	Focal CNS lesion, mononeuritis multiplex
Musculoskeletal	Intense arthralgia ± myalgia, arthritis, myositis
Vascular	Hypertension, pulmonary haemorrhage
Laboratory	↑ ESR & CRP, eosinophilia, anaemia, ANCA, factor VIII-related Ag (vWF), haematuria, cryoglobulinaemia

KAWASAKI DISEASE

This is an infantile polyarteritis of unknown cause.

Diagnostic criteria

Fever > 38.5°C for > 5 days and *four* of:

- Bilateral non-purulent conjunctivitis
- Oral mucosal changes (red cracked lips, bright red tongue)
- Cervical lymphadenopathy with one node > 1.5 cm
- Hands and feet red, swollen and then peeling of the skin
- Polymorphous generalized rash

The child is usually *extremely irritable*, has coryzal symptoms, cough and sometimes watery diarrhoea. The coronary vessels are affected by the vasculitis and significant cardiac complications can occur.

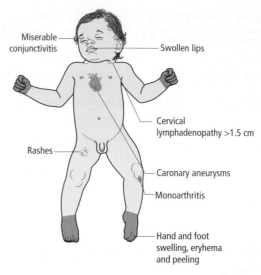

Miserable conjunctivitis

Swollen lips

Cervical lymphadenopathy >1.5 cm

Rashes

Caronary aneurysms

Monoarthritis

Hand and foot swelling, eryhema and peeling

Figure 22.16 Clinical features of Kawasaki disease

Cardiac complications

- Coronary artery aneurysms (20–40% of untreated children)
- Myocarditis and myocardial infarction
- Pericarditis and cardiac tamponade
- Cardiac failure

Investigations

FBC	Marked thrombocythaemia (2nd–3rd week)
Acute phase proteins	ESR and CRP ↑↑
Cardiac investigations	ECG, CXR and 2D echocardiogram

Management

- High-dose IVIG over 12 h within 10 days of disease commencement prevents cardiac complications
- Aspirin for 6 weeks or until aneurysms have gone
- 2D echocardiography at follow-up to check aneurysms resolving

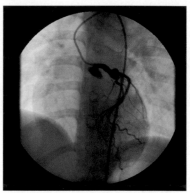

Figure 22.17 Cardiac angiogram showing coronary artery aneurysm in Kawasaki disease

NON-INFLAMMATORY PAIN SYNDROMES

These pains have characteristic patterns. The aetiologies are not well understood. Diagnoses are best made through a full history and examination and exclusion of other pathology.

Growing pains	Typically shin pain in evening and may wake from sleep Mostly young children Settles with gentle rubbing of the area
Benign joint hypermobility syndrome	Pain associated with hypermobility of joints Subtype of Ehlers–Danlos syndrome Management is reassurance and physiotherapy

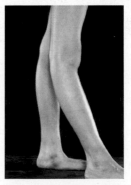

Figure 22.18 Hypermobility of the knee in benign joint hypermobility syndrome

OSTEOGENESIS IMPERFECTA

A group of disorders of fragile bones due to defective and/or reduced *type 1 collagen*. They are most commonly due to mutations in the genes *COL1A1* and *COL1A2*. The severity of the clinical features varies from mild to lethal.

Clinical features of type I

Skeletal	Multiple fractures pre-puberty; fewer post puberty
	Bowed limb bones
	May have vertebral crush fractures → hair, spine +/− scoliasis/kyphosis
	Soft brittle discoloured teeth (dentinogenesis imperfecta)
	Short stature
Skin	
Eyes	Blue–grey sclera
ENT	Deafness in 50% from age 20 years (most commonly conductive)
Other	Basilar invagination in a minority

Investigations

X–rays	Multiple fractures
	Bone deformities
	Wormian bones (skull)
Blood	Alkaline phosphatase ↑ or normal, acid phosphatase ↑ or normal
Urine	24–h hydroxyproline ↑

(a) (b)

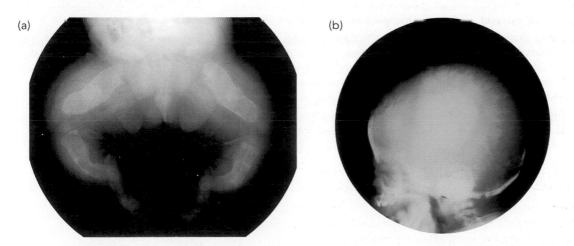

Figure 22.19 Type III and IV Osteogenesis imperfecta in a 9-day-old girl. (a) 'Ribbon bones' and multiple fractures. (b) Mosaic pattern of ossification is evident in the skull

Management

This is based on deformity and fracture treatment with expert occupational and physiotherapy, splints and corrective surgery. Bisphosphonates are commonly used to increase bone density, improve verterbral shape and reduce fracture frequency. Ensure good calcium and vitamin B status.

OSTEOCHONDRODYSPLASIAS

Developmental disorders of bone and cartilage are often associated with short stature, generally resulting from new gene mutations, although some are autosomal dominant and others have non–genetic causes.

ACHONDROPLASIA (DWARFISM)

This is the most common form of disproportionate short stature and most persons live independent, healthy, and productive lives, although lifespan may be limited by spinal stenosis and cord compression. A pure skeletal dysplasia, most features are a consequence of abnormal skeletal development. Specific growth charts have been designed for these children.

- Short limbs and trunk, with large head
- Exaggerated lumbar lordosis
- Genu varum
- Brachydactyly and 'trident' hands
- Mid–facial hypoplasia and relative prognathism
- Hydrocephalus (1–2%)
- Obstructive sleep apnoea
- Serous otitis media
- Hypotonia in infancy and delayed gross motor milestones

BACK DISORDERS

Causes of back pain

- Muscular spasm   – bad posture, stress, injury, overuse
- Chronic idiopathic pain   – no physical cause found
- Referred abdominal pain   – constipation, gastritis, pancreatitis, pyelonephritis
- Developmental: – kyphosis, scoliosis, tethered cord (cauda equina syndrome)
       – spondylolisthesis (slip of L5 on S1), Scheuermann, spondylosis
- Trauma   – vertebral (stress) fracture, herniated disc, pelvic anomaly
- Infection   – vertebral osteomyelitis, spinal abscess, e.g. TB
- Neoplasia: – 1° vertebral (osteogenic sarcoma), 1° spinal (neuroblastoma, lipoma)
       – marrow (ALL, lymphoma) metastatic
- Neuromuscular disease
- Osteoporosis

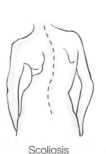
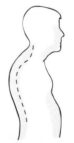
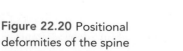

Figure 22.20 Positional deformities of the spine

Scoliosis   Kyphosis   Increased lumbar lordosis

KYPHOSIS

Postural   Bad posture (correctable by child, normal X-ray)
Idiopathic   Scheuermann disease
Congenital   Vertebral malformations, e.g. achondroplasia

Idiopathic kyphosis (Scheuermann disease)

- Osteochondritis of spine occurring during pubescent growth spurt
- Pain in mid-thoracic (75%) or thoracolumbar spine, or
- Painless around shoulders and kypho(scolio)sis
- Due to *wedging of vertebrae* caused by loss of anterior vertebral height

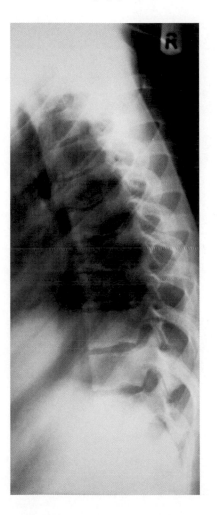

Figure 22.21 Scheuermann disease in an adolescent. Lateral dorsal spine film demonstrates mild disc narrowing, vertebral edge irregularities, anterior wedging (D7) and Schmorl's nodes (irregular endplates)

Management

Since this condition is generally self-limiting with good outcome, conservative management with physiotherapy is adopted. Plaster casts or surgical vertebral fusion may be necessary.

SCOLIOSIS

Structural   Curvature of spine with rotation of vertebral bodies and rib hump on spinal flexion
Congenital   Due to vertebral malformations

Idiopathic	Most common cause
	Mild disease (< 20°, M = F), often spontaneously resolves
	Severely progressive in 1 in 20 cases (F > M, associated with growth spurt)
Postural	No spinal rotation and normal alignment when flex spine
	May be secondary to:

- Neuromuscular disease, e.g. muscular dystrophy, unilateral paralysis
- Osteoid osteoma
- Leg length discrepancy

Enquire about bowel and bladder dysfunction and examine neurological system. *Management* is directed at any cause, plus brace for moderate deformity (20–40°) and surgical intervention if more severe.

INFECTIONS

SEPTIC ARTHRITIS

- Usually young child < 2 years, hip joint
- Generally from haematogenous spread, but also direct extension from osteomyelitis or abscess
- Serious joint destruction can occur if it is not promptly treated
- Neonatal disease may be multifocal

Causes

Children	*Staphylococcus aureus* and streptococci are the most common agents
	Haemophilus (now rare), enterococci, salmonella (in sickle cell disease)
	TB (prolonged indolent arthritis with stiff joint)
	Viruses and fungi
Neonates	*S. aureus*, Group B streptococcus, *E. coli*, gonococcus, enterobacteria

Clinical features

- Hot, red, tender, swollen joint
- Pain at rest and with movement
- Greatly reduced range of movement (pseudoparesis in infant)
- Joint position due to maximum joint relaxation or muscle spasm
- Toxic, febrile, may be irritable child

Investigations

Bloods	ESR, CRP, neutrophilia ($\uparrow\uparrow$)
	Serial blood cultures and antigens
X-rays	Normal initially, but helpful to eliminate trauma
	Widening of joint space and soft tissue swelling
Joint USS	Useful for hips in infants
Bone scan	'Hot spots' at involved joints
Joint aspiration	(Under USS guidance) for microscopy, culture and sensitivity and pain relief

Management

1. Antibiotics – prompt and prolonged course of appropriate IV antibiotics, then oral
2. Surgical – arthroscopic or open joint washout for hip disease and if delayed response to antibiotics
3. Physiotherapy – initially joint immobilization for pain relief, then mobilization to prevent deformity

OSTEOMYELITIS

- Acute, subacute and chronic depending on virulence of organism and efficacy of treatment
- Most commonly affects the proximal tibia and distal femur

- Usually due to haematogenous spread
- Occasionally multifocal
- Ineffective treatment results in discharging sinus and limb deformity

Causes

Similar to those of septic arthritis, with *Staph. aureus* the most common.

Clinical features

- Site dependent with point tenderness
- Overlying skin is warm, red and swollen
- Toxic, febrile child
- Painful immobile limb ± muscle spasm
- May have adjacent sympathetic joint effusion or extension to joint
- Older children may present with limp or back pain

Investigations

Bloods	CRP, ESR ↑↑, neutrophilia
	Blood cultures and rapid antigen tests
X-ray/USS	Normal initially
	Periosteal reaction > 2 weeks
	Subsequent lucent areas in bone
Bone scan	'Hot spots'
Aspiration	In atypical cases or immunocompromised child to identify organism

Management

1. Prolonged course (several weeks) of intravenous antibiotics
2. Surgical drainage/decompression if rapid response to antibiotics not seen

REACTIVE ARTHRITIS

Reactive arthritis comprises *viral and post-infectious arthritides* and includes acute rheumatic fever and arthritis following genitourinary tract and gastrointestinal tract infections. (Although described by a classical triad [arthritis, conjunctivitis, urethritis/cervicitis], Reiter syndrome is now considered synonymous.)

Clinical features

- Predominantly lower limb, asymmetrical, oligoarthritis
- Clear history of infection elsewhere during preceding 4 weeks (esp. diarrhoea)
- No clear clinical infection and no other known cause of arthritis present
- Yersinia, shigella, salmonella, campylobacter (adolescent – venereal infection)
- May last weeks–months with recurrences over several years

Investigations

- Stool culture
- Serology and PCR
- Synovial and urethral tests where appropriate

Clinical scenario

A 5-year-old girl develops a fever which is not resolved by antibiotics and lasts for 6 days until the GP suggests paediatric referral. When she is seen no infective source can be identified, and it is noted that she has marked cervical lymphadenopathy and glossitis. Two days later the tips of her fingers begin to peel.

1. What is the likeliest diagnosis?
2. What is the immediate treatment?
3. What is the ongoing treatment?
4. What is the most serious sequela from this diagnosis, and what is the usual incidence of this complication if the initial treatment is not given soon enough?

ANSWERS

1. Kawasaki disease
2. High dose intravenous immunoglobulin. High dose aspirin
3. Aspirin
4. Coronary artery aneurysms. Incidence of up to 10% potentially over many years, and therefore with the risk of sudden death from this complication, serial echocardiograms are necessary

FURTHER READING

Cassidy J, Petty R, Laxer R, Lindsley C. *Textbook of Pediatric Rheumatology*, 6th edn. London: Saunders, 2010.

Laxer R. *Pediatric Rheumatology: An Issue of Pediatric Clinics*. London: Saunders, 2005.

Luqmani R, Robb J, Porter D *et al*. *Textbook of Orthopaedics, Trauma and Rheumatology*. London: Mosby. 2008.

Reed A, Mason T. *Pediatric Rheumatology*. London: Manson Publishing, 2011.

Woo P, Laxer RL, Sherry DD. *Pediatric Rheumatology in Clinical Practice*. London: Springer-Verlag. 2007.

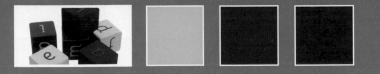

23 Ophthalmology

- Visual development
- Visual impairment
- Developmental abnormalities of the eye and adnexae
- Refractive error and squint (strabismus)
- Infections and allergies
- Retinopathy of prematurity
- Haemorrhage
- Further reading

VISUAL DEVELOPMENT

- Eye grows rapidly during the first 2 years of life
- Neonates have poor visual acuity (approx 6/200)
- By 6 months of age electrodiagnostic tests show that the vision improves to 6/6
- Any untreated obstruction or interference with focusing on objects during the first 7 years of life prevents normal development of visual acuity (**amblyopia**)
- **Binocular vision** develops in the first 3–6 months of life
- **Depth perception** begins at 6–8 months, is accurate at 6–7 years and improves during adolescence

Visual acuity

- Top number is the distance the subject is away from the chart in metres
- Bottom number is the number written by the side of the letter on the chart. This number indicates the maximum distance (in metres) that a normal sighted person can see that letter
- In the UK normal vision is 6/6 since metres are used; feet are used in the USA, i.e. 20/20 for normal vision

Visual Acuity Testing

Age	Test
Birth	Face fixation, preference for patterned objects
6 weeks	Fixes and follows a face through 90° (not to the midline until 3 months old) 90 cm away
	Optokinetic nystagmus on looking at a moving striped target
3 months	Fixes and follows through 180° 90 cm away
6 months	Reaches for a toy
10 months	Picks up a raisin
1 year	Picks up hundreds and thousands
2 years	Identifies pictures of reducing size (Kay's pictures)
3 years	Letter matching with single letter charts, e.g. Sheridan Gardiner, Stycar chart
5 years	Identifies letters on a Snellen chart by name or matching letters

VISUAL IMPAIRMENT

Causes

- Congenital – anophthalmos, optic nerve hypoplasia, cataracts
- Prematurity – retinopathy of prematurity
- Hypoxic–ischaemic encephalopathy
- Refractive error – amblyopia, myopia, hypermetropia
- Strabismus
- Optic atrophy
- Tumour, e.g. retinoblastoma
- Systemic condition, e.g. juvenile idiopathic arthritis (uveitis)
- Infection – orbital cellulitis, trachoma
- Delayed visual maturation (normal children with learning difficulties; they develop normal vision later)
- Cortical blindness (cortical defect, no eye abnormality)

Clinical presentation

- Lack of eye contact
- Failure to smile by 6 weeks of age
- Visual inattention, failure to track objects or fix on face by 3 months
- Nystagmus
- Squint
- Photophobia
- White pupillary reflex (**leucocoria**) (see below)

Investigations

Initial assessment by a paediatrician, an ophthalmologist and a neurologist is necessary:

- Ophthalmological assessment – general eye examination and visual acuity
- Full neurological assessment

Investigations are led by the individual case history and examination, but may include:

Electrophysiological tests	**Electro-retinogram (ERG)** (abnormal in retinal defects)
	Visual evoked response (VER) (abnormal in both eye and cortical defects)
Bloods	Serology for congenital infection
	Pituitary function tests
	Inborn error of metabolism, e.g. galactosaemia
Brain CT/MRI	

Management

- Treat any treatable cause
- Specialized regular developmental assessment with help from teachers from the Royal National Institute for the Blind (RNIB)
- Maximize non-visual stimulation
- Education:
  - Mainstream school or school for the blind
  - Braille (if blind)
  - Low vision aids (if impaired vision, e.g. high-power magnifiers, telescopic devices)
- Genetic counselling if appropriate

DEVELOPMENTAL ABNORMALITIES OF THE EYE AND ADNEXAE

LID ABNORMALITIES

Ptosis	Droopy lids
	Can cause amblyopia if obstructing the vision
Lid coloboma	Varies from a small notch to absence of lid (usually upper lid)
Dermoid	Smooth benign tumour
	May contain hairs and glandular tissue
Epicanthus	Vertical crescentic fold of skin between upper and lower lids
	May mimic *strabismus*
	Especially prominent in Asian children and seen in Down syndrome
Telecanthus	Wide interpupillary distance

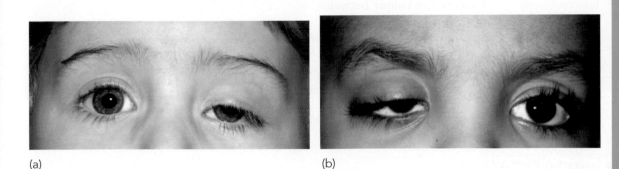

(a)   (b)

Figure 23.1 Congenital ptosis. (a) Left eye. (b) Congenital ptosis of the right eye with occlusion of the visual axis which has resulted in convergent squint developing (courtesy of Dr J Uddin)

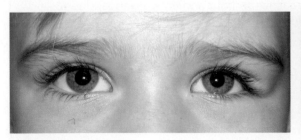

Figure 23.2 Dermoid on the outer left upper eyelid (courtesy of Dr J Uddin)

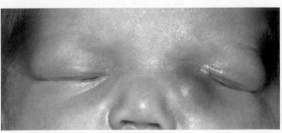

Figure 23.3 Left nasolacrimal duct obstruction in a neonate (courtesy of Dr J Uddin)

NASOLACRIMAL DUCT OBSTRUCTION

A persistent membrane across the lower end of the nasolacrimal duct is very common at birth, leading to a watery eye (about 5% of newborns). This normally disappears after the first year. If the problem persists beyond 12 months, the nasolacrimal duct is probed under general anaesthetic. This usually gives immediate resolution and, if not, the procedure is repeated.

IRIS ABNORMALITIES

Aniridia   **Iris hypoplasia**
Sporadic or autosomal dominant
Sporadic form – one-third develop
Wilms tumours (see ch. 19),
therefore yearly abdominal USS
and clinical evaluation for Wilms
tumour needed

Iris coloboma   **Notching of iris**
Associated with trisomy 13 and 18,
Klinefelter syndrome and Turner
syndrome

Brushfield's spots   **Iris stromal hyperplasia surrounded by hypoplasia**
Seen in 90% of Down syndrome

Heterochromia   **Variation in colour between the two irises**
Occasionally associated with Wilms tumour

Figure 23.4 Iris coloboma (courtesy of Moorfields Eye Hospital, London)

PUPIL ABNORMALITIES

Pupil sizes	
Small pupil	Common finding in babies that disappears in infancy May be associated with other eye abnormalities, e.g. congenital rubella syndrome Opiates
Large pupil	Iris trauma Drugs, e.g. ecstasy Parasympathetic neurological disorder: ■ Unilateral VI nerve palsy (seen in raised ICP) ■ Holmes–Adie pupil (slowly reactive to light and convergence, due to denervation in ciliary ganglion, seen in young girls)

Lack of red eye reflex (leucocoria, white pupil)

Causes

- Retinoblastoma
- Cataract
- Colobomas
- Infection – toxocara, toxoplasma
- Retinopathy of prematurity
- Uveitis
- Vitreous haemorrhage
- Retinal detachment

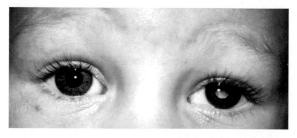

Figure 23.6 Leucocoria of the left eye (courtesy of Moorfields Eye Hospital, London)

CONGENITAL CATARACT

Causes

Bilateral cataract
- Idiopathic
- Any congenital infection, e.g. CMV, toxoplasmosis, rubella, varicella
- Hereditary – autosomal dominant (mostly), autosomal recessive or X linked (Down syndrome, Turner syndrome, trisomy 13 and 18, Marfan syndrome)
- Drugs – corticosteroids
- Metabolic:
  - Hypoparathyroidism
  - Galactosaemia ('oil-drop' cataract)
  - Neonatal hypoglycaemia

Unilateral cataract
Idiopathic
Trauma
Congenital rubella
Intraocular tumours
Anterior segment dysgenesis

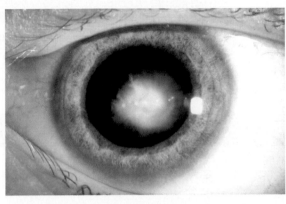

Figure 23.7 Congenital cataract (courtesy of Moorfields Eye Hospital, London)

CONGENITAL GLAUCOMA

Primary congenital glaucoma is seen in 1 in 10 000 births. Mostly sporadic, may be autosomal recessive. Males > females.

- Intraocular pressure rises due to a maldevelopment of the drainage angle in the anterior chamber
- May present at birth or develop later (usually < 3 years old)
- May be secondary to neurofibromatosis, congenital rubella syndrome, aniridia, retinopathy of prematurity and retinoblastoma

Clinical features

- Buphthalmos (excessive corneal diameter [> 13 mm] due to stretching of the eye from the constant elevated intraocular pressure). Cornea becomes white and hazy due to corneal oedema
- Other features include photophobia, lacrimation and eye rubbing
- Both eyes are usually affected but asymmetrically
- Eyes have a tendency to become myopic with disc cupping

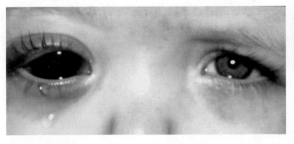

Figure 23.8 Buphthalmos of the right eye (courtesy of Moorfields Eye Hospital, London)

Management

This involves drainage angle surgery, along with topical antiglaucoma medication, with regular follow-up and refraction.

> ### Differential diagnosis of proptosis in children
>
> Malignant e.g. rhabdomyosarcoma, neuroblastoma
>
> Benign Inflammatory, e.g. orbital cellulitis
> Traumatic, e.g. haematoma
> Metabolic, e.g. Graves disease
> Infiltrative, e.g. glioma
> Developmental, e.g. dermoid cyst
>
>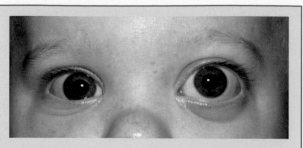
>
> **Figure 23.9** Proptosis of the left eye (courtesy of Moorfields Eye Hospital, London)

REFRACTIVE ERROR AND SQUINT (STRABISMUS)

REFRACTIVE ERROR

Hypermetropia

- Long-sightedness
- Most common childhood refractive error
- Early correction (with glasses) necessary to prevent amblyopia

Myopia

- Short-sightedness
- Uncommon in childhood, often hereditary

Amblyopia

- *Permanent impairment of visual acuity* in an eye that has not received a clear image while vision is developing
- Usually only one eye affected, known as a '**lazy eye**'
- Results from *any interference* with visual development:
  - Refractive errors
  - Squint
  - Obstruction of vision, e.g. haemangioma occluding vision, ptosis

Management

- Patching the good eye for periods of time during the day to force the affected eye to work and therefore develop
- Treat underlying cause, e.g. correct any refractive error with glasses, treat squint
- *Treatment while young is very important.* After age 7 years, improvement is unlikely (see p. 410)

SQUINT (STRABISMUS)

Squint is a common condition and is due to misalignment of the visual axes. Squints may be:

Features

- **Real** or **apparent**, e.g. unilateral epicanthic fold

- **Convergent** (esotropia), **divergent** (exotropia) or **vertical**

414

- **Constant** (manifest, -tropia), **intermittent** (latent, -phoria – only present during inattention, ocular alignment is maintained with effort) or **alternating**
- **Concomitant** *(angle of deviation is constant)* or **non-concomitant** *(angle of deviation changes on direction of gaze)*
- **Non-paralytic** or **paralytic**

Convergent squint

This is the most common type of squint in children. It is usually related to **accommodation**, caused by an *imbalance* of stimulation for accommodation and convergence. Eyes accommodate and converge when looking at near objects. Convergent squints in children are usually constant.

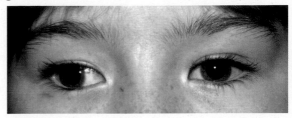

Figure 23.10 Divergent paralytic squint secondary to right III nerve palsy (courtesy of Moorfields Eye Hospital)

Accommodation is the process of altering the shape of the lens to focus the incoming light onto the retina.

Accommodative convergent squint

This is usually due to a child being long-sighted. Due to difficulty in focusing on near objects, the stimulation for convergence is increased when the eyes try to accommodate to focus on a near object, causing a squint. This may also occur with normal sightedness if the stimulation for convergence is disproportionately high during accommodation.

Essential infantile convergent squint

This is an idiopathic squint which presents in the first 6 months of life; the infant *alternates* fixation between the two eyes. This is usually corrected surgically by the age of 2 years.

Divergent squint

Intermittent divergent squint	Usually presents around the age of 2 years as an intermittent squint With tiredness or inattention may become constant
Constant divergent squint	This may be congenital, due to underlying visual impairment in older children, or happen after surgical over-correction of a convergent squint

> **!** **NB: Young babies often have a squint at times (particularly on convergence looking at a close object) as they have not yet developed binocular vision. There should be no squint by age 4 months.**
>
> *Any squint present after 2–3 months of age should be referred to the ophthalmologist as binocular vision should have developed by this time.*

Tests

Visual acuity must be assessed first (see p. 409).

- **Corneal light reflection test** — Simple test in which a pen torch is shone to produce reflections in both corneas. If the reflection is in different places in each cornea, a squint is present

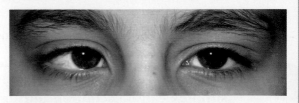

Figure 23.11 Corneal light reflection in convergent squint (courtesy of Moorfields Eye Hospital, London)

- **Eye movements** Child is asked to look at an object/toy which is moved in a horizontal, vertical and diagonal direction at one-third of a metre
- **Cover test** Eyes are covered individually with a card using a toy for visual fixation
    If the fixing eye is then covered, the squint eye moves to take up fixation
    On removal of the cover the eyes move again as the normal fixing eye takes up fixation (manifest squint)
    Used to detect a **latent squint** where the eye squints when covered
    An **alternating squint** is where each eye moves in turn when covered

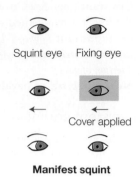

Squint eye   Fixing eye

Cover applied

Manifest squint

Figure 23.12 Cover test in a manifest squint of the right eye

Children should have fundoscopy and a refraction test for glasses if there is any history of squint. This should be repeated yearly as their refraction may change.

INFECTIONS AND ALLERGIES

CONJUNCTIVITIS

Clinical features

- Conjunctival injection
- Pus in the eye
- 'Gritty' or irritating eye
- Otitis media is commonly associated with bacterial conjunctivitis, and should be examined for

Causes

Neonatal (ophthalmia neonatorum)	(Notifiable disease in the UK)
	Staphylococcus aureus – usually present early
	Neisseria gonorrhoea – florid pus on first day
	Chlamydia trachomatis – presents late (after 1st week)
	Escherichia coli
	Haemophilus influenzae } Uncommon
	Streptococcus pneumoniae
	Aseptic causes, i.e. chemical irritants
Infant/child	*Staphylococcus aureus*
	Haemophilus influenzae
	Streptococcus pneumoniae
	Moxarella catarrhalis
	Viral
	Allergic

Ophthalmia neonatorum is any purulent conjunctivitis occurring in the first 3 weeks of life.

> **!** **NB: Chlamydia,** *Neisseria gonorrhoea,* **streptococcus, chemical and herpes simplex can be acquired during delivery from the genital tract.** *Neisseria gonorrhoea* **is particularly dangerous as it can penetrate the cornea within 24 h.**

Management

Eye swab	Microscopy (Gram stain) and culture. (Chlamydia and gonorrhoea require special media)
	PCR for rapid detection
Frequent eye and lid hygiene	
Neonate	Chloramphenicol or neomycin eye drops hourly or 2 hourly
	Chlamydia – oral erythromycin (2 weeks) plus tetracycline eye drops
	Gonococcus – eye irrigation with crystalline penicillin hourly. IV penicillin 10-day course
Infant/child	Fusidic acid, chloramphenicol or neomycin eye drops

For *Haemophilus influenzae* type b, oral antibiotics are needed.

ORBITAL AND PERIORBITAL (PRE-SEPTAL) CELLULITIS

Periorbital cellulitis	Infection in the tissues anterior to the eyelid septum, with white conjunctiva, no diplopia, proptosis or loss of vision
Orbital cellulitis	Infection posterior to orbital septum, which is much more serious and can lead to loss of vision, ophthalmoplegia, cavernous sinus thrombosis, meningitis and septicaemia

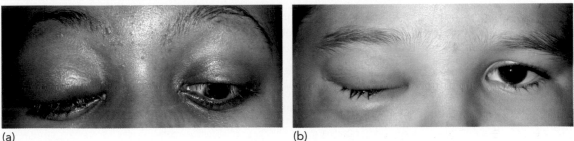

(a)   (b)

Figure 23.13 (a) Preseptal cellulitis – note good eye movements present (child looking down). (b) Right orbital cellulitis (courtesy of Dr J Uddin)

Clinical features distinguishing periorbital and orbital cellulitis

Periorbital cellulitis	Orbital cellulitis
Conjunctiva/sclera white	Inflamed oedematous conjunctiva/sclera
Normal ocular motility	Decreased/painful ocular motility causing diplopia
Normal acuity	Impaired acuity
Normal colour vision	Impaired colour vision
Normal pupillary reflex	Impaired pupillary reflex (if severe)
No proptosis	Proptosis
No fever, no/little systemic upset (usually)	Fever with systemic upset

!   **NB: The above features of orbital cellulitis are *danger signs*, indicating possible need for surgery.**

- An ophthalmologist should be contacted to help make the differentiation between orbital and periorbital (see previous page) cellulitis
- Orbital cellulitis may result from severe sinusitis, and therefore an ENT specialist should also be involved to assess the need for any urgent intervention
- Complications of orbital cellulitis include cavernous sinus thrombosis, meningitis, subdural and periosteal abscesses, and amblyopia/blindness if visual axis is interrupted for more than a few days

Investigations

- Eye swab
- If orbital cellulitis is suspected:
  - Blood cultures
  - FBC
  - Orbital and sinus CT or MRI scan always necessary to show any involvement of the sinuses and intraorbital complications necessitating surgical drainage

Treatment

Periorbital cellulitis	Oral antibiotics
Orbital cellulitis	Broad-spectrum IV antibiotics and possible surgical intervention

RETINOPATHY OF PREMATURITY

Retinopathy of prematurity (ROP) is seen in premature infants given oxygen therapy. It is thought to occur because of proliferation of blood vessels at the junction of the vascular and non-vascular retina due to high oxygen saturation in the blood of premature babies secondary to re-oxygenation after hypoxia. It results in:

- Decreased visual acuity
- Retinal detachment
- Blindness if very severe

Management

- Screening of all premature infants at risk (< 1500 g at birth or < 32 weeks' gestation) from 32 weeks by ophthalmologist
- Prevention by minimizing oxygen therapy to lowest necessary level
- Laser photocoagulation or cryotherapy if necessary
- Most lesions spontaneously resolve

HAEMORRHAGE

Causes

Conjunctival haemorrhage	Tussive injury, e.g. whooping cough
	Coagulation disorder
	Trauma
	Leukaemia
Retinal haemorrhage	Non-accidental injury
	Tussive injury, e.g. whooping cough
	Leukaemia
	Coagulation disorders
	Birth trauma (normally resolved by 1 month)

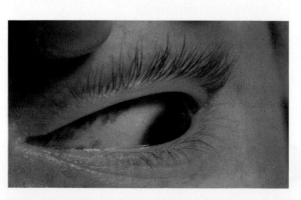

Figure 23.14 Subconjunctival haemorrhage

Clinical scenario

A 6-month-old infant girl is seen by the clinical nurse attached to the local general practice. It is apparent that her eyes do not look in the same direction.

1. The corneal light reflection test is useful – why?
2. What four components of a squint (strabismus) do you need to identify in its assessment?
3. After what age should a child with a squint be referred? (essentially because by this age binocular vision should have developed)

ANSWERS

1. Distinguishes between real and apparent squint
2. Real v apparent, Convergent v divergent, Latent v manifest, Paralytic (non-concomitant) v non-paralytic (concomitant)
3. 6 months of age

FURTHER READING

Olitsky S, Nelson L. *Pediatric Clinical Ophthalmology*. London: Manson Publishing, 2011.

Nelson L, Olitsky S. *Harley's Pediatric Ophthalmology,* 5th edn. London: Lippincott, Williams & Wilkins, 2005.

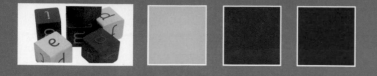

24 Behavioural Problems and Psychiatric Disorders

- Behavioural problems in infants
- Behavioural problems in toddlers
- Behavioural problems in school-age children
- Behavioural problems in adolescents
- Psychiatric disorders
- Further reading

BEHAVIOURAL PROBLEMS IN INFANTS

SLEEP DISTURBANCE

Infants have short sleep–wake cycles, needing to sleep every 2–3 h initially. Gradually they can remain awake for longer periods during the day and learn to get through the night without waking their parents. They will wake at intervals during the night, but will go back to sleep by themselves.

- By 3 months of age 70% do not wake their parents during the night
- By 6 months of age 90% do not wake their parents during the night

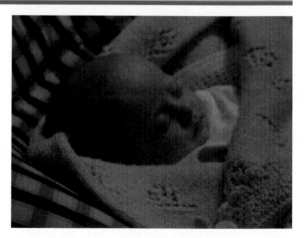

Figure 24.1 3-month-old baby sleeping

Techniques to improve sleep patterns

- Bedtime routine, e.g. bath, bottle, bed
- Putting the infant in the cot while awake, stay a while then leave them to fall asleep alone
- Making the cot fun – teddies and toys in the cot and nightlight
- Do not isolate the child (keep in the same room as the parents, or leave the door open and visit frequently)

BEHAVIOURAL PROBLEMS IN TODDLERS

Common toddler behavioural problems

- Aggressive behaviour, e.g. temper tantrums, breath-holding attacks
- Undesirable habits, e.g. prolonged thumb sucking, head banging, nail biting
- Overdependency, e.g. separation anxiety, shyness
- Daily routine problems, e.g. food refusal, sleep disturbance, toilet training problems

TEMPER TANTRUMS

- Universal in toddlers
- May be accompanied by breath–holding (see below)
- Due to immaturity of the developing brain
- Impossible to reason with them
- Management strategies include:
  - Try to divert their attention
  - Ignore the tantrum but set limits on when to intervene
  - Remove them from the situation temporarily
  - Praise good behaviour
  - Be consistent

BREATH-HOLDING ATTACKS

These are common between ages 6 months and 4 years.

Physical or emotional → Intense → Stops breathing → Pallor or cyanosis → Loss of → Generalized
upset causing   crying   in full expiration   and rigidity   consciousness   tonic–clonic
frustration or anger   seizure

> **!** **NB: Breath-holding spells are distinguished from seizures because the convulsion occurs before the cyanosis in a seizure.**

FOOD REFUSAL

- Common problem with the child being a 'fussy' eater or refusing to eat
- One way a child can begin to exert some control and independence
- Child is well nourished, with normal weight gain
- Strategies to help include:
  - Reassure parents the child will not starve him/herself
  - Regular mealtimes
  - Do not force feed
  - Keep relaxed
  - Introduce a wide variety of food early on when weaning so the child appreciates variety
  - Do not punish the child
  - Reward good eating by giving favourite foods for puddings
  - Do not expect the child to eat excessively large amounts or to finish every meal

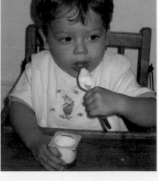

Figure 24.2 1-year-old child

421

NIGHT TERRORS

The child wakes in a very distressed state due to rapid emergence from deep non-REM stage IV sleep, and is difficult to arouse and difficult to console. They usually fall back to sleep if not fully awoken. **Sleep walking** is also due to disturbance from this stage of sleep.

Management

- Explain the phenomenon to the parents
- Advise them to try not to wake the child
- If they occur regularly at the same time, then waking the child prior to onset for a week can disrupt the pattern

> **NB: Nightmares are frightening dreams that take place during REM sleep, from which the child is relatively easily consoled.**

BEHAVIOURAL PROBLEMS IN SCHOOL-AGE CHILDREN

RECURRENT FUNCTIONAL ABDOMINAL PAIN

Features

- Most commonly age 6–9 years (school-age symptom)
- Girls > boys
- Pain para-umbilical and worse on waking
- Growth normal and good health otherwise
- No signs or symptoms of organic abdominal pathology
- High achiever personality (doing well at school, anxious)

Management

1. History and examination:
    - Pain: site, nature, timing, recurrence rate
    - Aggravating factors (? related to school)
    - Vomiting, weight loss, bowel habit, urinary problems, headache
    - Ask parent(s) and child what they think the cause is
    - Take thorough social history (family life, school life)
2. Any necessary investigations to exclude organic disease:
    - An MSU should be done to exclude a UTI
    - Other investigations only if indicated, e.g. FBC, ESR, CRP, AXR, endoscopy, etc.
3. Treatment:
    - Explain that, although a psychosomatic cause, the pain is *real*
    - Reassure parents, child and teachers that no organic cause was found. This can result in the symptoms improving
    - Try to avoid medications as these imply there may be something organic

> **NB: Other common recurrent pain syndromes are headache and limb pain.**

Features that suggest an organic cause

- Pain:
  - Localized away from the umbilicus
  - Awaking child at night
  - Radiates to back, legs or shoulders
- Bowel habit change
- Rectal bleeding or mucus
- Dysuria
- Child unwell (fever, weight loss, failure to thrive)

SCHOOL REFUSAL

School refusal may be:

Anxiety-related type	Separation anxiety from parents, insecurity, bullying
	Girls > boys, usually good students
Secondary-gain type	No anxiety, lazy, prefers to be at home
	Boys > girls, poor students

This is managed with a graded return to school (short days initially) and dealing with any underlying problems.

ANTISOCIAL BEHAVIOUR

Minor occasional antisocial behaviour is common – defiance, occasional disobedience, lying, stealing, minor vandalism.

More serious repeated antisocial behaviour:

- Frequent disobedience
- Fighting
- Stealing
- Destructiveness
- Lying frequently
- Truancy
- Running away

Conduct disorder is serious antisocial behaviour causing impairment of general functioning.

Associations

- Smoking and alcohol abuse
- Family violence, marital breakdown
- Boys > girls
- Educational retardation

Management is with family or individual therapy.

! **NB: These children have an increased risk of adolescent *delinquency* and maladjustment as an adult.**

Behavioural Problems and Psychiatric Disorders

NOCTURNAL ENURESIS

Nocturnal enuresis is involuntary passage of urine during sleep.

- *Primary* (always present)
- *Secondary* (beginning after continence was achieved for > 6 months)

It is due to:

- Inability to wake when the bladder is full
- Bladder overactivity and/or
- High nocturnal urine output

Urinary continence	
Daytime achieved in:	50% by 2½ years
	95% by 4 years
Night-time achieved in:	95% by 5 years, i.e. 5% of children have nocturnal enuresis
	97–98% by 10 years, i.e. 2–3% of children have nocturnal enuresis
	> 98% by 15 years, i.e. < 2% children have nocturnal enuresis
NB: Boys are slower than girls to achieve continence	

Causes

Psychological	(> 95%)
Organic	UTI
	Constipation
	Polyuria, e.g. IDDM, diabetes insipidus, polyuric renal failure
	Neurological, e.g. spina bifida
	Renal structural abnormality, e.g. ectopic ureter

> **!** **NB: Organic causes must be ruled out prior to dealing with this as a psychological problem. The history is most important and guides the investigations.**

Initial assessment and investigations

- History of onset and frequency
- Diet, fluid intake, stress and nocturnal access to the toilet
- Examination of abdomen, genitalia, spine, neurological assessment and growth
- Blood pressure check
- Urine sample – checking for glycosuria, proteinuria, infection and osmolality
- Renal USS if indicated (± AXR)

Management options

- Star charts and reward systems (positive reinforcement)
- Alarm pads (negative reinforcement)
- Behavioural programmes, e.g. retention control during the day to increase bladder capacity
- Drugs:
  - Anticholinergics, e.g. oxybutinin
  - ADH analogue (desmopressin) for short–term relief (intranasal)

BEHAVIOURAL PROBLEMS IN ADOLESCENTS

ALCOHOL AND DRUG DEPENDENCY

This is generally a problem of adolescents, although many children experiment earlier. Experimentation is common, but *regular use* with *dependency*, personality changes and *addiction* may develop.

Reasons for drug and alcohol use
- Peer pressure, perceived as a sign of maturity
- Rebellion
- Poor self-esteem, to boost confidence
- To escape from painful emotions
- Frustration and depression
- For pleasure, to gain an altered state of mind

Problems associated with dependency

Behavioural	Personality changes, antisocial behaviour, aggression and violence
	Relationship difficulties
	Problems at school and home
	Missing school
	Criminal activity, esp. stealing (with harder drugs and alcohol)
Physical	Medical problems associated with acute and chronic use and dependency
	Overdose (accidental or intentional) and withdrawal

Substances abused

Cigarette smoking
Alcohol
Hallucinogens, e.g. cannabis (marijuana), ecstasy (MDMA), solvents (glue sniffing)
CNS stimulants, e.g. cocaine
Narcotics, e.g. IV opiates

PSYCHIATRIC DISORDERS

ATTENTION DEFICIT HYPERACTIVIY DISORDER

Diagnostic criteria
- Inattention
- Hyperactivity
- Impulsivity
- Lasting > 6 months and commencing < 7 years, and inconsistent with the child's developmental level

These features should be present in more than one setting, and cause significant social or school impairment.

These children also have an increased risk of:

- Conduct disorder
- Anxiety disorder
- Aggression

Risk factors

- Boys > girls, 4:1
- Learning difficulties and developmental delay
- Neurological disorder, e.g. epilepsy, cerebral palsy
- First-degree relative with ADHD
- Family member with depression, learning disability, antisocial personality or substance abuse

A significant proportion of children with ADHD will become adults with antisocial personality and there is an increased incidence of criminal behaviour and substance abuse.

Management

Psychotherapy	Behavioural therapies
	Family therapy
Drugs	If behavioural therapy alone insufficient
	Stimulants, e.g. methylphenidate (Ritalin), amphetamines (dexamphetamine)
Diet	Some children benefit noticeably from exclusion of certain foods from their diet, e.g. red food colouring

DEPRESSION

Clinical features

- Persistent depressed mood, feeling unhappy
- Helplessness to change the situation (despair)
- Apathy
- Self-blame and lack of self-worth
- Hopelessness for the future
- Social withdrawal
- School performance dropping
- Recurrent pain syndromes

Depression may be *endogenous* or *reactive*, i.e. in response to an environmental change, or a mixture of both.

Risk factors

- Boys > girls – pre-adolescent
- Girls > boys – adolescent
- Other behavioural disturbances, e.g. ADHD, eating disorders, conduct disorders
- Family history of depression
- Adverse life events
- Dysfunctional family
- Separation:
  - Infants separated from primary carer (withdrawn, apathetic, faltering growth)
  - Preschool children separated from parents (protest, despair, detachment)

Management
- Psychotherapy
- Drugs – antidepressants

PARASUICIDE AND SUICIDE

Suicidal thoughts are more common than attempted suicide, which is more common than completed suicide.

Risk factors

- Suicide is more common in boys, parasuicide more common in girls
- Rates increase throughout adolescence. Rare < 12 years old
- Associated with family breakdown and conflict with friends and family
- Attempt is often an impulsive reaction to a personal crisis, e.g. argument with boyfriend/girlfriend

Management

- Acute hospital treatment with admission if necessary
- Urgent psychological assessment of child and family to assess in particular:
  - Attempt and potential lethality
  - Premeditation
  - Reason for attempt
  - Family problems
  - Friend/boyfriend/girlfriend problems
  - Mood assessment (? depression)
  - Use of illicit drugs
- Psychotherapy ± antidepressants. Admission to psychiatric unit if necessary

ANOREXIA NERVOSA

This is predominantly a disorder of Western adolescent girls. Girls > boys, 10:1.

Diagnostic criteria

- Fear of becoming obese
- Disturbance of perception of body size, shape and weight
- Refusal to maintain body weight over the age/height minimum (via calorie restriction, obsessive exercise, vomiting, laxatives)
- Amenorrhoea

The typical psychological profile includes:

- Overachiever
- Poor self-esteem
- Strong willed, distrustful, uncommunicative
- Depression, irritability
- Obsessional (obsessive thoughts of food and body shape in particular)
- Family dysfunction with overprotection and conflict avoidance
- Control battles over food

Physical features

Bodyweight	Below expected for age/height
Skin	Dry skin, rashes, fine lanugo hair on body and face
Cardiac	Bradycardia, low BP with pronounced postural drop, long QT interval, arrhythmias (may cause sudden death)

Hormones	GH ↑, T3 ↓, rT3 ↑, hypothalamic–pituitary–ovarian disorders (amenorrhoea, LH and FSH ↓)
Electrolytes	K ↓, hypochloraemic alkalosis due to vomiting
Other	Hypothermia, cool peripheries, slowly relaxing reflexes, constipation

Management

A combination of expert psychotherapy and nutritional rehabilitation (at home or in hospital) is necessary. The prognosis is best if treated early, otherwise long term eating problems are common with a mortality of up to 10% in adulthood.

BULIMIA

This is also predominantly a disorder of adolescent girls, and is more common than anorexia nervosa.

Clinical features

- Episodic high-calorie binge eating
- Followed by self-induced vomiting, laxative abuse and/or episodes of fasting
- Weight is usually normal or mildly overweight
- Teeth enamel erosion, salivary gland enlargement and cheilosis may be seen from recurrent vomiting
- Electrolyte and cardiac abnormalities as in anorexia nervosa may occur

The *diagnosis* is made from the history. *Management* is with specialist psychotherapy.

OBSESSIVE–COMPULSIVE DISORDER

This disorder features obsessions and compulsions that may vary in intensity over time:

- Rituals, e.g. excessive cleaning, repeated motor rituals
- Repetitive checking behaviour, e.g. checking doors all locked

Treatment

- Cognitive behavioural therapy
- Serotonin-reuptake-inhibiting medications, e.g. fluoxetine, sertraline

AUTISM

Autism is a developmental behavioural disorder of **social interaction and understanding**, which is the endpoint of several organic aetiologies. Prevalence 5–6 in 10 000 (currently rising).

- Features and severity are very variable and thought to be part of a *spectrum*
- Recognized to be the endpoint of several organic aetiologies, e.g. prenatal insults, metabolic disorders, localized CNS lesions, postnatal infections, e.g. encephalitis. The specific organic cause is rarely found (< 10%)
- Genetic factors – siblings have a 2–3% prevalence, i.e. 50–100 × greater than average incidence; monozygotic twin concordance 60%
- Increased risk of epilepsy in teenage years

Clinical features

- Diagnosis made at 2–3 years. Features noticeable from 1 year
- Severity varies greatly between individuals and over time in a single child
- Impairment of social interactions:
  - Limited eye contact
  - Child relates to *parts* of a person not the whole person
  - Plays alone

- Narrow range of interests and repetitive behaviour:
  - Repetitive play, fascination with movement
  - Interest in detail
  - Poor concentration span
  - Early development of numbers
- Rigidity of thought and behaviour – difficulty in changing from one activity to the next or in stopping an activity
- Abnormal speech and language development:
  - Delay in speech
  - Echolalia
- Developmental stasis or regression – seen in 25–30% at 15–18 months of age
- Most have low IQ

Management

1. Assessment	Detailed medical and developmental history (focusing on development and core behaviours)
	Medical examination and play observation
	Hearing and vision testing
	Other investigations if indicated, e.g. lead, FBC and iron studies, chromosomes and fragile X, Rett gene, thyroid function, PKU test
	Neuroimaging only if specific neurological signs. EEG if epilepsy
2. Action plan	A written report is produced for parents and all relevant professionals and an action plan is made for the family
3. Interventions	Behavioural therapies and educational programmes (several approaches may be used, none of which has been shown to be more effective than others)

ASPERGER SYNDROME

These children have a severe impairment in reciprocal social interaction, but are otherwise relatively normal.

- No delay in language, but have unusual language development, e.g. interpret literally, have one-sided conversations
- Variable fine and gross motor delay (clumsy, walk later than they speak)
- Difficulty in understanding non-verbal communication
- Generally high level of intelligence
- Develop all-absorbing special interests
- May be able to memorize large amounts of information, though not necessarily fully comprehend it

Clinical scenario

A 13-year-old girl is found unconscious in a park and brought to accident and emergency where she is kept until she regains conciousness, and she says that she simply cannot remember what happened. After contacting her mother and step-father it transpires that she has a habit of staying out late, and there may be a pattern of behaviour to suggest drug use. The only other history of medical issues is that of prolonged enuresis and constipation as a younger child and school avoidance.

Examination by the paediatric doctor on call reveals a number of linear marks on her wrists which are scarred and have broken the skin surface at some point. Her body mass index, it is noted, is only 14.5 and she has a heart rate of 48. Subcutaneous fat stores are minimal.

1. Which allied health professionals would be most important in the management of this young girl?

She is admitted initially to the children's ward and observed – she appears to be a withdrawn individual, and exhibits a reluctance to eat with repeated and prolonged visits to the toilet, and nurses note some diarrhoea. Biochemistry reveals a low serum potassium.

2. What is her most likely problem?
3. Which drugs might she be abusing?

After a 2-week period of inpatient admission she admits that her stepfather has been sexually abusing her, and when she told her mother of this her mother became angry and threw her out of the house which is how she ended up in the park.

4. What would be the next most appropriate step?

ANSWERS

1. Psychologist; dietician
2. If inflammatory bowel disease is adequately excluded then the most likely scenario is laxative abuse
3. Lactulose; senokot or other laxatives
4. Involvement of the child protection team

FURTHER READING

Goodman R, Scott S. *Child psychiatry*, 2nd edn. Oxford: Wiley–Blackwell, 2005.

Taylor S, Nunn K, Lask B. Practical Child Psychiatry: The Clinician's Guide. Oxford: BMJ Publishing Group, 2003.

Dulcan M, Wiener J. *Essentials of Child and Adolescent Psychiatry*. Virginia: American Psychiatric Press, 2006.

Frith U. *Autism: A Very Short Introduction*. Oxford: Oxford University Press, 2008.

Chandler C. *The Science of ADHD: A Guide for Parents and Professionals*. Oxford: Wiley–Blackwell, 2010.

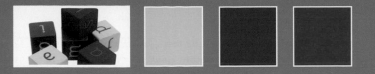

25 Surgical Conditions

- Urological surgery
- Abdominal surgery
- Neonatal surgical conditions
- Orthopaedic conditions
- Further reading

UROLOGICAL SURGERY

UNDESCENDED TESTES (CRYPTORCHIDISM)

- Testes descend through the inguinal canal to the scrotum in the third trimester of pregnancy
- Approximately 3.5% of boys have undescended testes at birth and 1.5% at 3 months of age (as some descend after birth)
- After 9 months of age they rarely descend spontaneously
- Undescended testes have an increased rate of malignant transformation *even after orchidopexy*
- They may be:
  - Bilateral or unilateral
  - Palpable or impalpable
  - Somewhere along the normal line of descent or ectopic
- Not to be confused with retractile testes, which can be massaged fully into the scrotum with no tension but retract back into the inguinal canal
- To examine the testis, it is massaged gradually down the inguinal canal into the scrotum if possible
- Karyotyping should be done if bilateral impalpable testes or bilateral/unilateral impalpable testes are associated with abnormal genitalia
- Check β–hCG if bilaterally impalpable

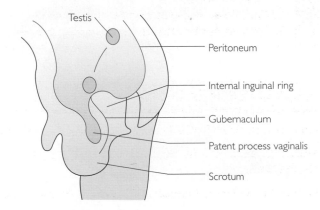

Figure 25.1 Line of normal testicular descent *in utero*

Investigations and management

Palpable	Inguinal orchidopexy
Impalpable	Laparoscopy to make the diagnosis and then proceed according to findings
	Present – orchidopexy (usually in two stages laparoscopically 3 months apart)

Dysplastic – excision laparoscopically and fix remaining testis (as for absent testis)
Absent – fix remaining contralateral testis in the scrotum to avoid the small risk of torsion

Orchidopexy (surgical correction)

This is usually done before the age of 2 years as a one- or a two-staged procedure, depending on the length of the testicular artery. It is done for:

- Cosmetic reasons
- To optimize testicular development and theoretically to increase fertility
- To allow early detection of malignant change

If the testis is abnormal or unilateral intra-abdominal and unable to be corrected, it is removed (orchidectomy).

> **!** **NB: Undescended testes most commonly lie in the superficial inguinal pouch.**

SCROTAL/INGUINAL SWELLINGS

Inguinal hernia

Inguinal hernia in children is usually *indirect*, i.e. due to a wide patent processus vaginalis which allows omentum or bowel to pass into it. Right side > left side; male > female.

Associations

- Undescended testes
- Prematurity
- Connective tissue disorders, e.g. Marfan syndrome

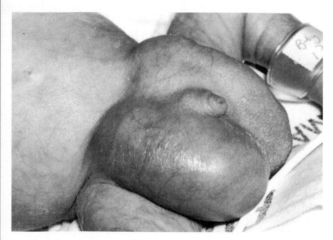

(a)

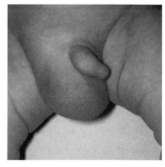

(b)

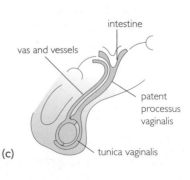

(c)

Figure 25.2 Hernias. (a) Bilateral inguinal hernia in a neonate. (b) Right inguinal hernia in a child (courtesy of Mr Peter Cuckow). (c) Patent processus vaginalis in indirect inguinal hernia

Clinical features

- Intermittent scrotal swelling, more prominent on crying or straining
- If an **irreducible hernia**:
  - Painful
  - Risk of bowel obstruction or strangulation
  - Must be reduced urgently by a combination of *firm* pressure on the fundus, combined with control of the neck of the hernia. Alternatively, analgesia and Gallow's traction may be effective

Management

Emergency repair	Indicated if incarcerated (irreducible), tender and any signs of bowel obstruction or bowel damage (perforation and peritonitis are rare but life-threatening complications) Children, especially babies, must be carefully resuscitated with fluids prior to the operation
Elective surgical repair	Once reduced (with *minimum delay* as incarceration may occur in the meantime)

Hydrocoele

A hydrocoele in infancy is due to a narrow patent processus vaginalis that only permits peritoneal fluid to drain to the scrotum. They are common after birth.

Clinical features

- Scrotal swelling, usually fluctuant (may be tense)
- Variation in size of testes
- Transilluminates with a torch
- In an older child, will characteristically increase in size during the day and reduce over night

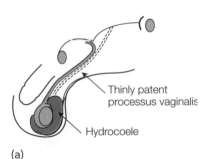

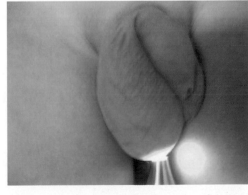

(a)   (b)

Figure 25.3 Hydrocoele. (a) Most common mechanism in infancy and childhood. (b) Hydrocoele of the right scrotum transilluminated from below (courtesy of Mr Peter Cuckow)

Management

Small hydrocoeles are usually observed for 1 year as most spontaneously resolve. Large and persistent hydrocoeles are treated with surgical ligation of the processus vaginalis (herniotomy).

Testicular torsion

Testicular torsion is a rotation of the testis which causes vascular compromise by kinking the testicular pedicle.

Clinical features

- Acute scrotal pain, nausea and vomiting
- Firm dusky red scrotal swelling
- Pain may be a dull abdominal ache
- Usually tender on palpation
- Testis may be high in the scrotum and the spermatic cord feels thickened

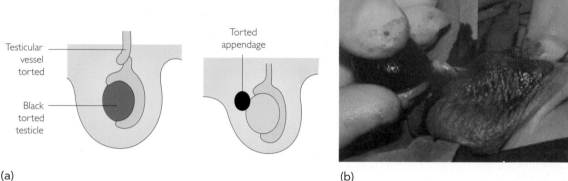

(a)

(b)

Figure 25.4 (a) Diagram showing testicular torsion and torted testicular appendage. (b) Testicular torsion at operation showing necrotic right testis (courtesy of Mr Peter Cuckow)

The diagnosis is *clinical*. Although Doppler ultrasound of the testes can demonstrate the blood flow, it is relatively inaccurate and should not be relied on.

Management

- Any suspected testicular torsion should be taken to theatre to be *explored*
- Torted testis is untwisted and fixed. If it is non-viable it is excised
- *Other testis* should be fixed at the same time to prevent future torsion

> **!** **NB: Testicular torsion is a surgical emergency and must be operated on within 6 h of onset of symptoms in order to save the testis.**

Torted testicular appendage (hydatid of Morgagni)

This is the commonest cause of acute scrotum in younger boys. It is due to torsion of the appendix testis – at the upper pole of the testis. As it mimics testicular torsion, diagnosis is often made at exploration.

Early examination may reveal the 'blue dot' sign – a visible lump at the upper pole of the testis. When this is seen by an experienced surgeon, it may be treated conservatively.

Epididymo-orchitis

This is inflammation of the epididymis and/or testis. It is associated with UTI or is secondary to viral infection, e.g. mumps or STD.

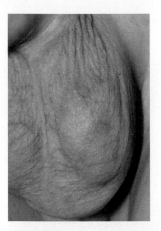

Figure 25.5 Torted left testicular appendage seen as bluish colour on the upper pole of the testis (courtesy of Mr Peter Cuckow)

Clinical features

The symptoms mimic testicular torsion but:

- More gradual onset of testicular pain
- Nausea and vomiting uncommon
- Usually associated with dysuria, pyuria and discharge
- Often febrile

Management

Treatment is with antibiotics. In equivocal cases, surgical exploration must be performed to exclude torsion.

HYPOSPADIAS

Hypospadias is a common congenital abnormality due to a failure in midline fusion of the urethral folds. Degrees of severity are described according to the position of the urethral meatus.

There are three problems:

Ventral urethral meatus	This may lie anywhere from the base of the penis to just below the normal opening on the tip of the glans
Hooded prepuce	Due to a failure of the foreskin to form completely on the under surface of the penis
Chordee	A ventral curvature of the penis

Hypospadias is associated with a higher incidence of inguinal hernia and undescended testis. Unilateral or bilateral impalpable testis and hypospadias raise the possibility of an intersex condition so a karyotype and specialist review is indicated.

Management

Surgical correction is based on straightening the penis and lengthening the urethra to the tip of the penis. More severe forms are often repaired in two stages. The foreskin hood is often used in the repair and boys are usually left with a circumcised appearance. Surgery is usually performed in the second year of life with a good long term outcome from specialist centres.

> **!** **NB: Parents must be told not to have their son circumcised as the foreskin may be used in the repair.**

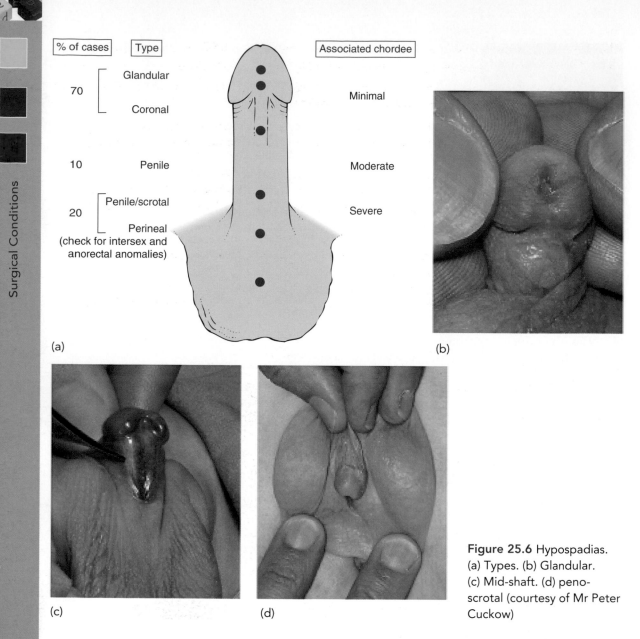

% of cases	Type		Associated chordee
70	Glandular		Minimal
	Coronal		
10	Penile		Moderate
20	Penile/scrotal		Severe
	Perineal		

(check for intersex and anorectal anomalies)

(a)

(b)

(c)

(d)

Figure 25.6 Hypospadias. (a) Types. (b) Glandular. (c) Mid-shaft. (d) peno-scrotal (courtesy of Mr Peter Cuckow)

FORESKIN AND CIRCUMCISION

A non-retractile foreskin is *normal* in infants and young boys. In its early development, the foreskin is *conical* in shape and cannot be retracted over the glans. In addition the under surface of the foreskin is *adherent* to the outer surface of the glans (physiological adhesions).

During childhood the tip of the foreskin widens and the adhesions resolve at a variable rate leading to retraction for around 70% by 5 years of age. Parents of young boys can be reassured and advised that gentle retraction in the bath may help produce a retractile foreskin.

Phimosis

Phimosis (meaning muzzling) describes a tight foreskin which is non-retractile. Non-retraction may persist at **puberty** in around 1% of boys. In most of these there is a secondary scarring of the tip preventing its retraction. This is no longer a physiological narrowing but a pathological entity of the skin known as **lichen**

sclerosus et atrophicans (also known as balanitis xerotica et obliterans [BXO] or posthitis [XO, PXO]). This is the only true indication for medical circumcision, which cures the condition.

Other foreskin problems tend to be transient, with no long term sequelae for foreskin development or general health, so they are only relative indications for circumcision:

Balano-posthitis	Inflammation of the glans (*balano*) and foreskin (*posthitis*) is self-limiting
	Rarely, severe cases may result in urinary retention but most resolve in a few days with bathing
	Systemic or topical antibiotics and antifungals are non-contributory
Ballooning	Seen during voiding in young boys – foreskin distends due to turbulence of urine beneath it. Although it may appear spectacular, it is rarely painful and resolves with foreskin retraction
Paraphimosis	A narrow foreskin becomes stuck behind the glans and restricts the venous and lymphatic drainage of the distal penis. The glans and inner prepuce swell and become quite painful
	Urgent reduction is needed and is achieved after prior compression of the oedema, usually without anaesthetic. Foreskin may continue to develop normally after this

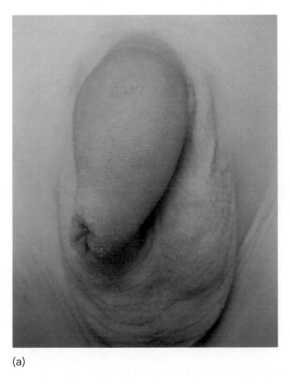

(a)

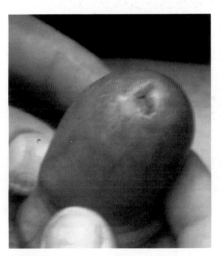

(b)

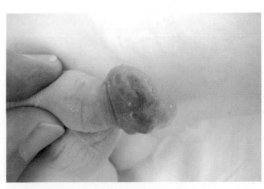

(c)

Figure 25.7 Phimosis. (a) Physiological phimosis. (b) Lichen sclerosus (true phimosis). (c) Paraphimosis (courtesy of Mr Peter Cuckow)

Circumcision

Circumcision is performed for medical reasons and also by some religious groups. In addition, recurrent UTIs may be resolved by circumcision, due to reduction of paraurethral organisms, and it is indicated in boys with severe urinary tract anomalies.

Medical reasons for circumcision

- True phimosis – usually BXO and an absolute indication due to the abnormal foreskin
- Recurrent balano-posthitis – dependent on severity and frequency of symptoms
- Symptomatic ballooning
- Paraphimosis (rare)

ABDOMINAL SURGERY

THE ACUTE ABDOMEN

An acute abdomen is a clinical diagnosis indicating serious intra-abdominal pathology. It requires urgent management through resuscitation and, usually, surgical intervention.

Clinical features

General	Unwell, fever, rigors (sometimes)
Abdominal	Abdominal pain – location, duration, severity, intermittent or constant?
Other	Anorexia, nausea, vomiting, dysuria, haematuria, altered bowel habit (diarrhoea, blood in stool, constipation)

Examination signs

Fever

Vital signs	Pulse (tachycardia), BP (hypotension?), RR (tachypnoea)
	Peripheral shutdown with capillary refill time < 2 s
Abdominal signs	Tenderness (location and severity)
	Guarding
	Rebound tenderness
	Rigid abdomen (unable to 'blow out' abdomen to meet examiner's hand when held a few cm above)

} Features of **peritonitis** (inflammation of the peritoneum)

	Abdominal mass
	Rectal examination to be done by experienced paediatric surgeon or physician (tenderness, blood, mucus)
General signs	Jaundice (gallstones)
	Anaemia (bleed)

Investigations

These will depend on the probable cause, but important investigations are:

Urine	Urinalysis, and microscopy and sensitivities if indicated. Pregnancy test
Blood	FBC, U&E and creatinine, amylase, glucose, sickle cell status if indicated
	Arterial blood gas, LFT, bone profile (Ca and PO_4)
CXR	Erect (chest infection – usually lower lobe, gas under the diaphragm)
AXR	Supine (dilated loops of bowel)
USS abdomen	(Pyloric stenosis, intussusception, ovarian pathology)

Surgical causes of an acute abdomen

Upper GIT	Perforation (oesophageal, gastric or duodenal)
Hepatobiliary	Cholecystitis
	Ruptured liver, spleen or gallbladder (trauma)
Lower GIT	Acute appendicitis
	Inflamed Meckel's diverticulum
	Incarcerated hernia causing ischaemia or obstruction
	Ischaemic bowel, e.g. intussusception, volvulus
	Inflammatory bowel disease causing obstruction, perforation, severe exacerbation or megacolon
Retroperitoneal	Pancreatitis
	Ureteric obstruction (renal colic from stones, trauma)
Pelvic	Testicular torsion
	Ovarian cyst rupture or torsion
	Pelvic inflammatory disease
	Ruptured ectopic pregnancy

Medical causes mimicking an acute abdomen

Respiratory	Lower lobe pneumonia
Gastrointestinal	Mesenteric adenitis, gastroenteritis, constipation
Liver	Acute viral hepatitis
Haematological	Sickle cell disease crisis
Renal	Urinary tract infection (especially pyelonephritis)
	Henoch–Schönlein purpura (see p. 236)
Metabolic	Diabetic ketoacidosis
	Acute porphyrias

INTESTINAL OBSTRUCTION

Causes

Infants	Older children
Pyloric stenosis	Appendicitis
Intestinal atresia or stenosis	Inguinal hernia
Malrotation/volvulus	Malrotation/volvulus
Inguinal hernia	Inflammatory bowel disease
Intussusception	Intussusception
Appendicitis	Gastrointestinal malignancy (rare)
Hirschsprung disease	

Clinical features

- Features of an acute abdomen
- No passage of faeces or flatus per rectum

- Vomiting:
  – Non-bile stained (high obstruction above bile duct entry)
  – Bile stained (obstruction below bile duct entry)
  – Faecal (very low obstruction large bowel)

ACUTE APPENDICITIS

Peak age 10–20 years; rare < 5 years.

Clinical features

- Abdominal pain:
  – Commencing para-umbilically and then moving to the right iliac fossa (McBurney's point)
  – Worse on movement, gradually worsening
  – Guarding indicates peritonitis
- Nausea, vomiting and anorexia
- Low-grade fever, flushed, tachycardic, foetor
- Perforation (common in younger children)
- In young children the pain is poorly localized and features of peritonism may be absent
- A retro-caecal and pelvic appendix may present with atypical signs

Investigations

Diagnosis is *clinical* and difficult as often classical signs are not present. All the above causes of an acute abdomen (both medical and surgical) are in the differential diagnosis.

- FBC (neutrophilia)
- Urinalysis (to exclude UTI). NB: Pyuria may be seen in appendicitis, and so misdiagnosis of UTI should be avoided

Complications – Appendix mass, abscess or perforation.

Management is with urgent appendectomy.

Mesenteric adenitis

This inflammation of the mesenteric lymph nodes can mimic appendicitis with non-localized abdominal pain and is thought to be due to a viral, e.g. adenovirus, or bacterial infection, e.g. *Yersinia enterocolitica*.

INTUSSUSCEPTION

Intussusception is invagination of a dilated segment of bowel into an adjacent proximal segment, usually just proximal to the ileo-caecal valve. The blood supply to the intussuscepted bowel is compromised and may become necrotic if not reduced rapidly. Most common at 6–9 months of age.

Associations

- Male > female
- Meckel's diverticulum
- Henoch–Schönlein purpura
- Intestinal polyps
- Lymphoma

Clinical features

- Episodic abdominal pain with screaming and pallor, and infant draws his/her knees up. Often well in between attacks

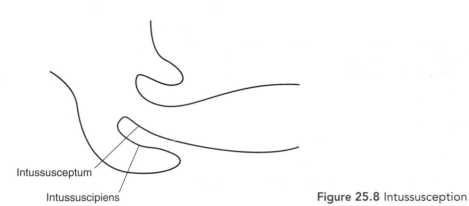

Intussusceptum

Intussuscipiens

Figure 25.8 Intussusception

- Abdominal distension, abdominal tenderness, sausage-shaped abdominal mass
- Blood stained mucous on rectal examination ('redcurrant jelly stools') – a late sign
- Vomiting and diarrhoea
- Infant may be very unwell, dehydrated and progressing to shock

Investigations

Abdominal USS	May reveal the mass if the radiologist is skilled ('target' appearance)
Abdominal X-ray	Signs of small bowel obstruction (fluid levels, dilated loops of small bowel)
Air enema	May be therapeutic as well as diagnostic

Management

- Initial fluid resuscitation as needed
- Air (or contrast) enema reduction (successful in 75%)
- Contraindications to enema:
  – Rectal bleeding
  – Peritonism
- Surgical reduction ± resection if enema contraindicated or unsuccessful

MALROTATION

This is due to *incomplete rotation of the intestine* around the superior mesenteric artery during the third month of gestation. It may present as:

- Intestinal obstruction – neonatal or intermittent childhood obstruction
- Midgut volvulus

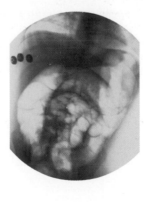

(a)

(b)

Figure 25.9 (a) Air enema of an ileo-colic intussusception in a 1 year old. The leading edge of the intussusception is seen within the air column of the transverse colon (arrow). (b) Successful pneumatic reduction of the intussusception (courtesy of Dr Simon Padley and Dr Kapila Jain)

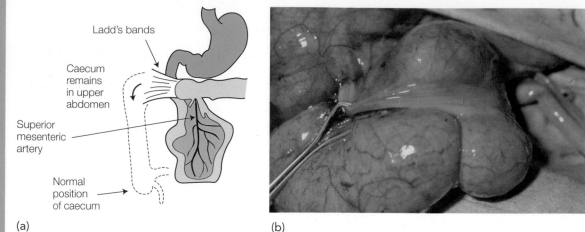

Figure 25.10 (a) Malrotation. (b) Ladd's bands in malrotation seen at operative correction

- A protein-losing enteropathy secondary to bacterial overgrowth
- May be asymptomatic to adolescence (up to 50%)

This should always be treated surgically even if asymptomatic to avoid a volvulus in the future.

MECKEL'S DIVERTICULUM

Meckel's diverticulum is a remnant of the vitellointestinal duct (approximately 2 inches long, and 2 feet from the ileo-caecal valve). It may contain ectopic gastric or pancreatic tissue. Approximately 2% of people are affected.

Clinical features

- Mostly asymptomatic
- May present with rectal bleeding, intussusception, volvulus or acute appendicitis

Investigations

A technetium scan (increased uptake by gastric mucosa) identifies 75%. NB: This should be performed 4 weeks post-bleed to avoid false-negatives (as the gastric mucosa is often ulcerated post-haemorrhage).

Management is surgical resection.

CONGENITAL HYPERTROPHIC PYLORIC STENOSIS

This is due to hypertrophy of the circular muscle layer of the pylorus, and is of unknown cause. Usually presents at 4–6 weeks in first-born males

Associations

- Males > females
- Positive family history (especially maternal)
- Turner syndrome

Clinical features

- Persistent vomiting (may be projectile, not bile-stained)
- Thin but hungry infant
- Visible peristalsis on examination
- *Olive-shaped* tumour in the right upper abdomen

Investigations

Diagnosis is made on a *test feed* or *USS*, both of which are operator-dependent.

Test feed   Palpate the abdomen while infant feeding (milk) for olive-shaped tumour and observe for peristalsis across upper abdomen from left to right ± vomiting

Abdominal USS This may outline the tumour as a 'dough–nut' ring (muscle thickness > 4 mm, pyloric length > 14 mm)

Blood electrolytes and pH must be done to look for signs of dehydration, jaundice (5–10%) and **hypochloraemic hypokalaemic metabolic alkalosis** (due to vomiting).

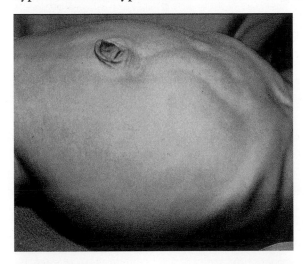

Figure 25.11 Visible wave of peristalsis in a 6-week-old infant with congenial hypertrophic pyloric stenosis

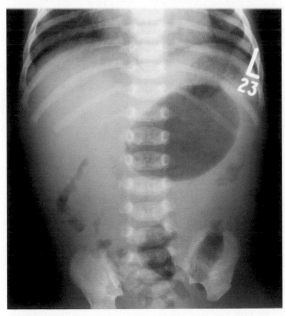

(a)

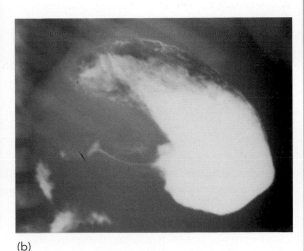

(b)

Figure 25.12 (a) Plain film in a child with congenital hypertrophic pyloric stenosis showing marked dilatation of the stomach with little gas in the distal bowel. (b) Characteristic findings of barium study. The pyloric canal is narrowed and elongated with indentation of the hypertrophied muscle on the lesser curvature

Management

Resuscitation	Initial resuscitation with IV fluids is essential
	0.45% dextrose saline with 40 mmol KCl/L is given over the first 12 h until the bicarbonate is corrected and then standard fluid replacement
	Nasogastric tube with suction
	Regular U&E and blood gas measurements
Surgery	When rehydrated and the alkalosis is corrected, a **pyloromyotomy** (Ramstedt's procedure) is performed

NEONATAL SURGICAL CONDITIONS

CHOANAL ATRESIA

This is a failure of the bucconasal membrane to cannulate during development. As babies are obligate nasal breathers, unless the baby is crying, it presents as breathing difficulties from birth. It may be unilateral or bilateral.

Diagnosis	Inability to pass a nasogastric tube in the affected nostril(s)
Management	Provide an airway (pharyngeal or ETT) until surgery performed (urgently)

> **!** **NB: Babies are obligate nasal breathers unless they are crying.**

OESOPHAGEAL ATRESIA AND TRACHEO-OESOPHAGEAL FISTULA

Oesophageal atresia is usually associated with tracheo–oesophageal fistula, and there are five different types. Overall incidence is 1 in 3000 live births.

The presentation varies depending on the type:

- Maternal polyhydramnios (60%)
- Recurrent aspiration pneumonia
- Coughing episodes with cyanosis
- Abdominal distension (air passes into the gut from the lungs)
- In H-type fistula, intermittent choking with feeds (NB: These are notoriously difficult to diagnose)

Investigations

- Inability to pass a radio-opaque catheter into the stomach (except for H-type)
- AXR – no gas in stomach (types A and B)
- CXR – areas of collapse
- Non-irritant radio-opaque contrast study (to define the lesion)
- Cine contrast swallow with prone oesophagogram (for H-type fistula)

CONGENITAL INTESTINAL ATRESIAS

These may occur anywhere along the gastrointestinal tract. The features are those of obstruction and vary depending on the level of obstruction.

Clinical features of obstruction

- Polyhydramnios
- Bile-stained vomiting

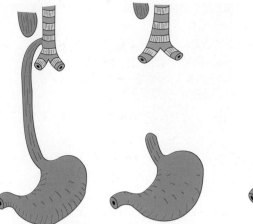

Proximal oesophageal atresia, distal tracheo-oesophageal fistula

Pure oesophageal atresia

H-type tracheo-oesophageal fistula

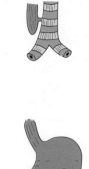

Oesophageal atresia, proximal tracheo-oesophageal fistula

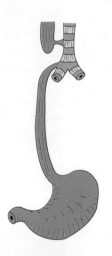

Oesophageal atresia, double tracheo-oesophageal fistula

Figure 25.13 Types of oesophageal and tracheo-oesophageal atresia

■ Abdominal distension
■ Visible peristalsis
■ Delayed or absent passage of meconium
■ Features of dehydration

Investigations

Diagnosis is made on imaging studies, in particular:

Duodenal atresia   'Double bubble' of air seen beneath diaphragm on plain AXR
Imperforate anus   Air bubble seen on AXR after first 12 h with baby held inverted

Duodenal atresia is associated with Down syndrome.

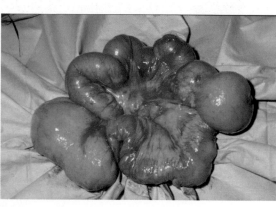

(a)

Figure 25.14 (a) Ileal atresia seen intraoperatively. Note the pre-stenotic dilatation before the section of ileal atresia. (b) Plain X-ray showing jejunal atresia

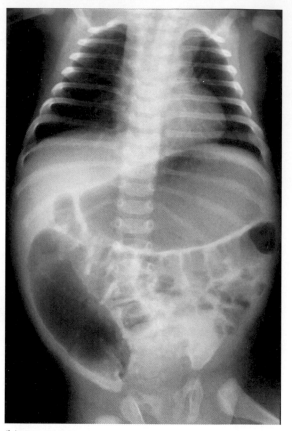

(b)

Imperforate anus

- Incidence 1 in 2500
- Low and high forms exist ± fistula to the urethra or vagina
- Management is often with an initial colostomy with further repair later
- Rectal inertia is a long term problem (see VATER syndrome)

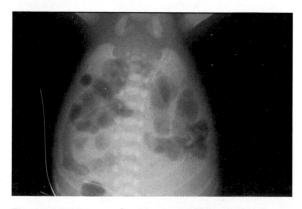

Figure 25.15 Imperforate anus. Abdominal X-ray, taken with the child in the inverted position, showing a gasless rectum

CONGENITAL DIAPHRAGMATIC HERNIA

This sporadic condition is seen in 1 in 4000 live births.

Clinical features

- Severe respiratory distress at birth
- Cyanosis
- Scaphoid abdomen (as intestine in chest)
- Apex beat displaced to the right
- Complications of pulmonary hypoplasia and PPHN may be present (due to lack of space for fetal lung development)

Investigations

CXR and AXR   Loops of bowel in the thorax

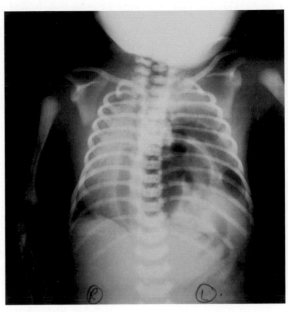

Figure 25.16 Newborn infant with a typical congenital diaphragmatic hernia (Bochdalek) of the left hemidiaphragm. Note the intra-thoracic gas-filled herniated loops (courtesy of Dr Simon Padley and Dr Kapila Jain)

Management

Resuscitation   NG tube and aspiration, intubation and ventilation (IPPV) and circulatory support
Surgery   Correction when fully resuscitated

GASTROSCHISIS AND EXOMPHALOS
Exomphalos

Exomphalos is evisceration of the gastrointestinal contents *through the umbilicus covered by peritoneum.* Incidence 1 in 5000. Associated abnormalities include trisomy 13, trisomy 18, renal malformations and congenital heart disease.

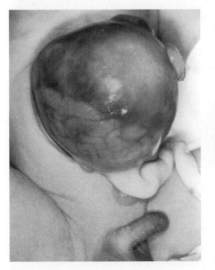

Figure 25.17 Exomphalos

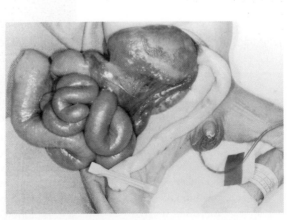

Figure 25.18 Gastroschisis

Gastroschisis

Gastroschisis is evisceration of gastrointestinal contents *through a right paraumbilical defect*. No covering. Incidence 1 in 30 000. Associated abnormalities include bowel scars and adhesions, atresias, strictures and stenosis.

The abdominal contents are wrapped in a moist antibiotic-soaked gauze, and the infant is resuscitated. Small lesions can be repaired directly, but larger lesions need a staged repair.

ORTHOPAEDIC CONDITIONS

OSTEOCHONDRITIDES

Clinically, osteochondritides are idiopathic, acquired, localized disorders of bone and cartilage, typically affecting ossification centres and characterized by localized pain. Some forms are listed below and are possibly related to trauma.

	Osteochondritis	Clinical features
Osgood–Schlatter disease	Tibial tubercle	Tenderness and swelling
Perthes disease	Femoral head	Painless limp (see below)
Freiberg disease	Second metatarsal head	Pain on weight bearing and swelling
Scheuermann disease	Mid-thoracic or lumbar spine	See Kyphosis, p. 401

Perthes disease (Legg–Calve–Perthes)

This is idiopathic avascular necrosis of the *femoral head*, often due to compromise of the nutrient artery. Males > females. Usually aged 4–10 years at presentation.

Clinical features

- Intermittent referred pain to anterior thigh or knee
- Limp (may be painless)
- Reduced internal rotation, abduction and extension of hip (at rest semi-flexed and externally rotated)
- Leg length inequality
- 10–20% bilateral

Investigations

Hip X-rays	Fragmented, flattened femoral head often of increased density Subchondral fracture
MRI hip	May better illustrate early changes
Radionucleotide scan	Reduced femoral head uptake (but increased when neovascularization)

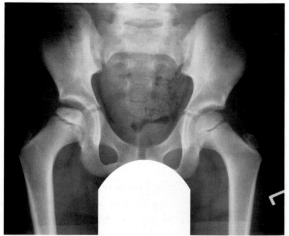

Figure 25.19 Advanced Perthes disease in a 5-year-old boy. The right femoral head is flattened and irregular with subluxation of the right hip and increased joint space suggestive of hypertrophy of the cartilage of the femoral head and the adjacent acetabulum (courtesy of Dr Simon Padley and Dr Kapila Jain)

Management

Varies between centres and depends on severity. Typically conservative (splints and bed rest) if < 6 years old; femoral osteotomy may be required in over 6s.

Causes of limp	
Painless	**Painful**
Missed congenital dysplasia of the hip (CDH)	Infection (septic arthritis, osteomyelitis)
Talipes	Trauma
Perthes disease	Neoplasia
Short limb	Slipped upper femoral epiphysis (SUFE)
Muscular weakness	Irritable hip (transient synovitis)
Neurological, e.g. ataxia, cerebral palsy	Juvenile idiopathic arthritis

> **!** **NB: Any child with knee pain may have *hip pathology* presenting with *referred pain to the knee*.**

CONGENITAL DISLOCATION OF THE HIP

Congenital dislocation of the hip (CDH) (also known as developmental dysplasia of the hip) is due to *incomplete shallow development of the acetabulum*, allowing the femoral head to dislocate. Optimal hip development *in utero* and postnatally requires abduction and external rotation. The following factors affect such positioning:

- Breech position (especially extended breech)
- Oligohydramnios
- Muscular or neurological problem, e.g. spina bifida
- Positive family history

Incidence 2 in 1000. Female > male.

Diagnosis

- Emphasis on screening by identifying risk factors and from examination (Ortolani and Barlow tests; see Neonatal section) at birth and 6-week check
- USS to confirm diagnosis ± orthopaedic examination (and screening of high-ripple infants)
- Clinically obvious when walking develops, by which time diagnosis is too late

Management

Detected early, the hip is immobilized by casts or splints in abducted position with hips and knees flexed to keep the head of the femur in the acetabulum and allow development of the acetabulum and ligaments. Late diagnosis often requires major orthopaedic surgery.

> **!** **NB: Thorough screening for CDH by history and examination is essential to allow early conservative management to be effective. Late detection is difficult to correct surgically and may result in pronounced deformity with limp, pain and early onset of osteoarthritis.**

SLIPPED UPPER FEMORAL EPIPHYSIS

In this disorder the femoral head 'slips' off the femoral neck. It is seen in adolescence, when the growth plate is thought to be at its weakest due to excess growth hormone relative to sex hormones. *Characteristically* either:

- Fat boys with relative hypogonadism (small testes) but normal growth, or
- Tall thin girls with increased growth hormone and normal sex hormone

Associated with hypogonadism, hypothyroidism and pituitary dysfunction.

Clinical features

- Acute presentation with pain (possibly knee pain) and limited hip movement
- Chronic presentation with antalgic limp, hip externally rotated
- On examination – *decreased internal rotation of hip*
- 25% bilateral
- Complications include chondrolysis (articular cartilage degeneration), osteonecrosis and early osteoarthritis

Investigations

Hip X-ray   Widened growth plate
                   Femoral neck anteriorly rotated
                   Femoral epiphyses slipped down and back (in frog legs view)

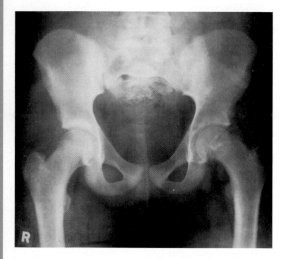

Figure 25.20 Slipped femoral capital epiphysis in a 10-year-old girl who had begun to limp a few weeks earlier. In the AP view the epiphyseal plate of the left femur is widened with caudal slipping of the femoral head in relation to the femoral neck. The right femur head is in normal position (courtesy of Dr Simon Padley and Dr Kapila Jain)

Management is surgical pinning of the femoral head.

IRRITABLE HIP

This is self-limiting transient reactive tenosynovitis associated with, e.g., gastrointestinal illness, EBV, influenza, mycoplasma, streptococcus (see reactive arthritis). It is a common cause of acute hip pain in children aged 2–12 years.

Clinical features

- Sudden onset joint pain (possibly referred to knee, but *no pain at rest*) or limp
- Decreased range of movement
- Child is well ± mild fever

Investigations

This is a diagnosis of exclusion and if there is doubt regarding septic arthritis, aspirate the joint.

- ESR/CRP/neutrophils normal or mildly elevated
- Blood cultures negative
- Joint X-ray – small effusion may be present

Management is bed rest and NSAIDs

PULLED ELBOW

- Distal dislocation of radial head through the annular ligament
- Common injury in toddlers
- Caused by rapid pull on child's forearm, e.g. when lifting child by one arm
- Pseudo-paralysis at the elbow with arm extended, forearm pronated and held at the side
- Often non-tender
- X-rays – radial head away from socket and no fracture
- Treatment is manipulation back into socket (hold flexed elbow in one hand and forearm in other hand, supinate forearm and place thumb over radial head and push it into the elbow)

POSTURAL VARIANTS IN TODDLERS

Postural variants of the developing skeleton are attributable to different load bearing at different ages and so resolve with time. Pathological skeletal variations are fixed and associated with identifiable pathology.

Feature	Normal postural variant	Pathological
Flat feet **(pes planus)**	Normal in toddlers, due to a fat pad under foot and ligamentous laxity	Arch support if persists (hypermobility) ± pain CTDs, e.g. Ehlers–Danlos syndrome
Out-toeing In-toeing	Common throughout childhood **Flat feet** **Metatarsus adductus** – mobile forefoot with adduction deformity Resolves by 5 years **Medial (internal) tibial torsion** esp. in toddlers and corrects by age 4–5 years Bow legs or knock knees **Femoral anteversion** (ligamentous laxity) generally resolves by 8 years Spasticity	Metatarsus varus may need surgery Persistence > 8 years may need surgery
Toe-walking Bow legs **(Genu varum)**	Common and affects Achilles Common in toddlers (May have medial tibial torsion)	Cerebral palsy and Duchenne MD Rickets Idiopathic (Blount disease – abnormal growth of medial proximal tibial epiphysis) Skeletal dysplasia, e.g. neurofibromatosis
Knock knees **(Genu valgum)**	Common in young children, usually improves with age	

TALIPES

Talipes is a positional deformity of the foot of which there are two types.

Talipes equinovarus Most common form
         May be positional or fixed
         Foot supinated with heel inwardly rotated
         Forefoot adducted
Talipes calcaneovalgus Foot everted and dorsiflexed

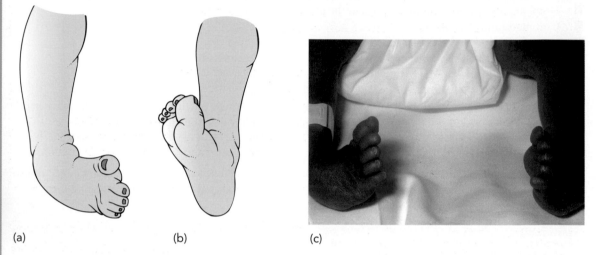

(a)   (b)   (c)

Figure 25.21 (a) Talipes equinovarus. (b) Talipes calcaneovalgus. (c) Talipes equinovarus in a newborn infant

Positional talipes will correct to normal anatomical position during manual examination and responds to physiotherapy. *Fixed talipes* requires diagnosis of underlying cause, e.g. muscular or neurological problems, oligohydramnios, and genetic conditions, and correction by conservative (serial plasters) or surgical means.

> **!** **NB: Congenital vertical talus causes 'rocker bottom' feet and is seen in Edwards syndrome.**

Clinical scenario

A 4-year-old girl is seen by her family practitioner with episodic screaming, pallor, and bowel motions which episodically contain mucous that has been noted to be red on occasions over the last 3 days. In between these episodes she is apparently well. She has a family history of gastrointestinal polyps and she has freckling on her lips.

1. What is the diagnosis and what is the most likely precipitating lesion that would lead to it in this girl?
2. What does the red mucus possible signify and what is it traditionally called?
3. How is the diagnosis arrived at in a non-invasive manner?
4. What are the three available treatment options?

ANSWERS

1. Intussusception and a Peutz–Jegher polyp in the small bowel
2. Possible bowel ischaemia and the 'redcurrant jelly' sign
3. Abdominal ultrasound is preferable to AXR
4. Air insufflations, i.e. pneumo-reduction under radiological surveillance. Gastrograffin reduction under radiological surveillance. Surgical reduction either laparoscopically or via laparotomy. Subsequent polypectomy and investigation for other GI polyps would be needed.

FURTHER READING

Luqmani R, Robb J, Porter D *et al. Textbook of Orthopaedics, Trauma and Rheumatology*. London: Mosby. 2008

Sponseller P. *Handbook of Pediatric Orthopedics*, 2nd edn. Stuggart: Thieme, 2011.

Walsh P, Retik A, Vaughan E, Wein A. *Campbell's Urology*, 8th edn. London: Saunders, 2002.

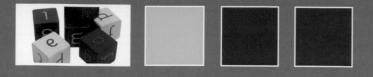

26 Emergencies, Accidents and Non-Accidental Injury

■ Resuscitation
■ Reduced consciousness and coma
■ Major trauma
■ Head injury
■ Status epilepticus
■ Shock
■ Apparent life-threatening event
■ Sudden infant death syndrome
■ Childhood accidents
■ Non-accidental injury
■ Further reading

RESUSCITATION

■ Whatever the underlying cause, in a seriously unwell child the basic initial management is the same (see below)
■ Any compromise of the airway, breathing or circulation must be attended to immediately using basic resuscitation measures
■ Advanced resuscitation is proceeded to when necessary and the equipment is available

The procedures for basic and advanced life support are regularly updated by the European and the UK Resuscitation Committees, and thus the current guidelines should be checked.

MANAGEMENT OF A SERIOUSLY ILL CHILD

Rapid primary assessment and resuscitation

Check area is SAFE	**S**hout for help **A**pproach with care **F**ree from danger **E**valuate ABC	

Assess responsiveness
Assessment and resuscitation:
    A Airway
    B Breathing
    C Circulation
    D Disability:
        Pupillary assessment (size and reaction)
        Conscious level – **AVPU** (see p. 459)
    E Exposure
		Basic life support

Secondary assessment
Detailed history
Detailed examination
Emergency investigations

Emergency treatment
Definitive further treatment (including investigations, monitoring and management as appropriate)

BASIC LIFE SUPPORT

	Infant (< 1 year)	Younger child (< 8 years)	Older child
Check area is SAFE	**S**hout for help **A**pproach with care **F**ree from danger **E**valuate ABC		
Responsiveness		Shake gently and ask if alright	
A – Airway (open and check):			
Head tilt position **Chin lift**	Neutral	Sniffing	Sniffing
Check patency	LOOK for chest and/or abdominal movements LISTEN for breath sounds FEEL for breathing		

	Infant (< 1 year)	Younger child (< 8 years)	Older child
B – Breathing			
Initial slow rescue breaths	Mouth to *mouth-and-nose* 5 breaths	Mouth to *mouth* 5 breaths	Mouth to *mouth* 5 breaths
C – Circulation			
Check pulse	Brachial or femoral	Carotid	Carotid
Start chest compressions (cardiopulmonary resuscitation, CPR) and ventilate if no or inadequate (< 60 beats/min) pulse			
Chest compressions	Two fingers or two thumbs One finger breadth below nipple line Compress to one-third depth of chest	Heel of one hand One finger breadth above xiphisternum	Heel of one hand Two finger breadths above xiphisternum
Rate	100 compressions/min		
Ratio (chest compressions: breaths)	15:2	15:2	15:2

Go for help after 1 min if no one has arrived (take a small child with you)

Adapted from *Advanced Paediatric Life Support*. London: BMJ Publishing Group, 2001[IM123].

Important differences in resuscitation for infants and children

- Head position in *neutral* in infants (not sniffing) as this will keep the airway open (due to their different anatomy)
- Mouth to *mouth-and-nose* in infants – because they are so small this is the easiest way to get air into them
- Check *brachial or femoral pulse* (radial pulse is too difficult to feel in infants)

ADVANCED LIFE SUPPORT

This involves the basic life support with the addition of:

Airway   Oral airway or
Nasal airway (not if risk of basal skull fracture) or
Endotracheal intubation if necessary

$$\text{ETT internal diameter (mm)} = \frac{\text{Age of child}}{4} + 4$$

$$\text{ETT length} = \frac{\text{Age of child}}{2} + 12$$

Suctioning and nasogastric tube insertion
Breathing   Bag and mask/mechanical ventilation with 100% oxygen
Monitor with pulse oximeter and ECG leads
Circulation   Assessment of cardiac output and rhythm (clinically and on ECG monitor)
Give drugs and defibrillate as per protocols
Fluid replacement (intravenous or intraosseous)

Cardiac arrest protocols

Most cardiac arrests in children are *respiratory* in origin with a secondary cardiac arrest.

Three basic cardiac arrhythmias are seen in cardiac arrest (see below):

- Ventricular fibrillation (and pulseless VT)
- Asystole
- Pulseless electrical activity

The blood sugar must be monitored during cardiac arrest as children have low glycogen stores and thus rapidly become hypoglycaemic.

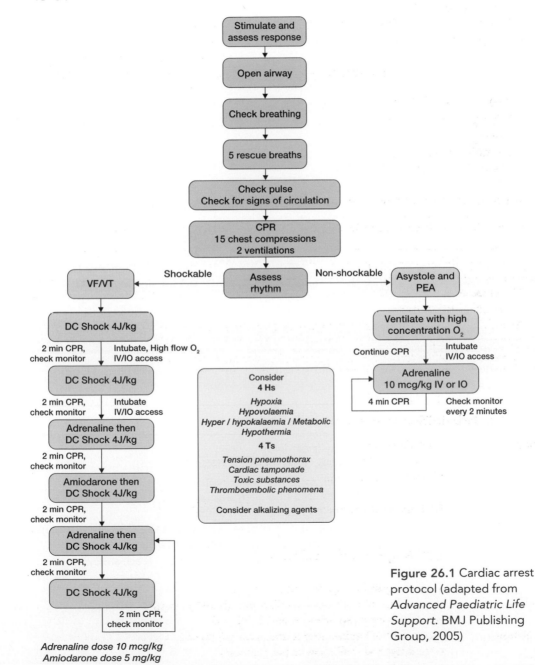

Figure 26.1 Cardiac arrest protocol (adapted from *Advanced Paediatric Life Support*. BMJ Publishing Group, 2005)

> **!** **NB: Almost all cardiopulmonary arrests in infants and children are respiratory in origin.**

CHOKING

If a child is choking (foreign body aspiration suspected) then use:

- Back blows and chest thrusts in an infant
- Back blows, chest thrusts and abdominal thrusts in a child > 1 year

(A finger sweep in the mouth, as used in adults, is not recommended in children as the soft palate can easily be damaged or foreign bodies can be forced further down the airway.)

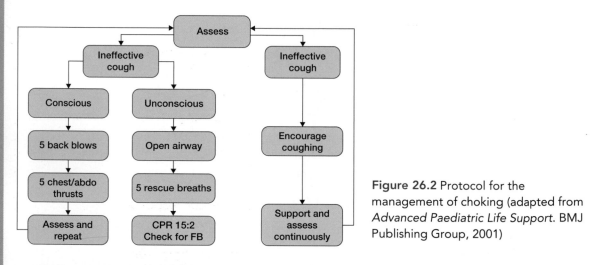

Figure 26.2 Protocol for the management of choking (adapted from *Advanced Paediatric Life Support*. BMJ Publishing Group, 2001)

REDUCED CONSCIOUSNESS AND COMA

Consciousness is awareness of oneself and surroundings in a state of wakefulness. **Coma** is a state of unrousable unresponsiveness.

Causes of reduced conscious level/coma	
CNS	Epilepsy (post-ictal)
	Traumatic brain injury (accidental or NAI)
	Infection, e.g. meningoencephalitis
	Subarachnoid haemorrhage
	Hypoxic–ischaemic brain injury
	Acute raised ICP, e.g. intracranial mass, CSF obstruction; coning
	Brain stem neoplasm, trauma or infarction
Toxins	e.g. alcohol, glue, carbon monoxide, lead, salicylates, accidental ingestion
Metabolic imbalance	e.g. glucose, calcium, sodium ($\uparrow$ or $\downarrow$)
Systemic organ failure	e.g. sepsis, liver failure, Reye syndrome, renal failure, respiratory failure
Temperature instability	Hypothermia or hyperthermia
Inborn error of metabolism	

COMA SCALES

These are important for the rapid assessment of depth of coma in a consistent way. A very rapid assessment is the AVPU coma scale, and the Glasgow and Children's Coma Scales are more comprehensive. The Children's Coma Scale (unlike the Glasgow Coma Scale) has not been validated.

AVPU – Rapid consciousness assessment in primary assessment

A Alert
V Voice responsive
P Pain responsive
U Unresponsive
And pupillary size and reaction should be noted
If P or U intubate and ventilate

Children's Coma Scale (< 4 years)		Glasgow Coma Scale (> 4 years)	
Response	**Score**	**Response**	**Score**
Eye opening		**Eye opening**	
Spontaneous	4	Spontaneous	4
To speech	3	To speech	3
To pain	2	To pain	2
None	1	None	1
Best motor response		**Best motor response**	
Spontaneous or obeys command	6	Obeys command	6
Localizes pain	5	Localizes pain	5
Withdraws from pain	4	Withdraws from pain	4
Abnormal flexion to pain	3	Abnormal flexion with pain	3
Abnormal extension to pain	2	Abnormal extension to pain	2
None	1	None	1
Best verbal response		**Best verbal response**	
Alert, babbles as usual	5	Orientated and converses	5
Fewer sounds/words than usual, irritable cry		4	
Disorientated and converses	4		
Cries to pain only	3	Inappropriate words	3
Moans to pain	2	Incomprehensible sounds	2
None	1	None	1

MANAGEMENT OF DECREASED CONSCIOUS STATE

The initial management of an unconscious patient is to assess and stabilize the child. While this is being done, further history, examination and investigations to establish the *cause* of the coma can be performed.

Rapid primary assessment (ABCDE) and resuscitation

Pay particular attention to:

- Securing the airway (give 100% oxygen and intubate and ventilate if necessary)
- Establish IV access, check glucose stick (and treat any hypoglycaemia)

- Initial blood samples.
- Give IV fluids 20 mL/kg initial bolus if in shock
- Give broad-spectrum antibiotic if meningitis or sepsis suspected or no cause found
- Rapid coma scale (AVPU), pupillary assessment, posture
- Check all over for other signs including temperature and rash

Secondary assessment

History (specific points)	Where discovered and by whom. Any witnesses?
	Resuscitation history with accurate timings
	Enquire about trauma, poisons, possible self-harm, infectious disease exposure, travel, preceding fit, febrile illness, pre-existing disease (neurological, metabolic) and social history (NAI)
Further examination	Check for any 'medic alert' bracelet.
	Detailed neurological examination (full coma scale score, pupil size and reactivity, fundi, posture and tone, deep tendon reflexes)
	Signs of injury (including nasal discharge. See Major Trauma, p. 461)
	Signs of meningism (fundi – retinal haemorrhages, papilloedema, neck stiffness)
	Skin rash (petechial rash, bruising, jaundiced)
	Abnormal smell, e.g. ketones, organic solvents, metabolic disorder
	General examination – signs of other systemic disease

Investigations

Blood	BM stix, blood cultures, FBC, clotting studies, cross-match, U&E, creatinine, LFT, glucose, CRP, toxicology, lactate, ammonia and blood gas
Urine	Glucose, protein, microscopy and culture, toxicology, amino and organic acids
	Keep sample for rarer inborn errors of metabolism especially if hypoglycaemic at time of presentation (store at − 70°C)
Brain scan	(CT or MRI) if no identifiable cause found
CXR ± AXR	(Post intubation)

Lumbar puncture should *not be done* on a comatose child. It can be performed later when the condition allows.

Further management

- Monitor vital signs (pulse, temperature, BP, respiration, oxygen saturation, neurological observations)
- Treat on paediatric intensive care unit if GCS < 8.
- Site nasogastric tube. Aspirate (keep initial contents for analysis)
- Catheterize
- Monitor and stabilize blood sugar and electrolytes
- Treat any epileptic seizures with anticonvulsants
- Consider aciclovir (if herpes encephalitis a possibility)
- Monitor and treat any raised ICP (mannitol IV ± hyperventilation to induce hypocapnoea)
- Further detailed investigations to establish the cause and treat specific conditions as necessary

BRAIN DEATH

Brain death is the irreversible *loss of consciousness* and the *capacity to breathe*. This is accepted to occur when there is permanent functional death of the brain stem.

- Diagnosis of brain death requires the absence of brain stem function (no brain stem reflexes) for at least 24 h
- Child must be unconscious with no drugs acting that affect consciousness or respiratory function

- Coma state must:
    - Be apnoeic despite hypercapnoiec drive (PaCO$_2$ > 6.7 kPa)
    - Be of diagnosed cause
    - Exclude drugs, poisons, hypothermia (< 35°C) and biochemical disturbance
    - There must be no treatable metabolic or endocrine cause
- Assessment of brain stem reflexes, tested by two senior physicians working independently. The reflexes must be retested at least ½ h apart

Brain stem reflexes in brain death	
Pupils	Fixed, dilated. No direct or consensual reflexes
Corneal reflex	Absent
Oculocephalic reflex	Absent ('doll's eye reflex')
Caloric tests	(vestibulo-ocular reflexes). Absent
Painful stimulus	No response to central and peripheral stimuli (primitive reflexes may be present)
Gag reflex	Absent
Apnoea	10 min disconnected from the ventilator, with 100% high flow oxygen, and arterial blood gas PaCO$_2$ > 6.7 kPa (50 mmHg)

MAJOR TRAUMA

1. Primary survey and resuscitation (ABCDE)

Life–threatening conditions are identified and treated immediately. Pay particular attention to:

- Securing the airway with **cervical spine** control (assume spinal injury until examination and adequate investigations found to be normal)
- Check for **pneumothorax and haemothorax**
- Estimation of **blood loss** (heart rate, BP, capillary refill, respiratory rate, temperature, skin colour and mental status)
- IV access, and give 20 mL/kg fluid bolus, repeat if necessary
- If > 40 mL/kg needed, give blood and obtain urgent surgical opinion
- Rapid **neurological status** assessment (AVPU, pupillary size and reactivity)
- Complete examination to check for **other injuries** (and then cover with blanket)

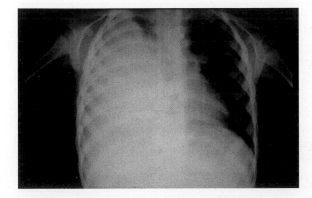

Figure 26.3 Chest X-ray showing right haemothorax in a child involved in a road traffic accident

During the resuscitation take a more detailed history (of accident and medical history) and do basic investigations:

Detailed history	**A**llergies
	Medications
	Previous illness/injury (PMH)
	Last oral intake
	Environment in which the injury occurred
Investigations	X-rays – CXR, pelvis, C-spine
	Blood tests – ABG, FBC, cross-match, glucose, U&Es

Also:

- Catheterize if necessary
- Nasogastric tube and aspiration (pass tube orally if basal skull fracture suspected)
- Give analgesia if necessary (IV morphine)

2. Secondary survey

When the child has been stabilized a detailed secondary survey can be done, from top downwards:

- Head ⎫
- Face ⎭ Assess for injuries
- Neck – assume spinal injury until proven otherwise
- Chest – open wound, tension pneumothorax, haemothorax
- Abdomen – ruptured organs (kidneys, liver, spleen, bowel)
- Pelvis ⎫
- Spine ⎭ Assess for injuries
- Extremities – open wounds, fractures

3. Emergency treatment

Treatment of any injuries discovered during the secondary survey.

4. Definitive care

HEAD INJURY

This is the single most common cause of trauma death in children. Minor head injuries are common.

Forms of head injury

Concussion	Brief reversible impairment of consciousness
Extradural haematoma	Bleed in the middle meningeal space due to rupture of the middle meningeal artery or dural veins
	A convex lesion is seen on CT scan
Subdural haematoma	Bleed between the dura and cerebral mantle, due to rupture of cortical veins
	Seen in *shaken infants* (non-accidental injury)
	May be *chronic*, with gradual enlargement and a history of irritability, poor feeding and lethargy
	A concave lesion is seen on CT scan
Intracerebral contusions	An insult to the brain substance

Causes

- Road traffic accidents
- Falls, e.g. windows, trees, walls
- Non-accidental injury (usually infants)

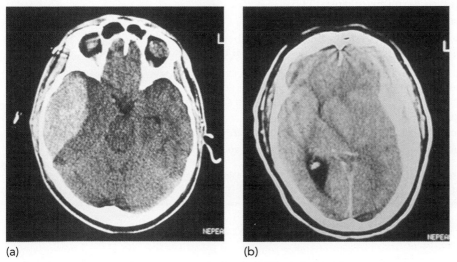

(a)   (b)

Figure 26.4 CT scans showing (a) extradural and (b) subdural haematomas

> **!** **ND:** A skull fracture is not always present with severe cerebral injury. Subdural haematoma is most common in head injuries without skull fracture.

Suspect severe head injury if:

- Substantial injury, e.g. RTA, fall from great height
- Loss of consciousness at time of injury
- Impaired level of consciousness
- Neurological signs
- Penetrating injury

STATUS EPILEPTICUS

Primary assessment (ABCDE)

Pay particular attention to:

- Airway maintenance and high flow oxygen
- Check glucose stick and treat hypoglycaemia
- IV fluids if signs of shock
- Give antibiotic if sepsis or meningitis suspected

Emergency treatment of convulsion

IV lorazepam if IV access quickly established. Rectal diazepam if no IV access

↓

If convulsion continues after 10 min repeat lorazepam. Rectal paraldehyde in olive oil if no IV access. If seizure continues:

- Get senior help (and liaise with anaesthetist/ITU)
- Give rectal paraldehyde if not already given

↓

- IV phenytoin infusion given over 20 min (phenobarbitone if on phenytoin for epilepsy)

↓

If seizure continues after phenytoin:

- Re-check ABC
- Have anaesthetist present
- Take blood, correct any metabolic abnormality and treat pyrexia. Consider mannitol
- Rapid sequence induction of anaesthesia with thiopentone and short-acting paralysing agent

SHOCK

Shock is the failure of adequate perfusion of the tissues.

Causes

- Hypovolaemic, e.g. blood loss, gastrointestinal fluid loss, ketoacidosis, skin loss (burns)
- Distributive, e.g. **septicaemia**, anaphylaxis, spinal cord injury
- Cardiogenic, e.g. arrhythmias, cardiac failure, myocardial infarction
- Obstructive, e.g. tension pneumothorax, cardiac tamponade, pulmonary embolism
- Dissociative, e.g. profound anaemia, carbon monoxide poisoning

Three stages of shock

It is important to recognize the early stages (compensated) shock because early treatment of shock is vital.

1. Compensated shock   Perfusion to vital organs is maintained at the expense of non-essential tissues (capillary refill time [CRT] may be normal or poor, core–peripheral differential of < 2°C)

Clinical features of the stages of shock

	Compensated	Uncompensated	Preterminal
Heart rate	↑	↑↑	↑ then ↓
Systolic BP	N	N or ↓	Falling
Respiratory rate	N or ↑	↑↑	Sighing
Pulse volume	N or ↓	↓	↓↓
Capillary refill time	N or ↑	↑	↑↑
Skin	Pale, cool	Mottled, cold	Pale, cold
Mental status	Agitation	Lethargic	Deeper coma
Urine output	↓	Absent	Absent
Peripheral temperature	Low	Low	Low
Core–peripheral temperature differential	< 2°C	>2°C	>2°C
Estimated fluid loss	< 25%	25–40%	> 40%

Estimated blood volume (EBV)	
Age	**EBV (mL/kg)**
Neonate	90
Infant up to 1 year	80
> 1 year	70

2. Uncompensated shock	Mechanisms start to fail, tissue hypoxia and acidosis occur
	Core–peripheral differential of > 2°C, poor CRT
3. Preterminal	Situation is becoming irreversible

Management

Immediate management is the same for all types of shock:

- **Primary assessment and resuscitation** (ABCDE). Pay particular attention to cardiovascular status:
  - Pulse rate, pulse volume, capillary refill, blood pressure
  - Effects of circulatory compromise on other organs (sighing respirations, pale skin, mental status, urine output)
  - Features of heart failure
- Give 100% oxygen via face mask
- Obtain IV or intra-osseous access. Fluid replacement in boluses of 20 mL/kg (crystalloid or colloid, then blood) as required
- Low threshold for broad-spectrum antibiotics as *sepsis is the most common cause in children*
- **Secondary assessment** (including detailed neurological status) with detailed history and examination

If there is no improvement, or if improvement requires > 40 mL/kg fluid, then consider mechanical ventilation, inotropic support, intensive monitoring, catheterization and correction of any biochemical and haematological abnormalities as necessary.

ANAPHYLAXIS

This is an IgE-mediated acute reaction to an allergen. The clinical features and severity are variable and include:

Airway and breathing	Bronchospasm, upper airway obstruction (stridor, wheeze, cyanosis), respiratory arrest
Circulation	Tachycardia, shock, collapse, cardiac arrest
Skin	Urticaria, conjunctivitis, facial swelling

Management

- Primary assessment and resuscitation
- Removal of the cause
- Airway:
  - If obstruction or stridor call for anaesthetic and ENT help
  - Give epinephrine (adrenaline) 10 μg/kg **intramuscular** and nebulized epinephrine (adrenaline) (5 ml of 1:1000)
  - Give 100% oxygen. Intubation or surgical airway if necessary
  - Monitor saturations and for wheeze
- Breathing – if bronchoconstriction give nebulized salbutamol ⎫ Epinephrine (adrenaline)
- Circulation – if in shock give colloid bolus(es) IV or IO ⎭ if not already given
- Further emergency management – as necessary consider intubation, treatment for asthma, further fluid boluses, further epinephrine (adrenaline), antihistamine and steroids

APPARENT LIFE-THREATENING EVENT

Apparent life-threatening events (ALTEs) are unexpected episodes in infants, which may involve:

- Apnoea
- Unresponsiveness
- Choking
- Central cyanosis or pallor

There are often no other obvious symptoms. A serious underlying disorder needs to be excluded but no cause may be found.

Causes

- Infection – sepsis, viral infection
- Seizure
- Gastro-oesophageal reflux
- Hypoglycaemia
- Central apnoea
- Cardiac – arrhythmia, cyanotic spell
- Encephalopathy – metabolic upset
- Suffocation (fictitious or induced illness)

Management

- Initial survey (ABCDE) and resuscitation as necessary
- Secondary survey:
  - Thorough history (in particular check social situation)
  - Full examination
- Admit to hospital for close monitoring (oxygen saturations, ECG, respiration)
- Investigate further as appropriate:
  - ABG, glucose, FBC, U&E, creatinine
  - Infection screen
  - Reflux investigations (pH study)
  - Cardiac screen (CXR, ECG, echocardiogram)
  - Metabolic screen
  - Toxicology screen
- Teach parents resuscitation

SUDDEN INFANT DEATH SYNDROME (OR SUDDEN UNEXPECTED DEATH IN INFANCY)

Sudden infant death syndrome (SIDS) is the sudden unexplained death of a previously well infant in which no cause is found after postmortem examination.

- It most commonly occurs at 2–4 months
- Risk of SIDS for subsequent children is increased

There has been a significant decrease in the number of SIDS cases with the advice:

- Put the baby on his/her back to sleep
- Avoid overheating the baby
- Tuck the baby in with his/her feet to the base of the cot (so the risk of slipping under the cover is reduced)

- Use blankets with holes in them and not duvets for infants
- Avoid smoking while pregnant and after pregnancy
- Avoid smoking in the house
- Have the baby sleep in the parents' bedroom for the first 6 months at least
- Do not put the baby in the parents' bed when they are tired or have taken drugs or alcohol

Basic resuscitation skills should be taught to parents of children at risk. Home apnoea monitoring for infants at risk may be considered, though in some cases this can prove anxiety-provoking for the parents and has not been proven to be of benefit.

CHILDHOOD ACCIDENTS

Accidents are the commonest cause of death in children aged 1–14 years, and they are broadly predictable and therefore often preventable.

Causes of fatal accidents

Road traffic accidents	50%
Fire	30%
Drowning	10%
Suffocation and choking	
Falls	
Poisoning	

ROAD TRAFFIC ACCIDENTS

Road traffic accidents are the most common cause of accidental childhood deaths in the UK. They may involve:

Car passenger	Well fitting car seat and seatbelts are preventative
Pedestrian	Young school boys are at most risk. Environmental measures are most preventive
Bicyclist	Most common in boys. Crash helmets are significant in reducing severity

For management see Major Trauma and Head Injury above, p. 461 and 462.

NEAR DROWNING

Drowning is the third commonest cause of accidental death in children in the UK. Up to 70% will survive if basic life support is provided at the scene. Termed **near drowning** if any recovery following immersion, and **drowning** if no recovery after immersion.

- Effects of submersion
  - Breath-holding → bradycardia (diving reflex) → hypoxia → tachycardia, BP ↑, acidosis
  - Then breathing movements occur (< 2.5 min) → laryngeal spasm and secondary apnoea
  - Then involuntary breathing efforts, bradycardia, arrhythmias, cardiac arrest
- Hypothermia common (this protects against hypoxic brain damage)
- Fresh water and salt water both cause (via different mechanisms) pulmonary oedema and hypoxaemia, and have the same prognosis

BURNS

Causes of burns and scalds

- Hot liquids
- Fire
- Smoke inhalation
- Electrical injury
- Chemical burns

Assessment

Burns are assessed by:

Depth — *Partial thickness* (pink or mottled skin, blistering, painful)
Full thickness (white or charred skin, painless)

Extent — Expressed as a percentage of body surface area (see below)

Location — Airway involvement in smoke inhalation must be checked for
Hand and face burns are of particular cosmetic and functional significance

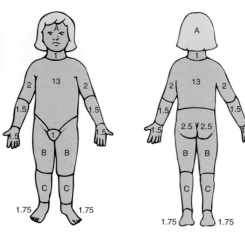

Figure 26.5 Assessment of burns

Percentage surface area at different ages					
Area	0 years	1 year	5 years	10 years	15 years
A	9.5	8.5	6.5	5.5	4.5
B	2.75	3.25	4.0	4.25	4.5
C	2.5	2.5	2.75	3.0	3.25

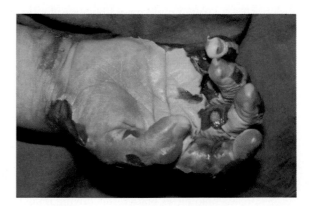

Figure 26.6 Scald of a child's hand

Management

Burn management is coordinated by the plastic surgical team, and if treated as an inpatient this should be on a burns unit.

- **Primary survey and resuscitation** (ABCDE). Pay special attention to:
  - Airway – if inhalation injury intubation by expert may be necessary
  - Exposure – rapid heat loss occurs from burnt areas
- **Secondary survey** – assess the burn (see above)
- **Emergency treatment**
  - **Analgesia** – burns are very painful and so strong IV analgesics are required for all but minor burns
  - **Initial shock**:
    - IV fluids via two large cannulae as skin fluid loss may be extensive
    - Burns > 10% body surface area will need additional IV fluid replacement:
    - *Additional fluid* requirement – percentage burn × weight (kg) × 4; monitor urine output
  - **Wound care**:
    - Removal of dead tissue, then placement of sterile dressings
    - Significant burns must be managed on a burns unit, e.g. full thickness burns, > 10% body surface area, inhalational burns, hand and face burns
- **Definitive care** – this is carried out on a paediatric burns unit

ACUTE POISONING

Poisoning in young children is usually accidental, though deliberate poisoning is seen in adolescents and in fictitious or induced illness (FII).

General management

- Take history including:
  - Substance(s) ingested
  - Amount
  - Exact timing
- Examination – ABCDE assessment and resuscitation. In particular:
  - Level of consciousness
  - Orophayrnx
  - Features specific to particular poisons (see below)
- Investigations:
  - Drug levels, e.g. salicylates, paracetamol
  - U&Es, creatinine, LFTs, clotting profile, ABGs, FBC
- *Elimination – contact the Regional Poisons Information Centre for advice*
- *Specific antidotes, investigations and therapy for particular poisons*

There are two methods of **elimination**:

Activated charcoal	Considered if ingestion is recent
	Charcoal is given orally (via nasogastric tube if necessary), and works by absorbing the drug itself, thereby reducing the intestinal absorption of drugs
Gastric lavage	Rarely indicated in children. Most effective < 1 h of ingestion
	Airway must be protected during the procedure
	Contraindicated after ingestion of corrosives and hydrocarbons due to potential for aspiration pneumonitis

Clinical features and possible causative drug

Small pupils	Opiates, organophosphates
Large pupils	Amphetamines, tricyclics, cocaine, cannabis
Tachycardia	Amphetamines, cocaine, antidepressants
Bradycardia	β-blockers
Hypotension	β-blockers, antidepressants, opiates, iron, tricyclics
Hypertension	Cocaine, amphetamines
Tachypnoea	Aspirin, carbon monoxide
Bradypnoea	Alcohol, opiates
Convulsions	Tricyclics, organophosphates

Specific poison remedies

Substance	Clinical effects	Specific management
Bleach	Local erosions	Give oral milk and antacids (may help) Avoid emesis Use of systemic steroids is contentious Ventilatory support if necessary Endoscopy to assess damage if necessary
Button batteries	Gastointestinal upset Gut wall corrosion Oesophageal stricture Mercury release if batteries broken	CXR and AXR to assess progress along the gut Remove if there are signs of disintegration or not moving, and consider if not passed within a few days Remove if in oesophagus within 6 hours
Paracetamol	Gastric irritation Liver failure after 2–3 days	Check plasma levels 4 hours after ingestion If plasma concentration high or > 150 mg/kg thought to have been ingested, IV acetylcysteine as per protocol Monitor liver function over next few days (PT prolongation is best predictor of need for liver support or transplant)
Salicylates	Nausea and vomiting Dehydration Tinnitus, deafness Disorientation Hyperventilation Respiratory alkalosis Metabolic acidosis Hypoglycaemia	Check plasma salicylate level Empty stomach if < 12 h of ingestion Correct dehydration, electrolyte and fluid imbalance Forced alkaline diuresis if severe Dialysis if severe
Alcohol	Hypoglycaemia	Monitor blood glucose regularly Give IV glucose if necessary

NON-ACCIDENTAL INJURY

Types

- Physical abuse
- Sexual abuse
- Emotional abuse and neglect
- Fictitious or induced illness (FII) (used to be termed Munchausen syndrome by proxy)

PHYSICAL ABUSE

Following accidental injury, parents would normally be very concerned and bring their child straight to medical attention and give a consistent and plausible history of events. The following features of the history should raise suspicion of physical abuse:

- Unexplained or multiple injuries
- Inconsistent history
- Late presentation
- Unusual parental behaviour, e.g. hostile, unconcerned
- Anxious withdrawn child (termed '*frozen watchfulness*')

Injuries seen in physical abuse

- Lacerated oral frenulum (due to carer forcing bottle into infant's mouth)
- Bruises:
  - Finger tip bruises
  - Posterior auricular bruising (from ear pulling)
  - Belt mark bruises
  - Bite marks
  - Unexplained multiple bruises (especially when *not* over bony prominences)
- Burns and scalds:
  - Unexplained burns or scalds
  - Cigarette burns
  - Buttocks scald (put in hot bath)
- Head injuries:
  - Retinal haemorrhages (caused by shaking injury 'shaken baby') (see p. 408)
  - Subdural haematoma (from shaking injury)
  - Wide skull fractures (> 3 mm displacement)
- Fractures:
  - Unexplained or multiple fractures
  - Spiral fractures
  - Old fractures not previously brought to medical attention

SEXUAL ABUSE

In most cases of sexual abuse the perpetrator is male and the abused child female, although all variations exist.

Features of sexual abuse include:

- Sexually transmitted infection
- Genital injury with no plausible explanation
- Urinary tract infection, enuresis
- Anal fissure, pruritis ani, constipation, encopresis
- Inappropriate sexual behaviour, i.e. sexualized behaviour
- Behavioural disturbance
- Direct allegation of abuse

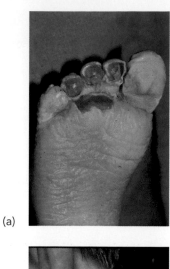

(a)

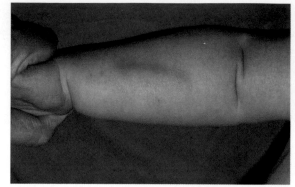

(c)

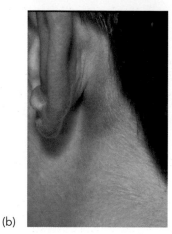

(b)

Figure 26.7 Physical abuse. (a) Scald to the foot of an infant can be due to being put in a hot bath. (b) Posterior auricular bruise can be secondary to pulling the ear. (c) Linear bruise on the arm of a child not overlying a bony prominence is suggestive of non-accidental injury

Differential diagnosis of physical non-accidental injury		
Bruising	Coagulation disorders (family history?)	
	Leukaemia	
	Immune thrombocytopaenic purpura (ITP)	
	Henoch–Schönlein purpura	
	Mongolian blue spot	
Fractures	Osteogenesis imperfecta	
	Copper deficiency	NB: All rare
	Rickets	
	Local bone tumour	

EMOTIONAL ABUSE AND NEGLECT

This can be difficult to identify. Features include general neglect, dirty child, scruffy clothing, a miserable child and faltering growth.

FICTITIOUS OR INDUCED ILLNESS

This is an uncommon form of abuse in which illness in the child is fabricated by the parent(s) or carer.

Features of the disorder include:

- Condition which is difficult to diagnose
- Features are only present when the parent is present
- Multiple hospital admissions
- Mother often has healthcare connections, e.g. a nurse

Examples are:

- Feeding salt to the child
- Putting blood in the urine, stool or vomit
- Putting sugar in the urine

The child can come to serious harm from these activities, not least from protracted unnecessary medical investigations to determine the source of the fictitious symptoms.

MANAGEMENT OF NON-ACCIDENTAL INJURY

There are the national guidelines regarding the management of NAI, emphasizing the team approach between hospital- and community-based professionals, and dedicated child protection teams including paediatricians, social workers, health visitors, GP, police, teachers and lawyers. Important points to remember in suspected cases are:

- Involvement of *senior child protection paediatrician early*
- *Detailed history* should be taken including direct 'quotes'. Remember to record date and time and sign notes. Include detailed family and social history
- *Full examination with consent* (ideally only once by senior paediatrician(s) and if necessary a forensic physician from the child protection team to minimize distress to the child). Observe child–parent interaction
- *Detailed documentation* of the injuries with chronology (if possible photographs with consent)
- Relevant *investigations* (X-rays, blood tests) and treatment of injuries
- In suspected or confirmed abuse, all cases are managed by a *dedicated multidisciplinary child protection team*. The team decides whether any emergency and/or long term action is needed
- If necessary *immediate protection* with admission to hospital for observation, treatment and investigation. (Parental consent usually obtained for this, but if not legal enforcement is necessary using a child protection order [see p. 477]
- A *child protection conference* is scheduled to decide if and what further action is necessary. From this there may be a decision to place the child on the Child Protection Register, and/or the development of a child protection care plan. In some cases placement in care is necessary (in severe cases long term foster care and/or adoption)

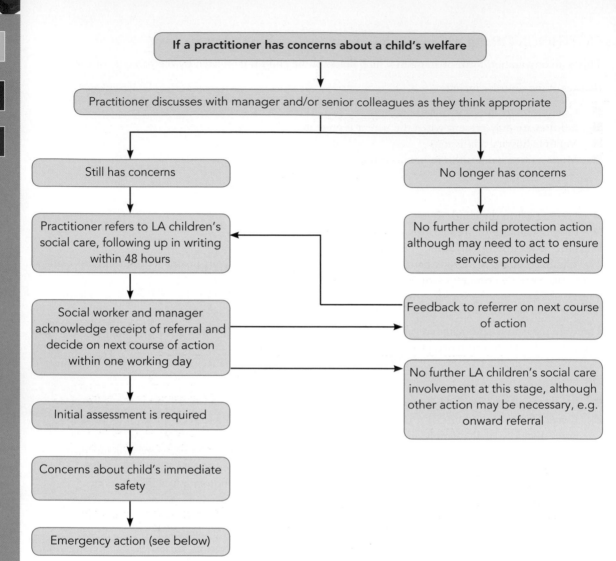

Figure 26.8 Management of non-accidental injury if a practitioner has concerns about a child's welfare (Department of Health Children's Services Guidelines 2006)

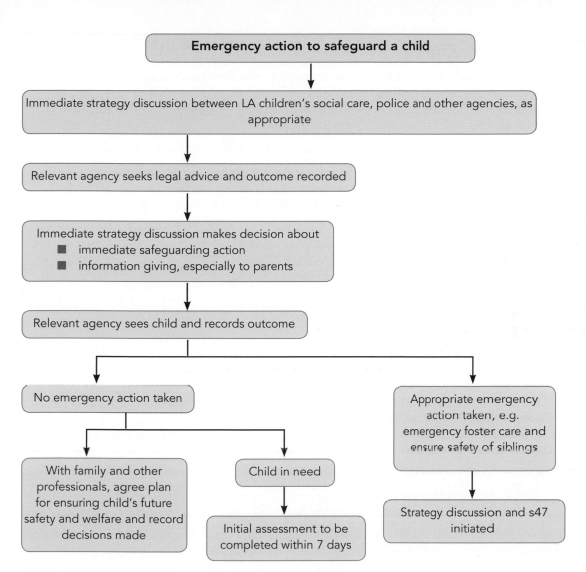

Figure 26.9 Management of non-accidental injury: emergency action to safeguard a child (Department of Health Children's Services Guidelines, 2006)

Clinical scenario

A 6-year-old boy is found at home and brought to the Emergency Department in an altered conscious state, unable to recognize his mother, and not able to obey simple commands. He has apparently been well that day until he was found by his step-father after he and his mother returned from a night out.

1. What are your first three priorities as he comes into the Emergency Department?

It transpires on rapid history taking that he is from a chaotic family background, that he has had no immunizations, and that grandmother is taking warfarin. A number of dark non-blanching skin lesions with some older linear-shaped bruises are evident on his limbs.

2. What four diagnoses are uppermost in your mind?
3. Suggest a first line treatment or approach for each.
4. How would you confirm or refute the diagnosis in each?

ANSWERS

1. ABC
2. 1. Meningococcal septicaemia
   2. Pneumococcal septicaemia
   3. Acute leukaemia
   4. Coagulopathy due to accidental warfarin overdose
3. 1 and 2. Immediate parenteral penicillin; 3. FBC, bone marrow aspirate and appropriate chemotherapy; 4. Vitamin K parenterally
4. 1 and 2. Blood culture + lumbar puncture; 3. FBC and bone marrow aspirate; 4. PT

FURTHER READING

Advanced Life Support Group. *Advanced Paediatric Life Support: The Practical Approach (Fourth Edition)*. London: BMJ Books. 2004.

Advanced Life Support Group. *Advanced Paediatric Life Support: The Practical Approach,* 5th edn. Oxford: Wiley-Blackwell, 2011.

Cameron P, Jelinek G, Everitt I *et al. Textbook of Paediatric Emergency Medicine*. London: Churchill Livingstone. 2005.

Crisp S, Rainbow J (eds.). *Emergencies in Paediatrics and Neonatology*. Oxford: Oxford University Press, 2007.

Tasker R, McClure R, Acerini C, Crisp S, Rainbow J (eds.). *Oxford Handbook of Paediatrics and Emergencies in Paediatrics Pack*. Oxford: Oxford University Press, 2009.

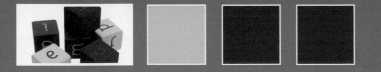

27 The Child and the Law

- The Children's Act
- Statementing
- Wardship
- Inherent jurisdiction
- Court orders
- Consent
- Further reading

THE CHILDREN'S ACT

The Children's Act is a document designed for the protection of children. It was fully implemented in 1991 (and given Royal assent in 1989). It includes the following features:

- Child's welfare is the court's paramount consideration, so any court order made should contribute positively to the child's welfare
- Prime responsibility for bringing up children lies with the parents
- Local authorities should provide supportive services to help parents in bringing up children
- Local authorities should take reasonable steps to identify children and families in need
- Every local authority should work in partnership with the parents

PROTECTION ORDERS

The Children's Act 1989 also provides protection orders for children 'at risk'. These are:

Emergency protection order (EPO)	Any person may apply to a magistrate's court for an EPO and then will have parental responsibility for the child if granted. The order lasts 8 days and an extension of a further 7 days is possible. An appeal can be made after 3 days
Police protection provision	Police may take a child into police protection without assuming parental responsibility. This lasts for up to 3 days only
Child assessment order	This allows proper assessment of a child to be done over a period of up to 7 days. (Removal of the child from the family home does not necessarily occur)
Care and supervision orders	These allow a child to be placed in the care of or under the supervision of the local authority. Maximum duration is 8 weeks

STATEMENTING

As part of the **Education Act 1981** (updated 1993) the local education authority must provide a statement for a child with special education needs to outline the special needs of the child and the consequent services that the education authority will provide.

- An **initial assessment** is made of the child's particular needs and disabilities by interested professionals (including, as necessary, teacher, paediatrician, educational psychologist, occupational therapist, physiotherapist and speech therapist)
- Then a **statement of special educational needs**, i.e. plan of help, of the child's educational and non-educational needs is made, which includes information given by the parents and professionals. The special services to be offered to the child are included within the statement, e.g. one-to-one tuition, special transport to school
- It is important that the statement be regularly reviewed and revised or cancelled as necessary

WARDSHIP

If a child is a '**ward of court**', 'the court is entitled and bound in appropriate cases to make decisions in the interests of the child which override the rights of its parents'. Wardship may not be invoked by the local authority or while the child is in care, but may be made by other interested parties, e.g. a health authority, and it ends when a child ceases to be a minor. This is a major step to take as, when evoked, 'no important step in the life of that child can be taken without the consent of the court'.

INHERENT JURISDICTION

This is most commonly used in medical law cases. The court only takes decisions on certain issues relating to the child's life, e.g. medical care. It can be invoked in an emergency and also by a local authority, even while the child is in care.

COURT ORDERS

The court has the power to make:

- **Prohibited step orders** – no step (specified in the order) can be taken by any person (including the parents) without the consent of the court
- **Specific issue orders** – give directions to determine a *specific question* in connection with any aspect of parental responsibility for a child

These orders cannot be made if a child is in care, or in an emergency, and are rarely made if the child is 16 years old. They do not represent a true order as they only allow a local authority to authorize and supervise a policy. As with all treatment, the final decision and duty of care still rests with the doctor in charge of the case.

CONSENT

THE COMPETENT CHILD

- Children over 16 years of age are regarded as though they are adult for the purposes of consent
- A child under 16 years may *give* consent if they are deemed *competent*. However, a competent child

cannot withhold consent (because a refusal to give consent can be countermanded by those with parental responsibility)

- A child under 16 years old will be considered competent to give consent to a particular intervention if they have 'sufficient understanding and intelligence to enable him or her to understand fully what is proposed' (known as *Frazer competence*)

THE INCOMPETENT CHILD

If a child does *not* have the *capacity* to provide consent a *proxy* may do so. The proxy is expected to act in the best interests of the child and they can include the following:

- A **parent** who has 'parental responsibility' for the child
- A **local authority** that has acquired '*parental responsibility*' and the power of consent. A local authority can only usurp this power by restricting their power as the parents
- The **court** can act as a proxy in wardship, under *inherent jurisdiction* or via *court orders*. In this way it can review a parent's decision, e.g. the refusal of a life-giving blood transfusion for a child of a Jehovah's witness

FURTHER READING

Cartlidge P. *Ethical, Legal and Social Aspects of Child Healthcare*. London: Elsevier, 2007.

Freeman M. *Children, Medicine and the Law*. Farnham: Ashgate Publishing, 2005.

Further reading

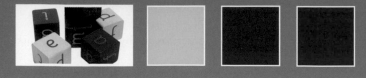

28 Paediatric Prescribing and Fluid Management

- ■ Fluid management
- ■ Paediatric prescribing
- ■ Clinical pharmacology of drugs in children
- ■ Further reading

FLUID MANAGEMENT

Normal fluid requirements

These are made up of:

- ■ Metabolic requirements, and
- ■ Loss from sweating, gastrointestinal tract, urine, respiration and tears

Maintenance fluid is the amount needed to keep the current hydration state balanced.

Table 28.1 Calculation of maintenance fluid requirements

Body weight (kg)	Fluid requirement mL/kg/24 h	mL/kg/h
0–10	100–120	(4)
10–20	1000 mL+ [50 for each kg > 10]	(2)
> 20	1500 mL+ [20 for each kg > 20]	(1)

DEHYDRATION

Causes of dehydration/increased fluid losses

- ■ Gastrointestinal upset
- ■ Polyuria
- ■ Increased sweating (fever, hot ambient temperature)
- ■ Increased metabolic rate (infection, illness)
- ■ Intravascular loss (capillary leakage, third space losses)
- ■ Trauma, e.g. burns

Clinical features

See p. 179.

Management

- Rapid volume expansion if in shock:
  - 20 mL/kg stat crystalloid or colloid
  - Repeat if required on reassessment
- Then rehydration fluid calculation:
  1. Deficit = % dehydration × weight (kg)
  2. Maintenance (calculated as above)
  3. Continuing losses (add continuing losses over maintenance losses) } Rehydration fluid

Intravenous fluids

Intravenous fluids can be divided into:

Crystalloid   Contain electrolytes ± dextrose

Used for the management of most fluid disturbances

4% dextrose and 0.18% sodium chloride is generally used for maintenance fluid therapy. However, 0.9% saline and 5% glucose, 0.45% saline and 5% glucose or Hartmann's solution are more physiologically appropriate. Potassium chloride is usually added to replace potassium losses

Normal saline is used for rapid volume expansion and to replace deficit

Colloid   Contain large molecules for volume expansion, e.g. blood, 4.5% albumin

Table 28.2 Intravenous fluid composition

Fluid	Na (mmol/L)	Cl (mmol/L)	K (mmol/L)	Energy (kJ/L)
0.45% saline 5% glucose	75	75	0	840
4% dextrose 0.18% saline	30	30	0	670
0.9% saline (normal saline)	153	153	0	0
Hartmann's solution	140	140	4	200

PAEDIATIC PRESCRIBING

Prescribing for children involves important differences from prescribing for adults:

- Dose must be individually **calculated** according to child's age and size (usually weight, or more accurately, body surface area)
- Certain **formulations** are better tolerated
- Many drugs are prescribed **unlicensed** or **'off-label'**
- Differences in the **pharmacology of drugs** in adults and children

Body weight and surface area (BSA) by age

Age	Weight (kg)	BSA (m²)
Newborn	3.5	0.25
6 months	7.7	0.4

Age	Weight (kg)	BSA (m²)
1 year	10	0.5
5 years	18	0.75
12 years	36	1.25
Adult	70	1.80

Formulations most suitable for children

- Liquids often better tolerated than tablets
- Inhalational medications useful (see p. 132)
- Flavoured oral medications can be helpful
- Intravenous better tolerated than intramuscular
- Rectal route if oral not tolerated

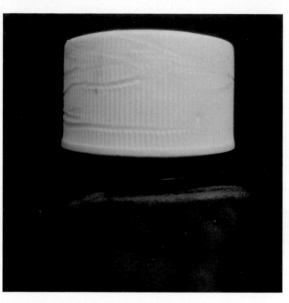

Figure 28.1 A child's teeth marks on a child-proof bottle

Unlicensed and 'off-label' medicines in paediatrics

- The **Medicines Act of 1968** was introduced following the problems of drug therapy in children with drugs such as thalidomide and chloramphenicol
- The **Medicines and Healthcare Products Regulatory Agency (MHRA)**, on behalf of the health minister with respect to clinical indications, age, suitable formulation, dosage and route, gives a drug its **marketing authorization** (formerly known as a **product licence**)
- A pharmaceutical company may make an application for a marketing authorization for the use of the medicine in adults, but choose not to make an application for the use of that medicine in children. If these medicines are given to children they are termed 'off-label'
- Most medicines currently available have been developed for use in adults and can be in forms that are unsuitable for use in children. This leads to problems for doctors and pharmacists to ensure the best quality of care is delivered to the child using the formulations currently on the market
- Use of unlicensed medicines, or of licensed medicines for unlicensed applications, is necessary in paediatric prescribing. Use of unlicensed and off-label prescribing is catered for in the Medicines Act
- Contrary to popular belief, it is not illegal for doctors either to prescribe or administer this group of drugs or for pharmacists to dispense or extemporaneously prepare them provided that the doctor is aware of his/her professional responsibilities. These responsibilities include having sufficient knowledge, experience and understanding of the pharmacology and monitoring of the treatment, and having the best interests of the child at heart

Why drugs remain unlicensed

- The reasons why suitable drugs are not licensed for children are often varied and complex

- There is a general agreement that for many drugs the paediatric market is small and the investment required for research and trials by pharmaceutical companies to gain a paediatric licence is not commercially attractive
- There is also a misconception that undertaking clinical trials in children is difficult and ethically inappropriate

Example of unlicensed and off-label prescribing in children	
Unlicensed	Magnesium glycerophosphate tablet – this drug has no marketing authorization and is used in an unlicensed manner in both adults and children
Off-label	Ranitidine – only licensed for the oral treatment of peptic ulceration in children but has an off-label use in the treatment of gastro-oesphageal reflux. This is using a licensed medicine for an unlicensed application

CLINICAL PHARMACOLOGY OF DRUGS IN CHILDREN

Various factors can affect the pharmacokinetics, pharmacodynamics, efficacy and toxicity of drugs in neonates and children:

- Age
- Race
- Organ maturity
- Drug formulation
- Compliance with therapy

Absorption

Oral	Drug absorption from the oral route is affected by *slower gastric emptying rates*. Gastric emptying rates of infants approach those of adults within the first 6–8 months of life First-pass hepatic metabolism for some drugs is faster in children than adults
IV and IM	The IV route for drug delivery is preferred over the IM route IM absorption of drugs can often be erratic due to *reduced muscle mass* and *variability in blood flow* to and from the injection site
Percutaneous absorption	This is *increased* the younger the patient due to the thinner stratum corneum and increased skin hydration

Drug distribution

- Dependent upon a number of factors, including protein binding, body compartment sizes, haemodynamic factors and membrane permeability
- **Albumin** has an increasing affinity towards acidic drugs from birth into infancy. Normal adult levels are reached at approximately 12 months of age
- **Binding of drugs to plasma proteins** is dependent upon a number of variables:
  - Amount of binding proteins available
  - Affinity of drug for proteins
  - Pathophysiological conditions which may alter the drug–protein binding interaction

Drugs that may have *greater unbound concentrations in the plasma* in children than adults include morphine, phenytoin, phenobarbitone, diazepam and furosemide

Relative strengths of glucocorticoids

Steroid	Relative potency
Cortisol	1
Hydrocortisone	1.25
Prednisolone	5
Dexamethasone	50

■ **Extracellular and intracellular volumes** (*as a percentage of body weight*) are greater in neonates than in children and adults

Approximately 65% of the neonate's bodyweight at birth is made up of extracellular fluid; this falls to approximately 30% by 1 year of age, and then falls slowly until puberty when it reaches an adult value (20%). This means that in order to achieve a comparable plasma and tissue concentration of a drug, *higher doses per kg of bodyweight* must be given to infants and children than to adults, e.g. aminoglycosides. (Faster hepatic metabolism for some drugs also contributes to this phenomenon.)

Metabolism

■ Difficult to predict the variability in the clinical pharmacology due to partially developed hepatic and/or renal function. Some pathways are well developed even in neonates, e.g. metabolism of paracetamol, whilst others mature over time, e.g. glucoronidation of morphine or the oxidation of diazepam
■ Drug metabolism, as in adults, follows two main processes:
  – **Phase I** involves the oxidation, reduction, hydrolysis and hydroxylation of drugs. Most phase I enzymes are at low levels immediately following birth but the oxidative enzymes show a rapid postnatal maturation
  – **Phase II** reactions involve the glucoronidation or sulphation of drugs. This helps to explain why the limited ability to conjugate paracetamol with glucoronide (a major pathway in adults) in neonates and children is more than compensated for by a well developed sulphation pathway

Excretion

■ Drug elimination via the renal route is reduced in premature neonates due to the *decreased glomerular filtration and tubular secretion*
■ Adult values for the glomerular filtration rate (GFR) are reached by 5 months of age. This increase is due to the combined effects of an increase in cardiac output, reduction in peripheral vascular resistance and an increased surface area available for filtration
■ GFR maturation is an important consideration when selecting dosage regimens for aminoglycosides in premature infants. Several studies have shown that newborns with a preconceptual age of < 34 weeks require either an individual dose reduction or a lengthening of the dosage interval

FURTHER READING

Costello I, Long P, Wong I *et al. Paediatric Drug Handling*. Pharmaceutical Press. 2007.

Rowe R, Sheskey PJ, Quinn ME. *Handbook of Pharmaceutical Excipients*. Pharmaceutical Press. 2009.

Thomas T. *Developing your Prescribing Skills*. London: Pharmaceutical Press.

British National Formulary for Children 2010–2011. London: Pharmaceutical Press, 2010.

For further questions after Clinical scenarios refer to:

Sidwell R, Thomson M. *QBase Paediatrics: Volume 1, MCQs for the MRCPCH.* London: Greenwich Medical Media, 2001.

Sidwell R, Thomson M. *QBase Paediatrics: Volume 2, MCQs for the Part A DCH.* Cambridge: Cambridge University Press, 2008.

Sidwell R, Thomson M. *QBase Paediatrics: Volume 3, MCQs for the Part B MRCPCH.* Cambridge: Cambridge University Press, 2008.

Further reading

Abbreviations

ABG	arterial blood gas		CGD	chronic granulomatous disease
ACTH	adrenocorticotrophic hormone		CML	chronic myeloid leukaemia
ADHD	attention deficit hyperactivity disorder		CMT	Charcot–Marie–Tooth
AE	airway entry		CMV	cytomegalovirus
A&E	accident and emergency		CNS	central nervous system
AGA	appropriate for gestational age		COM	chronic otitis media
AIDS	acquired immune deficiency syndrome		CPAP	continous positive airway pressure
ALL	acute lymphoblastic leukaemia		CPK	creatine cystokinase
ALT	alanine aminotransferase		CPR	cardiopulmonary resuscitation
ALTE	apparent life-threatening event		CRF	chronic renal failure
AMA	anti-mitochondrial antibody		CRP	C-reactive protein
AML	acute myeloid leukaemia		CRT	capillary refill time
ANA	antinuclear antibody		CSF	cerebrospinal fluid
APLS	advanced paediatric life support		CT	computed tomography
APTT	activated partial thromboplastin time		CVID	common variable immunodeficiency
AR	aortic regurgitation		CVP	central venous pressure
ARDS	acute respiratory distress syndrome		CVS	chorionic villus sampling
ARF	acute renal failure		CXR	chest X-ray
AS	aortic stenosis		DBP	diastolic blood pressure
ASD	atrial septal defect		DI	diabetes insipidus
ASOT	antistreptolysin O titre		DIC	disseminated intravascular coagulation
AST	aspartate aminotransferase		DPT	diphtheria and tetanus
AVSD	atrioventricular septal defect		DVT	deep vein thrombosis
AXR	abdominal X-ray		EAC	external auditory canal
BBB	blood–brain barrier		EBV	Epstein–Barr virus
BIH	benign intracranial hypertension		ECG	electrocardiogram
BMI	body mass index		ECMO	extracorporeal membrane oxygenation
BMT	bone marrow transplantation		EEG	electroencephalogram
BP	blood pressure		ELBW	extremely low birthweight
BPD	bronchopulmonary dysplasia		EMG	electromyelogram
BSER	brain-stem evoked responses		ERG	electroretinogram
CAH	congenital adrenal hyperplasia		ESR	erythrocyte sedimentation ratio
CAM	cystic adenoid malformation		ESRF	end-stage renal failure
CDH	congenital dislocation of the hip		EUA	examination under anaesthesia
CF	cystic fibrosis		ETT	endotracheal tube
CFRD	cystic fibrosis related diabetes		FBC	full blood count
CHD	congenital heart disease		FDP	fibrin degradation products

FFP	fresh frozen plasma
FII	fictitious or induced illness
FISH	fluorescent *in-situ* hybridization
FR	glomerular filtration rate
FSH	follicle stimulating hormone
GCS	Glasgow Coma Scale
GCSF	granulocyte colony stimulating factor
GFR	glomerular filtration rate
GI	gastrointestinal
GOLR	gastro-oesophageal-laryngo-respiratory
GOR	gastro-oesophageal reflux
GSD	glycogen storage disease
GVHD	graft versus host disease
hCG	human chorionic gonadotrophin
HDU	high dependency unit
HFOV	high frequency oscillatory ventilation
HHV	human herpes virus
HIE	hypoxic–ischaemic encephalopathy
HIV	human immunodeficiency virus
HMSN	hereditary motor–sensory neuropathy
HS	heart sounds
HSP	Henoch–Schönlein purpura
HSV	herpes simplex virus
HUS	haemolytic–uraemic syndrome
IBD	inflammatory bowel disorder
IBS	irritable bowel syndrome
ICP	intracranial pressure
ICS	intercostal space
IM	intramuscular
INR	international normalized ratio
IPPV	intermittent positive airway pressure
ITP	immune thrombocytopaenia
IRT	immunoreactive trypsinogen
UGR	intrauterine growth retardation
IV	intravenous
IVC	inferior vena cava
IVH	intraventricular haemorrhage
IVIG	intravenous immunoglobulin
IVU	intravenous urography
JCA	juvenile chronic arthritis
JIA	juvenile idiopathic arthritis
JVP	jugular venous pressure
LAD	left axis deviation
LBW	low birthweight
LCSC	lower segment Caesarian section
LDH	lactate dehydrogenase
LDL	low density lipoprotein
LFT	liver function test
LGA	large for gestational age
LH	luteinizing hormone
LHRH	luteinizing hormone releasing hormone
LIP	lymphocytic interstitial pneumonitis
LKKS	liver kidney kidney spleen
LP	lumbar puncture
LRTI	lower respiratory tract infection
LSE	left sternal edge
LVH	left ventricular hypertrophy
M, C & S	microscopy, culture and sensitivities
MCH	mean corpuscular haemoglobin
MCHC	mean corpuscular haemoglobin concentration
MCP	metacarpal
MCKD	multicystic kidney disease
MCUG	micturating cystourethrography
MCV	mean corpuscular volume
MDI	metered dose inhaler
MRI	magnetic resonance imaging
MSU	midstream urine
MSUD	maple syrup urine disease
NAD	nothing abnormal detected
NAI	non-accidental injury
NBT	nitroblue tetrazolium
NDT	neural tube defect
NEC	necrotizing enterocolitis
NG	nasogastric
NICU	neonatal intensive care unit
NPA	nasopharyngeal aspirate
NSAID	non-steroidal anti-inflammatory drug
NVD	normal vaginal delivery
OAE	otoacoustic emission
OCD	obsessive–compulsive disorder
ORT	oral rehydration therapy
PA	pulmonary artery
PCP	*Pneumocystis jejunii* (formally *carinii*) pneumonia
PCR	polymerase chain reaction
PCV	packed cell volume
PDA	patent ductus arteriosus
PDGF	platelet derived growth factor
PEF	peak expiratory flow
PHA	phytohaemagglutinin
PK	pyruvate kinase
PKU	phenylketonuria
PNM	perinatal mortality
PPHN	persistent pulmonary hypertension of the newborn
PS	pulmonary stenosis
PT	prothrombin time
PUJ	pelvo–ureteric junction
PVH	periventricular haemorrhage

PVL	periventricular leukomalacia	TAPVD	total anomalous pulmonary venous drainage
RAD	right axis deviation	TB	tuberculosis
RBBB	right bundle branch block	TFT	thyroid function test
RBC	red blood cell	TGA	transposition of the great arteries
RDS	respiratory distress syndrome	TM	tympanic membrane
RLL	right lower lobe	TMJ	temporomandibular joint
RR	respiratory rate	TOF	tetralogy of Fallot
RSV	respiratory syncytial virus	TPN	total parenteral nutrition
RUL	right upper lobe	TSH	thyroid stimulating hormone
RVH	right ventricular hypertrophy	TSS	toxic shock syndrome
SAH	subarachnoid haemorrhage	TT	thrombin time
SBE	subacute bacterial endocarditis	TTN	transient tachypnoea of the newborn
SBP	systolic blood pressure	U&E	urea and electrolytes
SBR	serum bilirubin	UMN	upper motor neurone
SCID	severe combined immunodeficiency	URTI	upper respiratory tract infection
SCT	stem cell transplantation	USS	ultrasound scan
SGA	small for gestational age	UTI	urinary tract infection
SIADH	secretion of inappropriate antidiuretic hormone	UVC	umbilical venous catheter
SIDS	sudden infant death syndrome	VER	visual evoked response
SLE	systemic lupus erythematosus	VLBW	very low birthweight
SMA	spinal muscular atrophy	VSD	ventricular septal defect
SOB	shortness of breath	VT	ventricular tachycardia
SSPE	subacute sclerosing panencephalitis	VUR	vesico-ureteric reflux
SSSS	staphylococcal scalded skin syndrome	VZV	varicella zoster virus
SUFE	slipped upper femoral epiphysis	WCC	white cell count
SVC	superior vena cava	WHO	World Health Organization
SVT	supraventricular tachycardia	XLA	X-linked agammaglobulinaemia
TA	tricuspid atresia	ZIG	zoster immunoglobulin

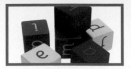

Index